The Embodied Performance of Gender

Norms of embodied behavior for males and females, as promoted in mainstream Western public arenas of popular culture and the everyday, continue to work, overtly and covertly, as definitive and restrictive barriers to the realm of possibilities of embodied gender expression and appreciation. They serve to disempower and marginalize those not inclined to embody according to such dichotomous models. This book explores the ramifications of the way our gendered, sexed, and culturally constructed bodies are situated toward notions of difference and highlights the need to safeguard the social and emotional well-being of those who do not fit comfortably with dominant norms of masculine/feminine behavior as deemed appropriate according to biological sex. The book interrogates gender inequitable machinations of education and performance arts disciplines by which educators and arts practitioners train, teach, choreograph, and direct those with whom they work, and theorizes ways of broadening personal and social notions of possible, aesthetic, and acceptable embodiment for all persons, regardless of biological sex or sexual orientation. The author's own struggles as a performance artist, educator, and person in the everyday, as well as the findings of empirical fieldwork with educators, performance arts practitioners, and high school students, are employed to illustrate and advocate the need for self-reflexive scrutiny of existing and hidden inequities regarding the embodiment of gender within one's own habitual perspectives, taste, and practices.

Jack Migdalek is a drama lecturer at Trinity College (Melbourne University) and Education Materials writer for the Arts Centre, Victoria, and has worked as a performer, writer, choreographer, director, and educator in Australia, the United Kingdom, and Japan.

Routledge Research in Gender and Society

For a full list of titles in this series, please visit www.routledge.com

12 **The Gender of Democracy**
Citizenship and Gendered Subjectivity
Maro Pantelidou Maloutas

13 **Female Homosexuality in the Middle East**
Histories and Representations
Samar Habib

14 **Global Empowerment of Women**
Responses to Globalization and Politicized Religions
Edited by Carolyn M. Elliott

15 **Child Abuse, Gender and Society**
Jackie Turton

16 **Gendering Global Transformations**
Gender, Culture, Race, and Identity
Edited by Chima J Korieh and Philomina Ihejirika-Okeke

17 **Gender, Race and National Identity**
Nations of Flesh and Blood
Jackie Hogan

18 **Intimate Citizenships**
Gender, Sexualities, Politics
Elżbieta H. Oleksy

19 **A Philosophical Investigation of Rape**
The Making and Unmaking of the Feminine Self
Louise du Toit

20 **Migrant Men**
Critical Studies of Masculinities and the Migration Experience
Edited by Mike Donaldson, Raymond Hibbins, Richard Howson and Bob Pease

21 **Theorizing Sexual Violence**
Edited by Renée J. Heberle and Victoria Grace

22 **Inclusive Masculinity**
The Changing Nature of Masculinities
Eric Anderson

23 **Understanding Non-Monogamies**
Edited by Meg Barker and Darren Langdridge

24 **Transgender Identities**
Towards a Social Analysis of Gender Diversity
Edited by Sally Hines and Tam Sanger

25 **The Cultural Politics of Female Sexuality in South Africa**
Henriette Gunkel

26 Migration, Domestic Work and Affect
A Decolonial Approach on Value and the Feminization of Labor
Encarnación Gutiérrez-Rodríguez

27 Overcoming Objectification
A Carnal Ethics
Ann J. Cahill

28 Intimate Partner Violence in LGBTQ Lives
Edited by Janice L. Ristock

29 Contesting the Politics of Genocidal Rape
Affirming the Dignity of the Vulnerable Body
Debra B. Bergoffen

30 Transnational Migration, Media and Identity of Asian Women
Diasporic Daughters
Youna Kim

31 Feminist Solidarity at the Crossroads
Intersectional Women's Studies for Transracial Alliance
Edited by Kim Marie Vaz and Gary L. Lemons

32 Victims, Gender and *Jouissance*
Victoria Grace

33 Gender, Development and Environmental Governance
Theorizing Connections
Seema Arora-Jonsson

34 Street Sex Workers' Discourse
Realizing Material Change Through Agential Choice
Jill McCracken

35 Gender, Ethnicity, and Political Agency
South Asian Women Organizing
Shaminder Takhar

36 Ecofeminism and Systems Thinking
Anne Stephens

37 Queer Women in Urban China
An Ethnography
Elisabeth L. Engebretsen

38 Gender and Rural Migration
Realities, Conflict and Change
Edited by Glenda Tibe Bonifacio

39 Gender and Neoliberalism
The All India Democratic Women's Association and Globalization Politics
Elisabeth Armstrong

40 Asexualities
Feminist and Queer Perspectives
Edited by Karli June Cerankowski and Megan Milks

41 Cross-Cultural Women Scholars in Academe
Intergenerational Voices
Edited by Lorri J. Santamaría, Gaëtane Jean-Marie, and Cosette M. Grant

42 Muslim Women, Transnational Feminism and the Ethics of Pedagogy
Contested Imaginaries in Post-9/11 Cultural Practice
Edited by Lisa K. Taylor and Jasmin Zine

43 The Embodied Performance of Gender
Jack Migdalek

The Embodied Performance of Gender

Jack Migdalek

Routledge
Taylor & Francis Group
LONDON AND NEW YORK

First published 2015
by Routledge

2 Park Square, Milton Park, Abingdon, Oxfordshire OX14 4RN
711 Third Avenue, New York, NY 10017

Routledge is an imprint of the Taylor & Francis Group, an informa business

First issued in paperback 2018

Library of Congress Cataloging-in-Publication Data

Migdalek, Jack.
The embodied performance of gender / by Jack Migdalek.
pages cm. — (Routledge research in gender and society ; 43)
Includes bibliographical references and index.
1. Sex differences. 2. Sex role. 3. Femininity. 4. Masculinity.
5. Human beings—Attitude and movement. I. Title.
HQ1075.M545 2015
305.3—dc23
2014025043

ISBN: 978-1-138-80983-3 (hbk)
ISBN: 978-1-138-37947-3 (pbk)

Typeset in Sabon
by Apex CoVantage, LLC

Contents

Figures

Acknowledgments

This book emanates from my PhD undertaken through Deakin University's School of Health and Social Development. I wish to express my heartfelt gratitude to my then supervisor, Maria Pallotta-Chiarolli, for her inspiration, insights, support, and cherished friendship.

I wish to express my appreciation to Miriam Sofer, Faye Bendrups, Bob Pease, Laurel Richardson, Michael Gard, Carl Leggo, Martin Mills, Wayne Martino, Shirley McKechnie, and Lynda Smerdon for their various academic, artistic, and/or technical inspiration, feedback, and support. Also to Deakin University's School of Communication and Creative Arts, the Arts Centre Melbourne, and Trinity College, Melbourne University.

My sincere thanks to the schools, arts organizations, and all the participants who played an essential role in my fieldwork, and without whom the research behind this book would not have been possible.

Finally, this book is dedicated to my beloved family, and especially to my mother, Eva (you know you are my hero), and to my adored partner, Ken.

Introduction

Norms of *fitting* embodied behavior for males and females, as promoted in mainstream Western public arenas of popular culture and the everyday, disempower and marginalize those not inclined to embody in gendernormative and heteronormative ways.

This book engages with concepts of embodiment, meaning the manner of physical deportment in which a physical practice is performed, and with concepts of gender as social constructions of femininity and masculinity. It investigates the demands and implications of dominant norms of gender embodiment for those whose embodied inclinations do not fit comfortably with such dichotomous models. It interrogates gender inequitable machinations of education and performance arts disciplines by which educators and arts practitioners train, teach, choreograph, and direct those with whom they work, and it theorizes ways of broadening personal and social notions of possible, aesthetic, and acceptable embodiment for all persons, regardless of biological sex or sexual orientation.

This research behind the book is grounded in two major qualitative methods of inquiry. First, through an autoethnographic lens, it focuses on the impacts that social constructions of masculinity have on me, both as a person in the everyday and as a performance arts practitioner/educator. Through a combination of academic and artistic means of expression, I analyze the delicacy of the relationship between social control/surveillance and personal agency over my embodiment of gender. Second, through empirical ethnographic fieldwork with some 400 high school students and 160 educators and performance arts practitioners, I speculate on the potential to challenge inequitable notions of gender embodiment.

This book will demonstrate that ideologies inherent in dominant discourses regarding the execution and display of feminine and masculine embodiment continue to work, overtly and covertly, as definitive and restrictive barriers to the realm of possibilities of embodied gender expression and appreciation in the everyday and in the performance arts. In order to safeguard the well-being of those whose embodied performance inclination is at odds with prescribed norms of behavior, social consciousness needs to be drawn to embodied gender inequities and enculturation processes, not ordinarily critiqued within mainstream society. Affecting such consciousness may be the realm of educators, carers, and also performance arts practitioners. However, this book explores and illustrates the need for these agents of positive social change to first scrutinize existing and hidden inequities regarding the embodiment of gender within their own habitus, perspectives, taste, and practices.

This book is divided into thirteen chapters. Chapter 1 draws attention to inequitable ways in which the young are positioned to view and do the embodiment of gender. It foregrounds the situations of those who are not inclined to enact and embody gender according to socially valorized norms, as well as the potential for individuals to deconstruct embedded notions pertaining to the embodiment of gender.

Chapter 2 relates the works of key theorists of habitus and embodiment to existing theories of gender, social development and performance, from areas of gender studies, sociology, education, performance arts, and queer theory. Reference to the work of Pierre Bourdieu, Angela McRobbie, Wayne Martino, Maria Pallotta-Chiarolli, Raewyn Connell, Judith Butler, Michael Gard, Alfred Schutz, Slavoj Zizek, Terry Threadgold, Helen Cahill, Emma Renold, Sande Zeig, and Patricia Leavy lays the groundwork for arguments and propositions that are raised in the body of the book.

Chapter 3 outlines my positioning and location to the research and the means of expression through which, as commentator, artist, and subject, I have chosen to express myself.

Chapters 4 to 8 draw on my lived experiences and consciousness as a male son, student, performance artist, educator, and person in the everyday. These five chapters comment on and analyze specific aspects relating to the embodiment of gender and feature the evocative media of autobiographical monologues, fictocritical narratives, dramatized scenarios, illustrations, and media analysis. In turning a mirror onto my own experiences and consciousness I also turn a mirror onto those who operate in situations and contexts that are sites of my own story: those who may be children (as I was); those who may be adults, educators, performance arts practitioners (as I am).

The focus of Chapter 4 is on enculturation processes through which individuals come to understand male and female bodies and masculine and feminine—and 'gay'—embodiment. Chapter 5 incorporates media analysis of embodied gendered representations as projected in advertising, sporting, and performance arts arenas. It examines the cultivation of taste and the aesthetics of valorized and subordinated embodied masculinities and femininities. The focus of Chapter 6 is the delicacy of the relationship between social control/surveillance and personal agency as regards an individual's perceptions and practices relating to the embodiment of gender. Chapter 7 puts the spotlight on the social and emotional well-being of the individual not inclined to embody gender according to socially valorized and often oppressive norms. It outlines and analyzes ways by which individuals can resist, comply with, or negotiate such norms. Chapter 8 delves into possibilities of social change and the potential to challenge embodied gender inequity, in both everyday and public arenas.

The material and commentary in Chapters 4 to 8 informs and connects to the fieldwork that is the focus of Chapters 9 to 11. Fieldwork sessions conducted with high school students are drawn on in Chapter 9 to shed light on social and emotional pressures pertaining to the embodiment of gender (and sexuality) that contemporary youth experience. Students' actions and responses are analyzed, and a case is argued for the need to challenge embodied gender inequities as they occur in performance arts, education, and everyday arenas.

Chapter 10 draws on and analyzes the outcomes of fieldwork with educators and performance artists. The chapter considers the potential role of practitioners in these areas in the deconstruction of inherent and inequitable gendered ideologies perpetuating the embodiment of masculinity and femininity, which are prevalent in mainstream Western societies. In addition, it highlights the need for these practitioners to self-reflexively question their own embedded and inequitable perceptions, blindspots, agendas, and practices concerning the embodiment of gender. Drawing on fieldwork with performance arts educators/practitioners, the latter part of the chapter focuses on performance arts arenas as powerful sites in and through which

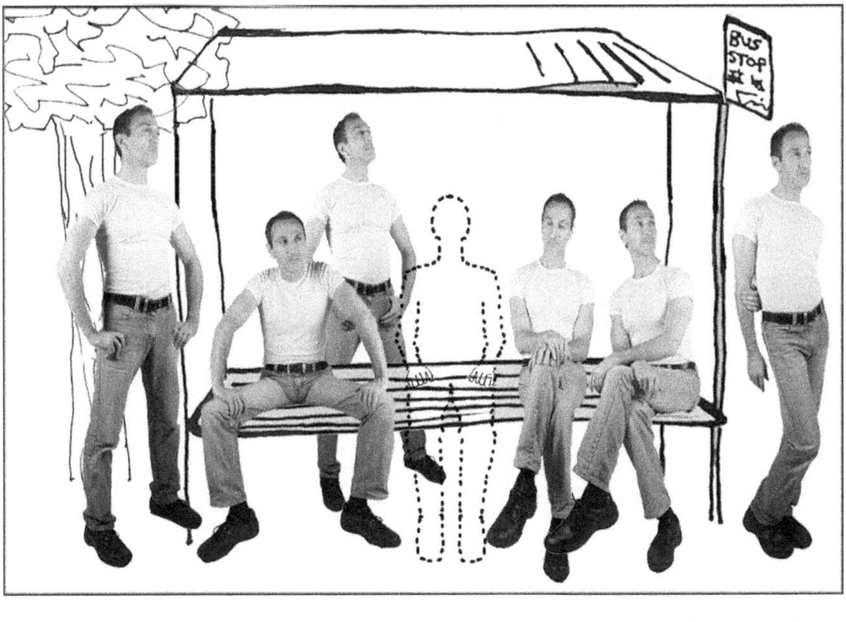

Figure Introduction.1 Waiting figures. Photograph by Rob Chiarolli (www.photosthattell.com). Artwork by Jack Migdalek.

deconstructive work pertaining to embodied gender inequity can occur, both cognitively and practically.

Chapter 11 restates the case for broadening personal and social notions of what is choreographically possible, aesthetic, and acceptable embodiment for all persons, regardless of biological sex or sexual orientation. Implications are also made regarding the need to destabilize inequitable social attitudes, behaviors, and practices in general.

The appendix of the book comprise a fictocritical playscript that can be read for reflection on issues of embodiment, gender, sexuality, homophobia, self-image, discrimination, and well-being, along with activity suggestions for course leaders that may be used in facilitating deconstructive work with educators, youth workers, trainee teachers/youth workers, and/or high school student groups.

This book is a personal and, I believe, artistic expression, intended to stir, stimulate, and interact with readers.

1 Embodiment

Learning, Viewing, Knowing, Doing

Episode

Night time. Two males walking along Utopia Road. A car approaches from behind. Male voices yell abusively from the windows, "*Ya poofs! Faggots!*"

> What brought this on?
> The backs of our bodies . . .
> were the basis on which those in the car decided to abuse us.
> The backs of our bodies . . .
> were the basis on which those in the car decided that we were faggots.

The above episode describes an event that occurred to me several years ago. I was one of the pedestrians. The episode hurled me directly into a multitude of questions regarding the embodied performance of gender, which form the backbone of this book.

This book is about embodied performance: performance that occurs on, with, through, around, and via bodies. It is concerned with bodies as matter that can be posed/reposed/actioned, bodies that through what they perform and the ways in which they perform come to signify and communicate meaning. Although the matter of the body—the flesh, shape, size, color, and even adornment—is a prominent component of a performance that can impact on cultural notions of femininity/masculinity, it is the choreography and manner of performance, coined by Marcel Mauss (1979) as 'bodily practice' and 'bodily technique', with which this book is primarily concerned. A bodily practice such as a simple walk can be perceived very differently according to the bodily technique or manner in which it is performed or executed. The technique, quality, style, or manner in which a person walks can make them appear to be alert, slovenly, aggressive, fragile, confident, and/or inhibited. The way in which a walk is performed can also make an individual appear to be feminine or masculine.

The book is motivated by personal experiences, exemplified by the episode narrated above. Although constructed around my own experiences as a Caucasian, homosexual, Jewish, Australian, biological male, son, student, dancer, actor, writer, teacher, choreographer, director, and civilian, this work also refers to the embodiment of the diverse, non-homogeneous range of biological males who identify and project as male, and of the diverse, non-homogeneous range of biological females who identify and project as female. I acknowledge that there are those for whom these dichotomous, binary categories of being do not fit and that issues of embodiment of gender and the opening and diversifying of possibilities of gender performance are also of relevance to transgender persons. I chose, however, to restrict the parameters of this book to the dominant binarily constructed and gendernormative categories of male and female, as they are categories by which so many individuals are defined and/or define themselves. As such, this study will not focus specifically on intersex, transsex, or transgender, nor on surgical manipulation, cross-dressing, or transvestism.

Using the episode presented above, the following is a brief explanation of how I interpret key terms used in this book.

EMBODIMENT: That which is manifest through the body and over which human beings have some form of corporeal government (see Goffman 1959, Turner 1984). Although the embodiment of the two males in the episode would include physical shape, size, form, color, adornment, and styling, in this book my focus is predominantly on physical deportment and action.

CHOREOGRAPHY: What a body does in finite terms such as bodily gestures and movements (see Foster 1998). The choreography of the two males in the episode included walking in the same direction, arms by sides, bodies 45 centimeters apart from one another, heads facing straight ahead and occasionally rotating toward one another.

PERFORMANCE: The style, disposition, or manner in which choreography is executed (see Foster 1998), for example, the *way* the two male bodies in the episode walked, swung their arms, swayed their hips, motioned with their heads. A performance need not necessarily be executed nor intended for an actual audience (see Butler 2004).

GENDER: The socially constructed aspects of femininity and masculinity—not biological sex. Like Judith Butler (1993) I am wary of and opposed to conflations between notions of gender and those of biological sex within public discourse (see also Kehily 2002, Paechter 2006). Likewise, a social tendency to couple readings of the embodiment of gender with understandings of sexual orientation is a recurring theme that is problematized throughout this book.

What is considered to be feminine and masculine, and how feminine or masculine embodiment may be perceived differently when performed by bodies of different size, shape, muscularity, or biological sex, is culturally dependent (Turner 1984, Shilling 2003). While gender categories of masculine and feminine may be dependent on culture, setting, and time, and as such are difficult to define (Butler 2004), I feel compelled to use these terms in order to draw attention to predominantly unproblematized social tendencies to align masculinities with male bodies and femininities with female bodies (Francis 2010). My definitions for 'feminine' are gentle, graceful, delicate, soft, pliant; and my definitions for 'masculine' are strong, forceful, powerful, unyielding. To utilize Laban movement analysis terminology (McCaw 2011), feminine styles of motion predominate in 'light effort actions' (dabbing, gliding, flicking, floating); masculine styles of motion predominate in 'strong effort actions' (punching, slashing, wringing, pressing).

Delving into the impact of frequently invisible hegemonic heteronormative ideologies on embodied performance of gender necessitates taking into consideration the inter-relationship between embodied performances in public arenas of popular culture and embodied performances in the everyday. By performances in public arenas of popular culture, I refer to performance as entertainment art, sports spectacle, or commercial advertising as viewed in theatres, cinemas, sports arenas, television, and print media. By performances in the everyday, I refer to performances that are not staged or produced specifically as entertainment art, sports spectacle, or commercial advertising. Embodied performances in the everyday include pose, repose, and action such as standing, sitting, and walking.

It can be argued that many performance arts practitioners are guilty of unknowingly reinforcing and reinscribing inherent gendered ideologies in the way that we/they teach, cast, direct, and choreograph (and design for) male and female bodies, and that these practices have a forceful impact on our/their students' and audiences' understandings of gender. In Chapters 4–7, I interrogate ways in which my thinking about 'feminine' and 'masculine' in certain ways has reinscribed, in my work as a performance arts practitioner/educator, the very stereo engendering of which I am critical. Fieldwork with performance arts practitioners/educators (Chapter 10) takes the interrogation further, attending to gender blindspots in others . . . and the potential, in mainstream culture, for social change in which embodied performance is not constricted or restricted according to an individual's assumed biological sex.

In cultural settings that I have experience of and membership in, bodies and certain styles of pose, repose, and action come to be perceived and classified as feminine or masculine. The identical motion can be read extremely differently according to (1) the biological sex of the performer and (2) the style or manner in which it is performed. My concerns center on situations where one's embodied choreography and performance style may mismatch or not conform to common culturally promoted norms of gender—gendernormativity—as prescribed to biological sex. In cultures with which I am familiar, gendernormativity incorporates masculine embodiment for males and feminine embodiment for females. These norms recurrently come to signify heterosexuality and can be referred to as heteronormativity (see Butler 1993, Martino & Pallotta-Chiarolli 2001). Frequently, embodied performances that oppose hegemonic gendered norms are perceived as indicators of homosexuality. This book concerns itself with how and why certain styles of embodied performance are perceived as indicators of sexual orientation, and it draws links with heteronormative and homophobic discourses that restrict and inhibit the physical embodiment of many individuals. When the individual not inclined to perform in gendernormative ways self-regulates and manages to *appear* normal, then, by virtue of their assumed attachment to society, the well-being of that individual and their struggles to conform tend to be easily overlooked.

Individuals should not be *unequal* if their embodied performances of gender do not align to socially prescribed norms. Yet those who pose, repose, and embody differently from gendered norms are marked as different or 'other'. My contention is that in a society that marks that which is other as subordinate to the norm, this has a negative impact on those whose embodied inclination differs from the norm.

I am not suggesting that all persons should perform in de-gendered, neutral ways. I have no objection to females embodying in a feminine manner or males embodying in a masculine manner, and I do not believe that these individuals need to modify how they embody their masculinity or femininity. Rather, what needs to be addressed is why those who are non-normative in their embodiment of gender might be regarded in negative terms. Why should performing in ways that are not gendernormative cause social disadvantage to the performer?

According to the *Oxford Dictionary*, 'symptoms' are manifestations or signs, and 'causes' are that which give rise to particular phenomena, conditions, or symptoms. In relation to the opening episode of this chapter, the symptoms can be seen to be the social 'dis-ease' we suffered as a result of being jeered at as "poofs". The cause or reason for the abuse was how 'the backs of our bodies' projected to those in the passing car. What needs to be addressed within the cause is the negative outlook toward *other* performances of masculinity/femininity as being tied up with a tendency to classify embodied performances as appropriate or inappropriate to males or females. What needs to be addressed is how those in the car might go beyond an either-or mindset that sustains that which is 'other' in binary opposition to that which is 'normal'. Rather than finding ways in which *victims* of this kind of abuse might defend themselves or get by, I contend that addressing the cause is the way to overcome or at least improve the lot of those who do not fit comfortably into societally prescribed norms of gender embodiment. Education and the performance arts may be sites through which such change may be instigated.

REFERENCES

Butler, J. (1993). *Bodies That Matter.* New York: Routledge.

Butler, J. (2004). *Undoing Gender.* New York: Routledge.

Foster, S. L. (1998). Choreographies of Gender. *Signs: Journal of Women in Culture & Society.* Vol 24, No 1, pp. 1–33.

Francis, B. (2010). Re/Theorising Gender: Female Masculinity and Male Femininity in the Classroom. *Gender and Education.* Vol 22, No 5, pp. 477–490.

Goffman, E. (1959). *The Presentation of Self in Everyday Life.* New York: Anchor.

Kehily, J. (2002). *Sexuality, Gender and Schooling: Shifting Agendas in Social Learning.* London: Routledge.

Martino, W., & Pallotta-Chiarolli, M. (2001). Gender Performativity and Normalizing Practices. In Haynes, F., & McKenna, T. (Eds.). *Unseen Genders: Beyond the Binaries.* New York: Peter Lang.

Mauss, M. (1979). *Sociology and Psychology: Essays.* London: Routledge.

McCaw, D. (2011). *The Laban Sourcebook.* London: Routledge.

Paechter, C. (2006). Reconceptualizing the Gendered Body: Learning and Constructing Masculinities and Femininities in School. *Gender and Education.* Vol 18, No 2, pp. 121–135.

Shilling, C. (2003). *The Body and Social Theory.* London: Sage.

Turner, B. (1984). *The Body and Society.* Oxford, UK: Basil Blackwell.

2 Contextualizing Embodied Performance of Gender

In his work as a social theorist, Chris Shilling (2003) is critical of existing sociology of the body for presenting the body as an item for discussion yet leaving it largely absent as an object of investigation. In a similar vein, feminist scholar and activist Gloria Anzaldua (1990) is critical of the separation of theory and lived experience. In general, theorists on gender and the body focus on action done to and on the body. In their discussion of action and embodiment, Iris Marion Young (1990), Raewyn Connell (1995), Chris Shilling (2003), Carrie Paechter (2003b), and Jon Swain (2004) focus largely on the *what* of bodies, such as aging, giving birth, growing, thinning, getting strong, working, playing, sweating, performing tasks, having sex. Where Bryan Turner (1984) and Swain (2004) focus on the *how,* they focus on embodied performances in regard to levels of speed and dexterity, revealing whether someone is gouty, blind, fit, crippled, or old. More attention needs to be given to the *how* in relation to the manner, demeanor, or disposition in which bodies perform and the signs that these elements reveal in regard to the projection of an individual's masculinity or femininity and, by default, sexuality. For example, the two males in the opening episode were abused as 'poofs', not because they were walking (the *what*), but probably because of the way they walked (the *how*). The how in this case does not hinge on quantitative measures of speed or dexterity.

What we embody (choreography) and *how* we embody (performance) can be differentiated. Using dance terminology, Susan Foster (1998) differentiates *choreography* and *performance* in much the same way that Mauss (1979) differentiates *bodily practice* and *bodily technique*. Choreography—or *bodily practice*—can be seen as a form of embodied text, for example, reaching for a grape and eating it. Performance—or *bodily technique*—can be seen as the execution of that text, for example, the way in which the grape is picked up, held, and chewed. Where Foster's focus is very much on the gendered reading, meaning, and impact of *choreography* pertaining to how we come to read male and female bodies, I will attend more closely to the gendered reading, meaning, and impact of *performance,* or in other words the style, technique, and manner in which choreography is executed.

Representations and images of gendered bodies are not universal to all cultures (Turner 1984, Burt 1995, Greer 2003, Paechter 2003a). What appears as masculine or feminine behavior in one society or localized community may not be so in another. Unless otherwise specified, theory put forward in this chapter pertains to Western society.

PERFORMANCE OF GENDER

Why Might Embodied Gender Behavior Vary according to Biological Sex?

While renowned movement theorist Rudolph Laban (see Davies 2006, McCaw 2011), claimed that men and women were both capable of exercising strength and delicacy, his movement analysis work of the 1940s grounded itself in the fundamental premise that women's movements and movement patterns were different from men's. Laban never pursued the possibility that these differences were the result of social conditioning as opposed to nature. Connell (1995) presents a historical overview of sociobiological perspectives on gender pertaining to masculinity and femininity. The main perspectives are as follows: the body is a natural machine that produces gender differently; the body is a neutral surface that is socially constructed; gender differences in behavior are the product of both biology and society. Looking back on the matter and manner of my embodiment in photographs and home movies from when I was growing up, I perceive—with a sense of loss—a shift in my deportment from feminine toward masculine, and I concur that neither biology nor society can be dismissed in explaining this shift in gendered behavior. While I acknowledge the impact of biology on gendered behavior, this book focuses on the impact of social norms of embodiment on the same.

It is problematic to assume that males or females think, learn, and/or perform in particular ways simply as a result of being male or female (Lingard et al. 2009). Social pressures to perform in certain gendered ways can act forcefully against an individual's biology. For example, girls and boys may be conditioned to pursue physical activities considered suitable for their biological sex. Regardless of physiology, sex-specific socialization is likely to impact on gender directive as well as sexual identity (Turner 1984, Zeig 1985, J. Butler 1990, Young 1990, Connell 1995). "The formation of human attributes and capacities cannot be confined to social, biological, or psychological functions per se, but is the effect of an ensemble of practices" (Martino & Pallotta-Chiarolli 2001, p. 89). This study, and the suggestions it proposes, emanates from an investigation of the effects that *ensembles of practices* may have had on my social development, gender directive, and sexual identity, and by inference on the social development of others.

Well-Being

Connell argues, "Not being fixed by the physical logic of the body, this practice-made world may be hostile to bodies' physical well-being" (1999, p. 97). I believe that prescribed practices in this practice-made world that are gendered can also be hostile to an individual's emotional and social well-being. Theorists such as Surya Monro (2005) bemoan the discrimination and social exclusion suffered by individuals who do not fit neatly or specifically into normalized categories of male or female. The workings of gendered practices in this world are frequently invisible. Ways in which individuals both view and live in their worlds can be seen to be patterns that are taught and that come to seem natural (Pratt 1991). People have become so used to playing the woman and playing the man that they are unable to recognize ways in which they have been conditioned (Zeig 1985). This oversight is likely to make the impact of habitual gendernormative practices all the more forceful.

THE READING AND DOING OF EMBODIED GENDER

How Are Subjects of Cultures/Discourses Predisposed toward Reading as Well as Doing Performances of Gender?

Learning to Read and Learning to Do Male and Female Bodies

SOCIALIZATION

Children are socialized into the patterns of culture necessary for survival and growth within the communities and environments in which they are raised (Crothers 2007). According to differences in biological sex or genitalia, males and females are subject to differential socialization from birth (Turner 1984, Goffman 1997, Rogers 1999, Gorely et al. 2003, Shilling 2003, Paechter 2006). Embodied practices and body training that we learn in our social upbringing as girls and boys—to the exclusion of the other—will impact on how we develop (Young 1990, Guillaumin 1993, Shilling 2003, Paechter 2007).

Masculinizing practices in the rearing of boys and feminizing practices in the rearing of girls can place great pressures on boys and girls to measure up to hegemonic forms of masculinity and femininity (Connell 1983). Ways of being male or female that come to be hegemonic, dominant, and/or revered are shaped on prevailing historical forms of selfhood, desire, masculinity, and femininity (Alsop et al. 2002), and, frequently, these ideals are formed on the back of heterosexist and homophobic shaming of that which is deemed to be the subordinate 'other' (J. Butler 1990, Frank 1993, Connell 1995, Kehily 2001, Mac an Ghaill & Haywood 2007, Paechter 2007).

Where biological sexuality tends to be transformed by societies into defining products of human activity this can be referred to as the 'sex/gender system' (as coined by Gayle Rubin in 1975). In such systems, assumptions are made that conflate biological sex, gender behavior, and sexual orientation. Taylor and Richardson (2005) argue that childhood is not an innocent, natural, or authentic state but a time during which these assumptions are taken on, along with adult-world agendas of gendernormativity and compulsory heterosexuality (see also Kehily 2001, Renold 2005, Paechter 2007, DePalma & Atkinson 2008). Masculine and feminine embodiment tends to be translated into matters of sex and sexuality (Pronger 1990). Where an individual's embodiment does not measure up to valued hegemonic norms, such as behavior that is gendernormative or heteronormative, the individual is at risk of being marginalized.

MODEL BODIES—TRANSGRESSIVE BODIES

An individual's awareness of the corporeal self can be seen to hinge on experiences and images of other people's bodies (Mauss 1979, Shilling 2003). Where learning is not formal or technical, a learner's principal agent is a model used for imitation (Hall 1959). This can be seen as an apprenticeship of sorts, wherein children come to respect and imitate actions that have been successfully performed by people in whom they have confidence. They learn as a result what it means to be a successful man or woman in the culture or community of practice in which they live (Mauss 1979, Paechter 2007). Particular qualities come to carry or are afforded social value, or what Pierre Bourdieu theorizes as social capital (Jenkins 2002), which can be afforded not only to qualities such as knowledge, possessions, or relations but also to physical attributes and performance. The same embodied action on a male or a female body does not always signal or mean the same thing (Grosz 1994), nor does it gain the same social capital. In subsequent chapters, I investigate the influences and impact that male models of success, as well as of failure, had on my embodiment and social development as a male subject. Models of masculinity and femininity can be found both in the everyday and also in arenas of popular culture. It can be argued that representations within theatre and other mass media influence, teach, and encourage particular gendered behaviors as much as they describe them (Bollen et al. 2008, see also Crothers 2007).

Usual ideals of heteronormal representation are masculine males and feminine females (J. Butler 1993). Such ideals of sexuality and gender are learned and imposed through socialization and enculturation long before children might be capable of discovering either (Shilling 2003). If social power can be derived from living up to ideals of normativity (Skattebol 2006), then, conversely, male and female bodies that do not project as successful must also exert an influence. Referring to German society in the 1970s, Marianne Wex (1979) contended that females who posed or strutted in masculine ways by taking more space and assuming broader poses—both in the media and in the everyday—were seen as improper and for the most part as proffering sex, just as males who posed or strutted in feminine ways were seen as socially weak or queer. In recent times too, effeminate embodiment on a male signifies homosexuality (Gard 2001, Gere 2001, Martino & Pallotta-Chiarolli 2001). Where there is fear or anxiety of being classified as gay, such coding is likely to condition males against effeminate behavior. In this book I investigate the effects that such sex-specific signification has on the well-being of individuals—regardless of sexual orientation—whose embodied performance inclination may not match prescribed norms, and I theorize on the contestation of such signification.

CHILDREN, SCHOOLS, AND SEXUALITY

> [C]hildren feel the need to draw strong boundaries between groups, expecting differences to be very clear-cut so that there is as little uncertainty as possible about their own and others' positions.
>
> (Paechter 2007, p. 155)

Childhood is a state that is affected very early on by the prevalent agendas of heteronormativity and gendernormativity in adult worlds (Taylor & Richardson 2005). DePalma and Atkinson (2008) argue that schools are sites of tacit instruction in the possibilities and limitations of gender and sexual identity (see also Kehily 2002, Renold 2005, Lingard et al. 2009). Through the parameters they set, schools, as social institutions, can be seen as key sites for the regulation and normalization of children's bodies and subjectivities, directing the bodies of boys and girls toward particular patterns of behavior (Kamler et al. 1994, Gard 2003a, Shilling 2003). Children come to learn that performances of self that are most closely aligned to established, traditional, and gendered norms continue to meet with the most success (Kamler et al. 1994). To be considered 'normal' involves the projection of a coherent and abiding heterosexual self (J. Butler 1990, Martino & Pallotta-Chiarolli 2005, Renold 2005, see also Mac an Ghaill & Haywood 2007, Lingard et al. 2009), and this includes embodied behavior. Even from an early age, those who transgress gendernormative stereotypes of masculinity for males and femininity for females—such as non-muscular males, muscular females, females engaged in stereotypical masculine pursuits such as weightlifting, and males engaged in stereotypical feminine pursuits such as dancing—risk being viewed in a negative light and risk having their (hetero)sexuality questioned (Mac an Ghaill 1994, Gard 2003a, Gorely et al. 2003, Francis 2010).

Mary Kehily (2002) makes reference to the 'hidden curriculum' as unofficial and unacknowledged teaching and learning that also takes place in schools. She argues that hidden curricula have the power to regulate clear-cut sex-gender categories and conforming attitudes and behaviors of individual bodies as well as collective bodies such as school populations. Despite sociologist Mark McCormack's (2012) claims that young males are now able to act in feminine ways without fear of being homosexualized (see also Anderson 2011), Kehily (2002), Epstein & Johnson (2008), and Hillier et al. (2005) found that the fear of being called 'gay' or 'sissy' in schools acts as a disciplinary technique regulating male behavior and embodied social practices. Forms of masculinity that align with notions of heterosexuality assume a dominant status in schools (Kehily 2002). Boys whose bodily actions, gestures, posturings, and tone of voice are not considered suitable for 'guys' become visible targets in the eyes of other boys (Martino & Pallotta-Chiarolli 2003).

Boys who see themselves as outside the hegemony of validated heterosexual masculinity can protect themselves from the implications of being seen as feminine—and, by implication, gay—via outward forms of bodily performance through participation in certain sports such as Australian rules football (Frank 1993, Nayak & Kehily 1996, Jackson 2002, Gard 2003b, Paechter 2006). Another way of ensuring that one projects as heterosexual—and by association 'normal'—is by labeling and harassing other boys who demonstrate transgressive masculinity as being 'gay' (Martino & Pallotta-Chiarolli 2003, 2005, Renold 2005, Pascoe 2007, Lingard et al. 2009). As a result of living in environments of hostility toward homosexuality, even homosexual students can develop anti-homosexual bias, commonly termed 'internalized homophobia' (Allen & Oleson 1999).

In upcoming chapters, I chart and comment on how I came to understand bodies that posed/reposed/moved in a masculine manner differently from bodies that posed/reposed/moved in a feminine manner, and how as a male subject within certain heteronormative cultural settings, such as home and school, I came to embody my male body in particular ways that marked, formed, and continue to resonate in how I project, perceive, and embody myself today. I investigate the desire—both conscious and unconscious—not to transgress socially prescribed gender norms in order not to be marginalized.

Physical Capital

As soon as a body is sighted, assumptions can be made concerning biological sex, race, physical ability, fitness, and health. Prior to speech or even motion, how a body is posed, reposed, clothed, or accessorized can lead to assumptions concerning personality, attraction, and sexuality. Indeed, the signification of the body "precedes its own action" (J. Butler 1993, p. 30).

Shilling (2003) views the body as central to the acquisition of status and distinction. Taking Bourdieu's notion of cultural capital (1977), wherein individuals are valued according to their competence in various social settings (social fields), Shilling speaks of physical capital, where the physical body itself is the bearer of value in society. "When social fields bestow value directly on a specific bodily form, activity or performance, they are effectively creating a category of physical capital" (Shilling 2003, p. 121). I argue that one's embodied performance of gender is a primary form of physical capital that can forcefully affect one's social and cultural standing (cultural capital) at any given time. Just as a certain embodiment may be highly valued, resulting in physical capital, other lesser-valued embodiment may result in physical poverty.

If certain masculinities and femininities—projected via male and female bodies respectively—project as heterosexual and normal (heteronormative), and if heteronormativity is valued (Martino & Pallotta-Chiarolli 2005, Vicars 2008), then it follows that other embodiment and embodied acts may project as abnormal and valueless (Monro 2005). So embedded are the values accorded to embodied behavior that transgressive gendered embodiment—such as feminine embodiment performed by males and masculine embodiment performed by females—is still for the most part viewed both in the media and in the everyday as comic, ludicrous, strange, and/or deviant.

Norms and ideals serve as signifiers that cast light on that which is 'other'. Slavoj Zizek's (1999) master-signifier theory (after Lacan) makes the point that when a signifier or that which carries meaning becomes stable in what it symbolizes, it can cause that which is different and the most removed from it to stand out as marked, other, and abnormal (see also Pickering 2001, R. Butler 2005). For example, where the signification of chewing with one's mouth closed becomes symbolic of good manners, it may have a degrading effect on the meaning of masticating with one's mouth open. Knowing that *difference draws attention to itself* is likely to exert pressure on individuals to embody or *not* to embody in certain ways. In cases where drawing attention has negative connotations, it is unlikely that an individual would want to stand out from the norm by embodying differently from others.

To alleviate anxieties around the masculinity and sexuality of male performance artists, bodies of males are frequently directed and choreographed in hypermasculine ways (Buchbinder 2004, see also Burt 1995, Gard 2001, 2006), with the male form depicted as being powerful, taking space, and using large, expansive, highly athletic movements. The cultural capital of a male—in formal public arenas and in the everyday—is at stake should his embodiment be soft or delicate, despite the fact that he is physically capable of performing in such ways. There is a tendency for males in the everyday to take up heteronormal ideals of masculinity and cultivate overt if not hyper-heterosexual behavior in order to prove their masculinity and heterosexuality (Connell 1983, 1985, Mac an Ghaill 1994, Mac an Ghaill & Haywood 2007) and as a means of escaping societal surveillance (Lanzieri & Hildebrandt 2011). In Chapters 5–7 I reflect, chart, and comment on my own sense of physical capital and poverty both as a performance artist and as a performer in the everyday.

PHYSICAL LIMITATIONS TO PERFORMANCE

A line of thought that concerns me is that the masculinities and femininities an individual can perform are partially dependent on the form of the individual's body. Does the form of our bodies delimit what and how we can perform? Carrie Paechter claims, "It is easier to enact superfemininity if you are slightly built, harder if you are six foot tall, overweight, have facial hair or muscular shoulders" (2006, p. 131). Such reasoning connects delimitations of gendered embodiment to physiology rather than to social conditioning, such as consciousness of how others will perceive one's performance. I argue that burly bodies with facial hair and muscular shoulders *are* capable of moving delicately and in a feminine way, and that what needs to be addressed is why social mores, socially constructed states of mind, and socially constructed senses of taste learned through models seen and commodified in public and everyday arenas tell us otherwise. Through autoethnographic investigation, I will demonstrate that what delimits our bodies are states of mind that become so habitual that their machinations are rendered invisible.

Regulation of Bodies

Our bodies are subject to choreographic regulation, from the lining up for service to the playing of sports. Such disciplines and repeated practices—at times varying according to biological sex—can be seen to produce bodies that are docile and valued by the societies that create them (Foucault 1977). In subsequent chapters, I reflect on my own embodied experience of being regulated, directed, and choreographed as a docile male dancer, actor, student, and citizen, as well as the regulatory work I have done—and do—on the bodies of others as a director, choreographer, and teacher.

PUNISHMENT

Michel Foucault (1977) charts the evolution of punishment in Western society from the corporeal and physically violent to what can be regarded as more lenient soft control mechanisms such as confinement, noting that central to each is the submission of perpetrators' bodies. Foucault's theories of punishment for perpetrators of crimes can be paralleled to the regulation that happens to bodies whose crimes may be transgressing prescribed norms of gender behavior within contemporary Western contexts. Later prison systems that Foucault refers to had benevolent aims of reforming criminals and bringing them back into society following the imposed punishment. Contemporary penalties or punishments that see the marginalization, alienation, ostracism, and harassment of those who do not embody gender as socially prescribed may also lead to reformed behavior on the part of perpetrators. However, it is difficult to identify benevolent intentions in the delivery of such punishment. For example, in the opening episode of this book, the males in the car may have found the style of the male pedestrians' walk unacceptable, yet I doubt that their verbal abuse (punishment) was delivered with the benevolent aim of correcting that walk. They may have wanted to point out the 'incorrectness' of the walk, but from my perspective—as one of the pedestrians—their intent was malevolent.

PANOPTICON AND SELF-REGULATION

Individuals who wish to fit into certain cultural settings may come to self-police their embodied performance of gender in order to do so. Foucault

(1977) outlines the mechanisms of self-policing via reference to Bentham's panopticon. Aware that they may be observed from a central tower at any time, prisoners in the panopticon are likely to regulate their behavior and behave *correctly.* "It is the fact of being constantly seen, of being able always to be seen, that maintains the disciplined individual in his subjection" (Foucault 1977, p. 187). Individuals who think they are under surveillance—be it walking down a street, sitting on a tram, or standing in a queue—are likely to self-police their actions in the knowledge that they may be the object of someone else's gaze or scrutiny, especially if they are aware of the possible social consequences or penalties for behavior that is considered transgressive. Through a postcolonial studies lens, Marta Savigliano (1995, after Franz Fanon [2008, originally published in 1952] and Albert Memmi [1967]) suggests that in order to get by, colonized subjects eventually come to colonize themselves. Males and females inclined to perform gender differently from prescribed norms can be regarded as colonized subjects when they are trained/educated in and adhere to hegemonic ways of 'normality'. Should they wish to fit in—or wish not to stand out—it is in their interest to self-regulate and conform to prescribed norms. Indeed, the imitation and replication of dominant hierarchies and modes can serve those in minority groups as a way of gaining equity if not power (see Kroeger 2003).

Schools can be regarded as panopticonic spaces where young persons not only are monitored by the institution but also learn to monitor themselves according to the culturally specific norms and expectations of the said institution (Martino & Pallotta-Chiarolli 2001, 2003, 2005, Paechter 2007, Pallotta-Chiarolli 2010). Many of these behavioral expectations are attached to mainstream notions of norms of gender and sexuality, resulting in mutual panopticism or public conformity to collectively constructed concepts of desirable and valued practices of masculinity and femininity (Paechter 2007). A person's "disciplinary history" (habitual patterns of movement and corporeal commitments undertaken in day to day life) will affect not only the person's body but also their thoughts and ways of being (Grosz 1994, p. 142, see also Kamler 1993). In this book I chart and comment on my own disciplinary history as a colonized subject of various gendernormative/heteronormative worlds and demonstrate ways in which they marked and formed me in the past and still inform and resonate in who I am today.

AGENCY

Individuals in everyday life can be equated to actors in performance (Goffman 1959). Like actors, individuals in everyday life can be seen to have agency over their own performances and the ability to present different versions of themselves according to the context, setting, and audience. In contrast, Foucauldian views regard the body as a malleable object determined by social structures and largely beyond individual control. Yet bodies can be seen as being both agents and objects (Turner 1984, J. Butler 1990, Connell 1999, Shilling 2003). In other words, despite social constraints on the body, control of bodies is also dependent, to an extent, on the actions and desires of the individual. Even from a young age, children can be seen to exercise a degree of agency through the placement and positioning of limbs in the pursuit of fitting desired identities (Skattebol 2006), such as those of male and female models viewed in the media and in the everyday.

The social success of an individual depends on the ability to manage the self, much of which hinges on the presentation of a socially acceptable body. In this regard Turner (1984) refers to the matter and adornment of the body in forms of plastic surgery, dentistry, hair, clothing, and manicure. Similarly, Shilling (2003) talks of individuals' control and maintenance of the body as their machine through means such as diet, medical procedures, and physical training (see also Bordo 1993). I will be focusing on agency and the managing of one's body more in terms of practice (choreography) and the manner in which practice is executed (performance). While theorists such as Turner and Shilling conjecture on bodily practices, their work does not adequately address the form and style of practice as prescribed or valued differently according to the biological sex of the individual performer.

The relationship between personal and social control of an individual's embodiment of gender is a delicate one. Cultural theorist Angela McRobbie (2009) argues that even where we appear to have agency, what we choose to do is framed, regulated, and contextualized to a large degree by cultural boundaries, influences, and parameters. Where neo-liberal sentiment may espouse a line of thinking in which individuals have agency to do anything, and as such to embody in any manner they choose, such lines of thought erase the influences of systemic inequitable frameworks such as patriarchal hierarchies of gender behavior that envelop us (McRobbie 2009). It is impossible not to take into account cultural influences such as the media and popular culture when contemplating ways in which individuals might choose, be inspired, or come to embody. As such, agency does not necessarily denote autonomy. Ironically, even when we operate with agency, our bodies may not always fulfill our intentions (Turner 1984, Shilling 2003). Indeed, how one thinks one is performing (*virtual* social identity) and how one's audience perceives the same performance (*actual* social identity) do not always or necessarily match (Goffman 1959).

Habitus and Taste

HABITUS

We are frequently unaware of habitual ways in which we come to perform certain embodied actions. Bourdieu theorizes about "habitus" as non-consciously performed practices that are "internalised as second nature and so forgotten" (1990, p. 56). According to Bourdieu, habitus manifests in "schemes of perception, thought and action" (p. 54). The first two forms, perception and thought, concern internal response and reaction. The third form, habitus in the form of action, manifests itself in and through the body. Theories on habitus are consistent with Judith Butler's theories on gender performativity, wherein gender is not a singular or deliberate act but rather the repeated stylization of the body (1990, 1993). Dancers talk about "body memory" where in performance dancers need not think, "What is the next step?" (Erskine 2005). The reason for this is that through rehearsal and repetition, the body remembers. In everyday performance too, individuals can be seen as dancers who through constant repetition embody learned styles and repertoires of everyday actions such as walking, sitting, and eating, without being particularly conscious of what or how they are performing. Drawing on my own experiences of perceiving and embodying gendered performance, I aim to demonstrate the interconnection of habitus as embodied action with habitual ways of thinking and perceiving.

Embedded practices that differ according to biological sex were an aspect of habitus that Bourdieu did not particularly delve into (Adkins & Skeggs 2004). To Bourdieu, gender was a lived social relation, whereas for Butler, it was a location within discursive structures (McNay 2004). Nevertheless, Bourdieu's theories of habitus can be applied to habitual and embedded ways of doing and perceiving that which is feminine and that which is masculine. Indeed, Bourdieu's work relating to habitus can provide an encompassing framework for the investigation of embodied performance of gender.

Bourdieu (1990) refers to fields as being the socially constructed settings in which we operate and argues that one needs a *feel for the game* in order to participate effectively and instinctively. Through autoethnographic data, I take these notions and signpost the problems involved when we are caught up in the game of gender performance in contemporary mainstream Western cultural settings; when we develop habitual ways of perceiving representations of sex-specific masculinity and femininity—as viewed in media, arts, sports, and everyday arenas—as desirable or undesirable; when we develop habitual ways of doing gender through our own bodies that may not align with the ways in which we desire or are inclined to embody gender; and when we may be unaware of the habitual ways in which we view and embody gender.

With regard to the performance of gender, I question the conceptualization that it is within individual agency to alter or change one's habitus (Schirato & Yell 1996). Reflecting on my own embodied experiences of gender, I question the ways in which one's embodied habitus, via one's own discursive location, limits what one can say and see (Threadgold 1994). The "active presence of past experiences . . . deposited in each organism . . . tend to guarantee the 'correctness' of practices and their constancy over time" (Bourdieu 1990, p. 54). Habitual practices rendered invisible by those who are located within cultures or discourses where the habitual feels and seems natural bring to mind Alfred Schutz's (1944) theories on phenomenology, where a 'stranger' or outsider viewing the everyday practices of a particular culture—for example, routines of greeting such as bowing, shaking hands, kissing, or rubbing noses—may find them questionable as a result of not sharing the same taken for granted assumptions about appropriate behaviors (see Brodersen 1971). Even those born into a culture or discourse who themselves may not be inclined to embody in socially prescribed ways may—as a result of effective colonization—accept and not question the dominant embodied habitual practices by which their culture operates.

TASTE

An individual's perceptions of certain practices as being right or comfortable or desirable may feel as though they are natural or instinctive. However, such perceptions are dependent on one's social location and can be defined as a person's taste (Bourdieu 1990, Turner 1992, Shilling 2003). Taste does not remain at the level of consciousness but is a manifestation of habitus that can cause people to take on or repel certain practices. Orientations of taste toward embodied practices can be gendered, affecting affinity with sports and other physical activities (Gorely et al. 2003, Shilling 2004). Our taste will affect how we view and perform embodied activity. What comes to feel right or wrong, pleasurable or disagreeable, becomes sedimented, fossilized, and is not easily upset or altered (Gorely et al. 2003, Migdalek 2009).

In arguing against the neo-liberal position that choice is within the power of the autonomous individual, McRobbie (2009) contends that what an individual comes to find aesthetic is very much influenced by externally promoted cultural subjectivities. What the individual takes to be their own essential or authentic sense of taste—devoid of social or other framings—can be understood to be imposed by external cultural forces and therefore rendered not authentic or essential at all. This contention is also relevant to habitual and favored ways of presenting and representing male and female bodies as taken up by performance arts directors, choreographers, and performers too. If aesthetic taste is understood to be a manifestation of habitus, then performance artists are unlikely to be aware of the relationship between their sense of aesthetics and their enculturation, nor are they likely to recognize gendered aspects that may be integral to their directorial/choreographic habitus, which to all intents and purposes feel natural and instinctive to them.

Dominant notions of what is aesthetic and un-aesthetic may also act forcefully on individuals who are marginal to the mainstream. In much the same way that colonized persons might come to adopt the values and ideology of the colonizer or oppressor (Memmi 1967), and in much the same way that those in minority groups might toe the hegemonic line through imitation and replication of dominant hierarchies as a form of passing or gaining power (Kroeger 2003, see also Freire 1990), it may be that colonized individuals also unknowingly come to take on as tasteful that which is valorized, and as distasteful that which is devalued, within the dominant cultures that oppress them. Examples of this can be found in studies that problematize reductionist discrimination against effeminate males within gay communities (see Payne 2007, Fisher & Shay 2009), and in tendencies of homosexuals to conform to heteronormative idealizations of masculinity (Lanzieri &

Hildebrandt 2011). These issues and what we unknowingly pick up from the media and other sources will be raised and explored in subsequent chapters.

CHANGE

Lecoq, a world-renowned drama training technique, strives to make actors aware of and then to strip away deeply ingrained behavior patterns by which they have been conditioned (Callery 2001, Lecoq 2002, Sears & Hollos 2002). The technique regards these patterns as a hindrance to neutrality and perfect balance. In a similar vein the Feldenkrais Method, an educational system centered on movement, is concerned with bringing awareness and mindfulness to limiting habits such as the ways in which we walk, stand, sit, and lie (Callery 2001, Feldenkrais Method 2008). Both techniques promote learning that enables one to know and do things in other ways, with change being seen as a matter of choice and agency:

> [H]uman dignity is dependent on freedom of choice. We rarely think of choice in relation to movement, assuming that our movements are automatic. Most of us accept the habitual ways in which we move without a second thought.
>
> (Callery 2001, p. 40, of the Feldenkrais technique)

The focus of the Feldenkrais Method (2008) is on combating damaging movement patterns and muscular habits such as hunching our backs or tensing our necks when working in front of a computer. I contend that habitual patterns of embodiment that are gendered can also be damaging but in ways that go beyond effects on muscular habit.

As people tend to reproduce the practices with which they are most familiar, change—regarding the reading and *doing* of embodied gender (in the interests of the social and emotional well-being of those whose gendered performance inclinations do not conform to mainstream gender norms)—is no simple process. Even though people may have a substantial degree of agency over their bodies (Goffman 1959, Turner 1984), it may be difficult for people to break out of the "corporeal trajectories assigned to them by their social location, habitus, and taste" (Shilling 2003, p. 128). Habitus and taste operate at a level of the subconscious and are therefore not necessarily open to change (Bourdieu 1990). Change, while within individuals' creative capacities, does not happen automatically, nor does it occur simply as a result of purely intellectual motivation (Shilling 2003, 2004, see also Pratt 1991, J. Butler 2004).

SEMIOTICS OF MASCULINE/FEMININE EMBODIMENT

Wex (1979), arguing for women to embody more freely, draws on images of male and female forms and focuses on the semiotics of embodied pose and how the same embodiment may come to signal and be understood differently according to who performs it and when. She claims that women in

1970s Germany were more restricted and limited in how they could move and pose their bodies than they had been in earlier eras. She also found that men in 1970s Germany enjoyed a greater range of acceptable embodied behaviors than did women, something I would claim is no longer so in contemporary Germany, or in other parts of the Western world. I believe that restrictive social pressures and limitations on how contemporary Western males may pose, move, and position their bodies have become embedded in the fabric of contemporary Western societies. In this book I suggest methods by which a more equitable state of gender semiotics may eventuate.

According to political scientist Lane Crothers (2007) the values, norms, and social practices embedded in the popular movies, music, and television programs of a dominant culture have the potential to shape and influence the values, aspirations, and lives of people of other cultures exposed to them via the mass media. Jacques Derrida talks of Western traditional orders of meanings as entities that seem unified and absolute even where they consist of discrepancies (Payne 1993). Through a plethora of cultural artifacts in the forms of media and entertainment, the values, norms, and social practices that appear to be representative of dominant social/cultural systems become globalized, leading toward cultural homogenization at the expense of cultural diversity. Popular entertainment—dominated by the US media—circulates dichotomous gender images that define notions of masculinity and femininity (Connell 1999). The transfer and dispersal of such "cultural commodities" (a term coined by Mac an Ghaill & Haywood 2007, p. 199) not only have the power to impose the norms and values of dominant cultures on local cultures but may also see the reconfiguration of gendered subjectivity and what it means to be a woman or a man in local cultures (Mac an Ghaill & Haywood 2007). Although in some societies these notions may not be taken up as ideals (Greer 2003) and even though fluid, hybrid, and/or transgressive gender images that oppose dominant norms exist (see Nixon 1996), I hypothesize that globalization of gendered images of the body limits the discursive space in which individuals in the everyday are easily able to define themselves.

A narrow range of embodied male and female representations in popular entertainment are so pervasive that their effect on and regulation of individuals—including directors and choreographers of male and female bodies—are all the more forceful. Indeed, it is a difficult thing for artists to defamiliarize themselves from what has become common practice within the art form (Trinh 1992). Change toward a more equitable state of gender semiotics may be an even greater struggle in practice than theorized by the sociologists, educators, artists, and critical linguists to whom I refer in later discussion on deconstruction.

Discourses and Ideologies

Discourse and ideology—which Neimes (2003) argues are ideas and values imbued in society as a part of the natural order—may predispose the mindsets of individuals toward gendered readings and performances of the body. The disciplining effects that enculturation via discourses of gender and sexuality have on a body's capacity for action can be used to explain the "astonishing gap between what bodies can do and what they 'choose' to do" (Gard 2003a, p. 219). Discourses and their workings are frequently rendered invisible and can be paralleled to the invisibility of a pane of glass that we might look through, which becomes perceptible only when the glass is shattered or broken (Davies 1993b). Discourses of sexism, difference, heteronormativity, homophobia, physical culture, and essentialism all impact on how performances of embodied gender are perceived and executed.

DISCOURSES OF SEXISM

Differences between men's and women's bodily comportment, motility, and spatiality in how they approach and perform some physical tasks are linked to powerful and embedded patriarchal models of how males and females should behave (Turner 1984, Young 1990, Threadgold 1994). These can be oppressive to those whose physical appearance and embodiment do not conform to those traditionally associated with women and men (Monro 2005).

DISCOURSES OF DIFFERENCE

Identification is built and consolidated at the expense of what it excludes (J. Butler 1990, 1993). Gloria Anzaldua theorizes about "borders" and "borderlands" as unnatural boundaries or dividing lines, set up "to distinguish *us* from *them*" (1987, p. 3). In this way, categories such as good/bad, male/female, masculine/feminine, straight/gay, and abled/disabled come to function as characterizing symbols and images of opposites, which tend to be classified as hierarchical dualisms (see Pallotta-Chiarolli 2010). Binary terms are the only way that many are able to engage with notions of gender and sexuality (Davies 1989, J. Butler 1990, 2004, Monro 2005, Mac an Ghaill & Haywood 2007). Even mainstream feminist theory—in contrast to postcolonial gender theory—has been guilty of universalizing men's issues and women's issues and has been rigid in its assumption that there is a clear distinction between male and female categories, and thus it has further reinforced notions of difference (hooks 2001, Said in Viswanathan 2004, Monro 2005).

Goffman talks of the phenomenon of "civil inattention", wherein people glance through one another as a sign of "trust, respect and apparent unconcern" (1997, p. 327). If we invert this point, the marked visibility of bodies that are seen to be in binary opposition to, transgressive of, or 'other' to the norm may signify in hierarchical terms as bodies to be mistrusted or disrespected. It is problematic that as a result of such "absolute despot duality"—between normal and 'other'—we are able to be only one or the other (Anzaldua 1987, p. 19).

Monro contends that "[g]ender diversity provides a challenge to the gender binary system" (2005, p. 11). Tierney (1997b) and Monro (2005) oppose the reduction and compartmentalization of complex concepts of gender, gender performance, and sexual orientation into either-or dichotomous categorizations. Rather, it is possible to appreciate the myriad of possibilities of gender and sexuality (Halberstam 1998) as points on a gender continuum in which identifications may be "fluid, transitory, fragmented, episodic" (Pallotta-Chiarolli 2010, p. 30) and not encumbered by imperatives to conform to the constraints of learned gender alignments (Taylor & Richardson 2005). Social systems that do not provide for identifications that are different or 'other' do damage to the lived realities of those who do not fit neatly into either-or standards of existence (Pallotta-Chiarolli 2010).

DISCOURSES OF HETERONORMATIVITY AND HOMOPHOBIA

Although gender can be enacted in a variety of ways, we are positioned to view and do gender according to the cultural confines of 'compulsory heterosexuality' (Rich 1987, J. Butler 1993) and 'hierarchical sexual dualisms' (Pallotta-Chiarolli 2010). Such ideology renders heterosexuality as uniform and normal, thereby positioning homosexuality as a binary opposite—that is, other and by default subordinate. As Monro states, "The representation of heterosexuality as foundational or natural . . . means that alternatives become constructed as abnormal or deviant" (2005, p. 29). In effect, heteronormative and homophobic regimes of bodily practice prescribe and regulate how *normal* bodies are to be moved and displayed (J. Butler 1993, Gard 2001).

Mainstream media and film plots are reflective of heteronormative discourses that marginalize the homosexual through stereotypical, one-dimensional depictions—usually comic or deviant—who frequently share common destinies (Russo 1981, J. Butler 1993, Jones 2003, Linne 2003, O'Connell 2012). Looking beyond scripts, plots, storylines, and narratives of dramas, I will discuss the signification of feminine/masculine embodiment itself as performed by bodies projected in the media, and how this impacts on the social mindset toward embodied transgression of heteronormativity.

DISCOURSES OF PHYSICAL CULTURE

Gender-appropriate sports and other physical activities serve as dominant standards for how male and female bodies should move, limiting and negating alternative bodily possibilities for both (Young 1990, Gard 2003b, Gorely et al. 2003, Paechter 2007). Those who violate gender norms in sports stand out as other and risk having their femininity/masculinity and their sexuality scrutinized and questioned (Gorely et al. 2003). The heritage of the classical ballet can be seen to have globalized certain aesthetic signals of gender identity in ways that are both sexist and homophobic in nature (Foster 1996, 2001, Stoneley 2007). Conventional and traditional signaling of gender continues to press forcefully on contemporary dance (Banes 1998, Stoneley 2007)—as well as other performance art forms—limiting and impacting on how commercial performance artists direct and choreograph male and female forms, and by association how mainstream audiences come to receive and perceive the same. However they might be abstracted, human forms in dance can never be separated from social constructions of meaning and significance (McKechnie 2002). How readily is delicate embodiment performed by a male perceived by mainstream audiences without evoking notions of homosexuality or humor? Oppositional icons of femininity and masculinity so prevalent and revered in the ballet tradition can be inscriptive of gender behavior in the everyday (Dempster 1988). These concerns will be explored through fieldwork with high school students and adult participants in Chapters 9 to 11.

ESSENTIALISM

Stephan Fuchs (2001) argues that when essentialist thinking occurs, individuals or groups consider their beliefs and values to be true and natural. Such thinking renders those individuals and groups blind to other possibilities. Even gender scholars, whose work is steeped in social constructionist theory, often retain a 'residual essentialism' that describes and upholds gender in dichotomous terms (Alsop et al. 2002). Notions such as these can become so established that they acquire the status of being authentic and unquestionable. In much the same way that individuals overlook the proposition that their sense of taste is culturally framed or imposed (McRobbie 2009), so too is there a tendency for individuals to take that which they understand to be their 'internal essence' as a given (J. Butler 2004). In this way individuals may overlook the proposition that what is understood to be one's sense of embodied self is also affected and/or formed by external cultural forces.

CONSEQUENCES: BODIES AND MINDS AT RISK

What Is the Impact of Oppressive and/or Dominant Discourses of Performance of Gender on the Social Well-Being of Those Whose Embodied Performance Inclinations Do Not Comply with Those Discourses? What Are the Consequences of Performing according to Desire?

Conforming or Being 'Other'

Foucault refers to the force of the "normalizing gaze" (1977, p. 184) as a form of surveillance that can regulate individuals' behaviors. Where an individual's behavior contravenes habitual perceptions and structures, they come to be understood as anything from suspicious to comic (Bourdieu 1990, Schirato & Yell 1996). These are qualities to be avoided, as failing to be 'in sync' with notions of normalcy tends to disable and marginalize those who may be different (Hall 1977). Those who perform masculinities and femininities that go against the norm frequently fit into the aforementioned categories of 'other' (Russo 1981, Flanagan 1982, Paechter 2003b).

"There are many oppressive aspects to the construction of bodies in line with gender stereotypes" (Shilling 2003, p. 97), and individuals whose appearance and actions do not conform to dominant norms—or recognizable standards of "gender intelligibility" (J. Butler 1990, p. 16)—may experience pressure to conform and censor their behavior in order to protect their personal security (Shilling 2003, Monro 2005). The threat of physical abuse (such as bashings), alienation, ostracism, marginalization, and/or exclusion for those who fail to perform their gender in socially appropriate ways may cause acute consciousness of how one's body projects (J. Butler 1993, Shilling 2003). There are pressures to not embody, let alone desire, that which the cultures we are part of distinguish as deviant (J. Butler 1993). Projecting normalcy is precarious and requires constant diligent maintenance work, as any slip in an individual's performance of self may alter the way that the individual is regarded or labeled (Goffman 1959, Shilling 2003, see also Davies 1989, Renew 1996, Swain 2004).

Signifiers—Straight or Gay

Males who project publicly as feminine and females who project publicly as masculine are commonly signified as homosexual (Mac an Ghaill & Haywood 2007) and—regardless of their sexual orientation—are at risk of expulsion from heteronormal circles of legitimacy (J. Butler 1990, Connell 1995, Gard 2003a, Renold 2003). That this classification is seen as a handicap that may lead to social marginalization is testimony to the inclination to safeguard children's social acceptance by raising them in a manner that maximizes the possibility of a heterosexual outcome (Kosofsky Sedgwick 1994). This brings to mind Zizek's theories of the "reflexive abbreviation" (R. Butler 2005, p. 51), where labeling someone X because they are Y leads to assumptions that because someone is Y they are X. Assumptions or concerns that an infant might be gay because he/she embodies in a feminine/masculine manner concur with reflexive assumptions that the male/female who moves in a feminine/masculine manner is gay.

In her work on discrimination, feminist bell hooks (1996) argues that the discourses of mass media have the power to do violence to people. If we relate this to gender and sexuality, public arenas of popular culture such as film, television, theatre, and sports present an abundance of representations of heterosexual males that are hypermasculine, homosexual males that are hyperfeminine, heterosexual females that are hyperfeminine, and homosexual females that are hypermasculine. These representations can be oppressive to male and female audiences in that they limit acceptable notions of alternative masculinities and femininities for heterosexual/homosexual males and females. Mark O'Connell (2012), a US psychotherapist concerned with negative social attitudes toward GLBT people, theorizes that the scarcity of empathetic, gender non-conforming characters in mainstream commercial movies effectively condones homophobia for audiences. O'Connell (2012) discusses case studies of children who on seeing typical trivialized images of characters that were perceived to be "faggots" experienced intense fears of being perceived similarly themselves, even by friends and family. As such, these prevalent portrayals are not benign. Even though it may be possible to achieve an oppositional reading of prevalent representations in popular culture of gay characters as being helpless, isolated, dangerous, or clownish, these representations can still be oppressive and damaging to the lives of those who are gay (Linne 2003) as well as those who are at risk of being perceived to be gay (see Crothers 2007). In Chapters 4–7 I will relate these points to my own history in order to demonstrate the debilitating effects of the limited set of options given and taken up as representative of male, female, heterosexual, or homosexual embodiment.

Pressures toward heteronormativity weigh equally heavily on heterosexual persons as on homosexuals (see Kirby & Hay 1997), for fear of what is at risk if their performance of heterosexuality does not measure up to what Turner terms "cultural criteria of appropriateness" (1984, p. 184). Turner discusses how criteria of appropriateness may cause anxieties that can impact on the body in conditions such as anorexia nervosa and bulimia. Inverting this line of reasoning, I believe that *inappropriate* embodiment may cause anxieties that impact on an individual's emotional and social well-being.

Research studies in which body gait and behavior are analyzed as being indicative of a person's sexual orientation (Sirin et al. 2004, Johnson et al. 2007) are problematic in that their focus tends to be on the subjects being analyzed rather than on the social and cultural conditioning of the people making discriminatory assumptions about the sexual orientation of others. The belief that a subject's sexual orientation can be assumed according to quantitatively definable body cues (Johnson et al. 2007) overlooks the possibility that individuals may willingly, or even subconsciously, embody against their inclination in order to comply with gender norms deemed socially/culturally appropriate to their biological sex.

School Students at Risk

Schools can be seen as sites where students who do not fit recognized norms of behavior can become marginalized and harassed. Social pressures to measure up to desirable heteronormative forms and versions of masculinity and femininity can impact significantly on the emotional and mental health and well-being of school students (Plummer 1999, Hillier et al. 2005, Martino & Pallotta-Chiarolli 2005, Ollis 2008). In their research into boys and schooling in Australia and the United Kingdom, Bob Lingard, Wayne Martino, and Martin Mills (2009) point out that differences between boys and girls continue to be essentialized, even in government policies on education, and that this further marginalizes boys and girls who do not fit traditional biologically determined homogenized notions of masculine and feminine behaviors.

The third in a series of national studies on the sexual health and well-being of same-sex attracted and gender questioning young people found that levels of homophobic abuse are on the rise in Australia, especially in school sites (Hillier et al. 2010). Despite laws that have become more inclusive in terms of sexual difference, positive media visibility of gay and lesbian adults, and work that has been done in schools to address homophobia, it is clear that other means of improving social attitudes toward gender and sexual diversity and expression need to be pursued. There are anxieties, especially for boys, about not measuring up as straight. Despite McCormack's (2012) claims of changing attitudes toward homosexuality among schoolboys, other researchers find that projecting as 'gay' is still one of the worst forms of denigration within school cultures (Frank 1993, Swain 2004, Martino & Pallotta-Chiarolli 2005, Pascoe 2007, Lingard et al. 2009). Part of such projection hinges on an individual's body and embodiment.

It should be noted that despite moves to encourage alternative constructions of masculinity, there continue to be pressures not only on male students but also on male teachers to meet dominant hegemonic constructions of masculinity such as being strong disciplinarians, being sporty, and engaging in normalized masculine activities (Lingard et al. 2009).

Males at Risk

Societies recognize and acknowledge femininity in men's personalities differently from the ways in which they recognize and acknowledge masculinity in women's personalities (Connell 1995). Similar differentiation also exists in the ways that societies recognize *embodied* performances of gender (see Halberstam 1998). "In most societies, there are far greater penalties for men who do not conform to local dominant configurations of masculinity, and these configurations are more closely specified and policed than is the case for their counterparts in femininity" (Paechter 2003a, p. 549). In regard to social acceptance, I believe that in contemporary mainstream Western societies there is more at stake for males whose bodies transgress prescribed norms of gender behavior than there is for women. This was not always so. Indeed, postures considered 'queer' or 'soft' for men were not associated with homosexuality until the 1900s (Wex 1979, Burt 2001, see also Greer 2003). As a result of taboos against male femininity, many males, including some homosexuals, experience 'femiphobia' (Ducat 2004). In order to measure up to desired forms of masculinity, and because of an unconscious dread of their own femininity, they resist and sometimes actively oppress homosexuals and effeminates (Martino & Pallotta-Chiarolli 2005, see Paechter 2007, Pascoe 2007, Risner 2007). Connell (1983) regarded antagonism toward gay men as a standard part of hegemonic heterosexuality in Australian culture. Adhering to hegemonic norms of behavior is a means by which to avoid such discrimination (McKenna 2001).

Tolls Exacted

There are bound to be tolls exacted on the social and emotional well-being of individuals whose inclinations for embodied gender performance do not match prescribed norms of behavior. Shilling speaks of the body as being either "attached to, or ruptured from society" (2003, p. 206). In regard to the embodiment of gender, individuals at risk include those whose physical embodiment goes against sex-specific rigid notions of appropriate gendered behavior—regardless of whether embodiment is consciously or unconsciously performed—and those who resist their inclinations and toe the hegemonic line via vigilant, lifelong self-policing of the body. The former group face being marginalized or oppressed. The latter group face lifelong strains of sustaining a mode of performance in order to maintain their attachment to society. They are also at risk of losing touch with ways in which they might otherwise desire or be inclined to perform. It is because of their very attachment to society that the well-being of the latter group is easily overlooked.

STRATEGIES: RESISTANCE/COMPLIANCE/NEGOTIATION

What Performative Strategies of Resistance, Compliance, or Negotiation Are Undertaken—or Can Be Undertaken—by Those Whose Embodied Performances Do Not 'Fit In' with Dominant Norms of Performance?

Transgressive Performance—Resistance

Gendered acts of resistance involve performing against biologically determinist, sex-specific norms of masculinity and femininity. Embodied performances of resistance can be consciously or unconsciously performed. While deliberate acts of resistance can be seen as a means of achieving social change for gender equity (Pratt 1991, J. Butler 1993, Connell 1995, Monro 2005), they may come at a cost. Embodied acts of resistance, such as a male walking in an effeminate manner, are visible and, because of their 'otherness', place transgressors at risk of marginalization, ostracism, ridicule, and abuse within cultures that are not accepting of such difference. Embodied performances that appear to toe the hegemonic line are less susceptible to this treatment. Individuals who are aware of the potential risks of transgressing norms of gender behavior may perform against what their inclinations might otherwise be, in order to avoid the possibility of negative consequences.

Mikhail Bakhtin (1968) refers to carnivals of medieval times as occasions when behaving in ways that deviated from the norm was acceptable and even encouraged. Carnivalesque behavior in which ordinary rules and regulations were suspended or reversed was allowed by church and other authorities as a release for otherwise suppressed voices and energies, usually immediately prior to seasons such as Lent. These occasions were a means by which people could let off steam in society but in a controlled way. Contemporary equivalents are Sydney's Mardi Gras parade, company casual dress days, or schools' dress-up days. In each of these cases the acceptability of carnivalesque behavior was/is only ever temporary. It can be argued that transgressive carnivalesque behaviors may set some questioning of norms of behavior in motion (Shields 2007). That said, transgressive behavior on carnivalesque occasions is also frequently framed and posited as grotesque and absurd. Ways in which the carnivalesque might serve as a deconstructive tool will be taken up in discussion on sites of education and critical inquiry toward the end of this chapter.

Passing—Compliance

It is possible to say, "I'm fine", and not feel well. It is possible to smile but not be happy. In much the same way that words and facial expressions can deceive, I believe that—contrary to claims that *movement never lies* (Graham 1991)—bodies too are highly capable of disguise, deception, and masking, passing for something that they are not.

We are able to construct different versions of ourselves to facilitate social interaction and advancement (Goffman 1959). Brooke Kroeger (2003) theorizes about 'passing' as a way of getting along in institutions, environments, or social settings that would otherwise exclude or marginalize the passer. Kroeger claims people pass in order to avoid conflict, danger, prejudice, discrimination, or rejection, or to fulfill certain aspirations that hinge on social acceptance. For example, school students are able to escape gender harassment or homophobic abuse if they pass or fit into normalized, appropriately heterosexual categories (Kehily 2002, Hillier et al. 2005, Martino & Pallotta-Chiarolli 2005, Paechter 2007).

Kroeger writes of passing in regard to race, religion, sexuality, class, age, and biological sex. She also argues that passing is a form of resistance when passers, on achieving their goals, *reveal* themselves for who they are. However, passing can also be understood to be a form of accommodation wherein the passer is complicit in keeping an oppressive system in place, a system that made it necessary to pass in the first place. I will apply Kroeger's theories on passing to embodiment and the signaling of masculinity and femininity and theorize that, with time, conscious agentic imitation of an embodied gender performance may become unconsciously performed, in other words, habitus (Bourdieu 1990). It must be noted that the effects or repercussions of habitus that are the result of imitation can vary dramatically according to context. For example, encouraging the foreign language speaker to perpetually imitate the habitus of native speakers as a vehicle toward fitting into a foreign language culture can be productive and empowering (Migdalek 2002). Perpetually imitating performances of masculinity or femininity in order to fit into certain gender categories—while potentially empowering—may cause the *passer* to lose touch with ways in which they might otherwise experience or express gender (see Zeig 1985, Allen & Oleson 1999, Ducat 2004).

Kroeger acknowledges the impact, strain, and conflict that must result from years spent editing out whole parts of one's thinking process. She concedes that these may cause depression, hostility, anxiety, and/or low self-esteem. "Passing never feels natural. It is a second skin that never adheres" (2003, p. 8). For these reasons I find it problematic to concede, as Kroeger does, that passing is a wondrous ability to create and recreate the self. Sometimes endeavoring to pass and behave according to gendernormative conceptions might be undertaken merely in order to achieve a more livable life (J. Butler 2004). More attention needs to be devoted to passing when performed as an ongoing means of getting by in accommodation to the status quo, where no tangible goal is reached and where no 'reveal' occurs.

Anzaldua (1987) suggests that those who do not feel psychologically or physically safe in the world develop an acute self-protective sensitivity toward danger. There are various strategies for dealing with unsafe worlds. Anzaldua (1990), whose work concerns differences and diversity of race and culture, speaks of individuals being able to construct or adopt masks, faces ("*hacienda caras*"), personas, or identities, as protective devices to hide behind in order to avoid being singled out, rejected, oppressed, or marginalized for being different. Anzaldua, like Kroeger, regards this ability to adapt as a strength that may serve as a means for survival. However, she also recognizes such behaviors as self-sabotaging in that an individual, through complying to social/cultural rules that differ from those of their native culture, may lose a sense of self. In this book I apply Anzaldua's and Kroeger's theories to investigate and theorize the impact of my own embodied performances of compliance as performances that went against aspects of how and who I wanted to perform and be.

Living between and/or on Borders—Negotiation

> Dominated and marginalized people have been socialized to see always more than their own point of view.
>
> (Trinh 1992, p. 140)

Those who inhabit subordinate categories and as such become attuned to performing in different contexts and settings—be it for sustained or discrete periods of time—can be seen to exist between or across borders. Border-dwellers both straddle and remain detached from their various worlds, and this positioning as both insider and outsider makes it possible for them to see the precarious, discursively constituted nature of identity (Anzaldua 1987, Davies 1993a, Pallotta-Chiarolli 2010). For example, while gays who pass as straight may be able to operate effectively and without discrimination in particular settings, they might also be well aware of who they are and the creative means through which they are able to advance themselves or facilitate passage between various settings and identities. Border-dwellers' sensitivity to social environments makes them well equipped to reflect on and critically examine social values, norms, and expectations (Pallotta-Chiarolli 2010). Strategic use of border-positioning can be used to one's advantage (Anzaldua 1987, Pallotta-Chiarolli 2004), wherein confrontation can be avoided through enacting different performances for particular settings and groups.

DECONSTRUCTION

How Might Subjects of Cultures/Discourses Learn to Deconstruct Embedded Readings of Gender in Embodied Performance in Order to Affect Social Change toward Gender Equity?

Toward Social Justice

On issues of social change and transformation, bell hooks (2001) has argued that sexist oppression can be successfully eradicated only if agents (such as males) who maintain and support such oppression are compelled to assume responsibility for transforming social consciousness. Similarly, it can be argued that if oppressive norms and attitudes toward the embodiment of gender are to change, then it is vital that those who maintain and support existing systems of gendered hierarchical binaries come to understand their complicity in sustaining those very systems of oppression. Bob Pease (2010) contends that this can be problematic, because where privilege is experienced as being natural and normal—such as by white, heterosexual, middle-class, able-bodied males—then there is also likely to be a blindness on the part of the privileged to ways in which they themselves sustain and reproduce systems of oppression and social division. A further problem here is that those who sustain existing systems of oppression are also frequently members of the oppressed (Freire 1990) who, as a result of their conditioning, are often unable to look critically at or cause changes within the social systems in which they are submerged and within which they are trying to gain some privilege.

Embodiment Revisioned

If norms of gender behavior are to be resisted, altered, or refashioned in order to alleviate oppression suffered for not fitting in with prescribed norms, it is likely to be open only to gradual change (Foster 1998). Choreographic norms of gender are so deeply embedded and routinized that they basically become visible only when transgressed. In advocating *re-embodiment* for men, Connell (1995) speaks of recomposing rather than negating cultural elements of gender in order to achieve transformation. Paramount to broadening acceptable gender behavior is an ability to take the viewpoint of the other, something ordinarily denied in hegemonic masculinity (Connell 1995). It may be that "[n]othing happens in the real world unless it first happens in our heads" (Anzaldua 1987, p. 87). How might we generate a mindfulness of embodied habitual ways of viewing, doing, and imagining bodies that may lead to uninhibited embodiment of gender in the *real* world?

Deconstruction and Formal Performance Arts

Derridean theories of deconstruction are concerned with the challenging and defamiliarization of inherited assumptions in our reading of texts, including visual and embodied texts (Payne 1993, Hill 2007). Anzaldua (1990) advocates creative acts as a form of political activism in resistance to dominant cultural norms (see also theatre practitioners/feminists; Zeig 1985, Case 1988). The arts are a powerful form of human discourse that may lead people to see themselves in new ways (Saxton & Miller 2009, Sinclair et al. 2009). Bell hooks (1996) argues that popular culture (cinema particularly) has the capacity to create new awareness and to transform culture. While drama theorists Jonathan Bollen, Adrian Kiernander, and Bruce Parr (2006, 2008) advocate the theatre's potential to challenge and destabilize existing social attitudes toward masculinity and gender, they also acknowledge that it can reinforce and stabilize the same. Their focus is predominantly on storyline and character portrayal, with inadequate attention paid to physical disposition and embodiment.

Historically, it seems that alternative representations of masculinity in the performance arts have been more or less acceptable in the mainstream only when presented as the exotic. Representations such as choreography performed by legendary Russian dancer Vaslav Nijinsky, which combined power and strength with sensitive and delicate movement, were accepted largely because these occurred within exotic settings that were far enough removed from an audience's contemporary ones (Burt 1995, Kolb 2009). That which is classified as exotic is easily commodified and maintained as that which is distant and other (Savigliano 1995, see also Said 2003). Despite making an impact, graceful and somewhat feminine alternative male embodiment as performed by artists such as movie star Rudolph Valentino and the aforementioned Nijinsky did not ultimately affect change our acceptance of different forms of male behavior. This is probably due to the very exoticism of the characterizations they depicted: Valentino as a sheik (in the 1920 silent movie *The Sheik*), as an Argentine tango dancer (in the 1921 silent movie *The Four Horsemen of the Apocalypse*), and as a rajah (in the 1922 silent movie *The Young Rajah*) and Nijinsky as the Rose (in the 1911 ballet *Le Spectre de la Rose*), as Puppet (in the 1911 ballet *Petrushka*), and as Faun (in the 1912 ballet *L'Après-midi d'un Faune*). Roles such as the sheik, rajah, or Argentine tango dancer link to histories of colonized locales that for Western audiences conjured images of males and masculinities that were constructed not only as exotic, glamorous, and mysterious but also as subordinate and inferior (see Said 2003). Had these somewhat effeminate male performances been presented as contemporary Anglo-Western characterizations, they may not have been embraced as they were, especially within storylines that positioned them as heroic as opposed to weak or ineffectual. An Anglo mindset that lauds the effeminate *exotic* male as that which is distant and 'other' but shuns the effeminate *Anglo* male implies a reflexive form of homophobia prominent within Anglo society. This is consistent with theories of colonialism wherein the colonizer firmly sustains hierarchical distance and distinction from that which is different (Memmi 1967, see also Said 2003).

Avant-garde dance and choreography that disrupt male/female conventions of embodiment may serve to challenge dominant and delimiting ways of representing masculinity (Burt 1995). Dance works such as Joe Goode's *29 Effeminate Gestures,* first presented in 1987—in which a masculine-looking man wielding a chainsaw performs in a feminine manner—may destabilize notions of masculinity and challenge audiences to deconstruct the rigid dichotomy between masculine appearance and feminine gesture (Gere 2001). While such performances may create for spectators "a detached and critical distance from which to perceive conservative gender norms, and challenge assumptions about 'natural' masculinity" (Burt 1995, p. 87), they do not ordinarily achieve significant mainstream exposure or acceptance. Although Goode's *29 Effeminate Gestures* remained in his company's repertoire for over ten years, its audiences were predominantly gay and queer-friendly (Burt 2009).

In mainstream performance arts, alternative embodied representations of maleness that are feminine and not detached from white, predominantly Anglo culture are ordinarily represented and perceived as comic, ludicrous, deviant, suspect, and/or homosexual. One exception that comes to mind is the slinky, feminine gait of John Travolta's Tony Manero in the 1977 movie *Saturday Night Fever* (Paramount Pictures), although it can be argued that this figure projects as exotic as a result of the character's ethnicity, class, and passion for what was an alternative dance scene. Nevertheless, the character's heterosexuality and desirability to women are clearly and powerfully presented in the film's first shots as Tony struts his way down the streets of Brooklyn (Buchbinder 2004). Either way, a positively accepted on-screen alternative embodiment, such as Manero's/Travolta's, has not effectively dented prevalent masculinist ideologies of embodiment for males as they manifest in the everyday (see Nixon 1996, Mac an Ghaill & Haywood 2007).

Judith Butler (1990) condones parodic practices that disrupt the categories of body, sex, gender, and sexuality and compel a reconsideration of the stability of the masculine and the feminine. She claims that such acts of subversion can serve to expose the regulatory force of dominant norms and disrupt expected embodied behavior according to biological sex. Parodic works such as those of the Trockaderos de Monte Carlo (Trocks), where male ballet dancers dress as and impersonate female ballet dancers, and *Priscilla, Queen of the Desert* (Polygram) have achieved great popularity with mainstream audiences. However, it can be argued that such parodic representations have not affected the ways in which people view gender. As Bronwyn Davies (1993b) argues, simply reversing what is is not necessarily effective deconstruction. Embodied parody is not only capable of challenging but also capable of reinscribing heterosexist norms (J. Butler 1990, 1993, Burt 1995).

Sexist and homophobic humor may serve as a way of managing discomforts (Gard 2003a), but in my view this does not necessarily lead to productive change in gendered mindsets or perspectives. In cases such as the Trocks, male bodies in tutus performing in hyperfeminine ways can be seen to reinforce established mainstream notions that femininity on a male body is bizarre and incongruous. The fact that the Trocks are popular in mainstream arenas is something I find disturbing, but at the same time it is also motivating toward finding and strategizing ways to destabilize and challenge binary gender frameworks that move beyond parody.

A recent dance work that had substantial mainstream exposure was Matthew Bourne's *Swan Lake*. The work (choreographed in 1995 and still touring internationally in 2014) establishes some gender disruption but not, in my view, in regard to norms of masculine embodiment for males. Although the work deconstructs iconic conventions of the balletic swan as delicate, fragile, and female, and challenges expectations that feminine movement is the only way to dance Tchaikovsky's swan creatures, for the most part Bourne's male swans move broadly, athletically, and powerfully (Foster 2001) in keeping with established norms of masculine embodiment for males (Gard 2006). Where delicate and feminine motion is performed by the character of the arguably homosexual prince, it serves to reinforce stereotypical connections of feminine embodiment in a male with homosexuality.

Education Sites and Critical Inquiry

Paulo Freire (1990, first published in 1968) contends that processes of education frequently integrate the younger generation into the logic of present systems. As such systems are social constructions, it can be debated that educational processes interfere with notions of childhood as an innocent or authentic state (see Renold 2005). Hooks (1994) and Tierney (1997a) claim the need for educators to reject the traditional belief that education and teaching are politically neutral. Modern mass school systems can be seen as non-neutral sites where males and females are disciplined to take up their assigned position in the discourses and narratives of the patriarchal order (Kamler et al. 1994, Threadgold 1994). Inversely, processes of education can also lead the young to deal critically within and actively engage in acts of transformation and change to their worlds (Freire 1990), with the classroom seen as a radical space of possibility (hooks 1994). Schools can be seen as sites of potential social transformation (Connell 1995, Martino &

Pallotta-Chiarolli 2001). Schools have potential as sites to promote multiple embodiments of gender rather than rigid binary categorizations of masculine and feminine, which can be oppressive to those who do not fit comfortably into the practices commonly associated with each. In Chapter 10, I examine the hesitation and discomfort of some educators in relation to the promotion of agendas that challenge or deconstruct inequities concerning the embodiment of gender.

Critical literacy may be a positive step toward gender equity (Threadgold 1994, see also Davies 1993a, 1997, Sinclair et al. 2009). Critical literacy is

> the ability to read behind the words, or whatever other units of meaning are presented (such as images, sounds, gestures, and actions) to discover the unspoken sub-texts—the attitudes, the political and philosophical ideologies, the world-view, the power relations and the emotions that give rise to every utterance, and shape it, but remain implicit or hidden from obvious view.
>
> (Sinclair et al. 2009, p. 34)

As such, critical literacy can be a means of exposing narrow and often oppressive definitions of what it is to be female and male (J. Butler 1990). Valuable educational materials exist such as *Reading Fictions* (Mellor et al. 1991) and *Gendered Fictions* (Martino & Mellor 1995), which teach readers to challenge existing gendered and sexist assumptions that occur in and through written text. There are also programs and resources such as *Pride and Prejudice* (Higgins et al. 2002), *Catching On* (Victorian Department of Education and Early Childhood Development 2004), *Beyond "That's So Gay"* (Witthaus 2010), and *Pridentity* (Women's Health in the North & Reidy 2011), which are designed to challenge homophobia and facilitate change in attitudes in schools toward gays and lesbians. While these materials challenge discrimination according to sexuality and sexual orientation, attention needs to be given more broadly to inherent and inequitable assumptions relating to the signification of the embodiment of gender—as a visual text—and how these relate not only to readings of sexuality and sexual orientation but also to readings of character. The same can be said for illustrated storybooks for young children such as *The Paper Bag Princess* (Munsch 1980), *One Dad, Two Dads, Brown Dad, Blue Dads* (Valentine 1994), *The Sissy Duckling* (Fierstein 2002), and *The Boy in the Dress* (Walliams 2008), which feature positive portrayals of individuals who do gender differently. While the focus of these storybooks is mostly on the protagonists' appearance or dress, whom they love, whom they are loved by, and/or what interests/occupations they pursue, they could go further in advocating their rights to *embody* gender broadly and freely.

At all levels, attention needs to be directed to why assumptions are made about an individual's personality being weak, strong, likeable, deviant, or pathetic, according to the manner in which they embody, and why it is that such assumptions differ according to an individual's perceived biological sex.

Whereas critical literacy is ordinarily used to disrupt, expose, and challenge inherent ideologies in spoken and written language, it can also be a useful tool to expose inherent ideologies—such as gendered ideologies—in embodied language. An overview of key theories of interest concerning sites and practices where embodied critical inquiry may occur follows. Many of these are based in and around the performance arts, and I draw on these in structuring ethnographic fieldwork described in Chapters 9 and 10.

Gard argues that dances can be treated as 'texts' to be analyzed in the performance arts as well as physical education sites in order to "make explicit modes of thinking which underpin Western cultural and social practices" (2004, p. 102). He speaks of raising questions for discussion and critical reflection concerning why it may feel good/bad to move in certain ways; why people do not more readily explore other bodily possibilities; how the ways in which we move may be influenced by the expectations of other people; and whether "bodily conformity" takes different forms for male/female, able/disabled, young/old, gay/straight, white/black people (2004, p. 95, see also Gorely et al. 2003).

Education researcher Helen Cahill (2010) emphasizes that in deconstruction work, discourses that normally escape our attention need to be made visible. She argues that if we want to shift patterns of behavior we must also detect and unravel the discourses that pattern our thinking and assumptions about what is 'natural'. She advocates the use of drama activities to position participants so as to be able to see and understand the constructed nature of the dominant discourses, storylines, and influences that serve to shape their desires and behaviors. This line of reasoning can be applied to exposing dominant discourses, storylines, and influences that shape socially common perspectives on aesthetic and fitting embodiments of gender. Cahill (2010) argues that it is only through embodying the possible, which is not yet part of reality, that we bring it into the realm of being considered, and toward becoming part of reality. In order not to simply duplicate our everyday realities, Cahill advocates working beyond usual patterns, positions, storylines, and dominant defining binaries in the drama classroom as a means by which to imagine, tell, and do things differently.

In reference to Bakhtin (1968), Carolyn Shields (2007) claims that carnivalesque experience in which individuals behave in different ways can be used to gain deeper understanding of issues and insight into possible alternatives. She proposes that the carnivalesque can be used in education to help students think about what we commonly reject as grotesque, ugly, or undesirable. Feminist theatre worker Sande Zeig (1985), who theorized that feminine sex/class gesture systems were contrived and unnatural, and assigned to females, argued that practical embodied experiences such as the drama workshop, in which participants could experience other ways of embodying, could interrupt such learned systems. She upheld that masculine embodiment was the natural form that females should aspire to, and that through changing their movement females could change their perception. While these claims are debatable, I admire her position that through practical experimentation one might analyze and deconstruct one's own sex/class gender system.

Through his work with boys in upper high school, Richard Sallis (2004) argues that the drama classroom can serve as a site in which students can try out and test roles associated with gender, a space where day to day identities can be transcended and alternatives explored (see also McDonald 2006). The hegemonic gender binds targeted in Sallis' practical research are very much steeped in verbal texts, storylines, and plots. I believe that embodied disposition and manner should be addressed in isolation from plot or storyline in order to pinpoint the culture-specific semiotic force of the body and embodied action as a fundamental entrée to exposing embedded gender inequities.

In 2005 Terry Threadgold was party to drama workshops with groups of children in which she observed how difficult it was for them to *perform*—and not just *tell* about what it might be to be 'other'. Threadgold noted that exploration via practical and embodied drama workshop activities shed light on "struggles with the body which are involved in the taking on of new stories and positions" (2005, p. 276). Threadgold stresses that through embodied experience one can not only understand and appreciate the experiences of others but also disrupt one's own habituated practices. For social change to occur, it is "a question of changing and rewriting habituated bodies and practices, not just stories—of learning to perform the self or the social differently" (Threadgold 2005, p. 256). Like Cahill (2010), Threadgold recognizes that locations such as the drama classroom can be sites where new embodied understanding may germinate. I take these theories with me into my ethnographic fieldwork with students and educators, which will be described and analyzed in Chapters 9 and 10.

Performance Arts Practitioners and Critical Inquiry

> [O]ur art is not about conserving but, rather, creating frameworks that reveal ambiguities, uncover complexities and raise questions so that we may see more clearly what lies at the heart of human actions.
>
> (Saxton & Miller 2009, p. 42)

Methods of critical inquiry can be used toward exposing biases in the ways in which many come to read and perform gender differently according to the biological sex of the performer. Drama Australia's *Drama Equity and Diversity Guidelines* (2005) for drama educators advocate critical exploration and analysis of gender roles and the means by which gender is and has been constructed and performed in works of drama and popular culture. Critical exploration of theatrical performances should necessarily include attention to embodied performance. As such, critical inquiry can also be used toward exposing biases in the ways in which many come to *direct* embodied action differently according to the biological sex of the performer (Migdalek 2009). It concerns me that the ways in which bodies are directed, choreographed, and designed for in formal performance arenas such as theatre and film serve to reinforce the gendered status quo and delimit options for transgression—even prior to and distinct from the storyline or plot. This is an area that warrants performance arts practitioners' self-reflection and exploration. In order to ensure that all students have a place and voice, drama educator Sharon Grady (2000) stresses that, given their positions of power, drama educators must look beyond their own ways of viewing the world and strive for more pluralistic and inclusive perspectives in their work. In my autoethnographic investigation and my fieldwork with performance arts practitioners/educators, I put forward questions concerning the degree to which their/our own practices of teaching, casting, directing, and choreographing male and female bodies may be gendered and inequitable, and how existing norms of representation might be challenged and deconstructed/reconstructed through embodied performance arts as well as performance arts education.

CONCLUSION

Despite rhetoric that argues for a future where multiple embodiments of gender are possible (Trinh 1992, Foster 1998, Martino & Pallotta-Chiarolli 2001, Paechter 2006), embodied performances of gender that transgress norms of behavior continue to be less valued by individuals and collective groups in mainstream sectors of Western (and other) society. Perpetrators are at risk of repercussions that may be detrimental to their social and emotional well-being. This chapter has signposted the impact that social norms of embodiment—as experienced in everyday settings as well as formal performance arenas—have on an individual's life, the various responses that individuals may have in reaction to norms of gender embodiment to which they are exposed, the links between embedded gendered norms of embodiment and social and emotional well-being, the need for social change wherein members of society learn to challenge and deconstruct embedded gendered norms of embodiment, and the vital role that performance arts practitioners/educators may play in affecting such change. These points of focus will be illustrated and explored in the chapters that follow.

REFERENCES

Adkins, L., & Skeggs, B. (2004). *Feminism after Bourdieu*. Malden, MA: Blackwell.
Allen, D. J., & Oleson, T. (1999). Shame and Internalized Homophobia in Gay Men. *Journal of Homosexuality*. Vol 37, No 3, pp. 33–42.

Alsop, R., Fitzsimons, A., & Lennon, K. (2002). *Theorizing Gender.* Malden, MA: Blackwell.
Anderson, E. (2011). Masculinities and Sexualities in Sport and Physical Cultures: Three Decades of Evolving Research. *Journal of Homosexuality.* Vol 58, No 5, pp. 565–578.
Anzaldua, G. (1987). *Borderlands, La Frontera: The New Mestiza.* San Francisco: Spinsters/Aunt Lute.
Anzaldua, G. (1990). *Making Face, Making Soul: Creative and Critical Perspectives by Women of Color.* San Francisco: Aunt Lute.
Bakhtin, M. (1968). *Rabelais and His World.* Cambridge, MA: MIT Press.
Banes, S. (1998). *Dancing Women: Female Bodies on Stage.* New York: Routledge.
Bollen, J., Kiernander, A., & Parr, B. (2006). *What's a Man Gotta Do? Masculinities in Performance.* Armidale: University of New England.
Bollen, J., Kiernander, A., & Parr, B. (2008). *Men at Play: Masculinities in Australian Theatre since the 1950s.* Amsterdam: Rodopi.
Bordo, S. (1993). *Unbearable Weight: Feminism, Western Culture, and the Body.* Berkeley: University of California Press.
Bourdieu, P. (1977). *Outline of a Theory of Practice.* Cambridge: Cambridge.
Bourdieu, P. (1990). *The Logic of Practice.* Oxford: Polity Press.
Brodersen, A. (1971). *Alfred Schutz: Collected Papers.* The Hague: Martinus Nijhoff.
Buchbinder, D. (2004). *The Sign of the Dancing Men: Negotiations of Masculinity in Film Musicals.* (Conference Presentation). Masculinities: Gender, Art and Popular Culture Symposium, The University of Melbourne. [Retrieved 4/4/06 from www.art-museum.unimelb.edu.au/events_transcripts]
Burt, R. (1995). *The Male Dancer: Bodies, Spectacle, Sexualities.* London: Routledge.
Burt, R. (2001). Dissolving in Pleasure: The Threat of the Queer Male Dancing Body. In Desmond, J. C. (Ed.). *Dancing Desires: Choreographing Sexualities On and Off the Stage.* Madison: University of Wisconsin Press.
Burt, R. (2009). The Performance of Unmarked Masculinity. In Fisher, J., & Shay, A. (Eds.). *When Men Dance: Choreographing Masculinity across Borders.* New York: Oxford University Press.
Butler, J. (1990). *Gender Trouble: Feminism and the Subversion of Identity.* New York: Routledge.
Butler, J. (1993). *Bodies That Matter.* New York: Routledge.
Butler, J. (2004). *Undoing Gender.* New York: Routledge.
Butler, R. (2005). *Slovoj Zizek: Live Theory.* London: Continuum.
Cahill, H. (2010). Re-thinking the Fiction-Reality Boundary: Investigating the Use of Drama in HIV Prevention Projects in Vietnam. *Research in Drama Education: The Journal of Applied Theatre and Performance.* Vol 15, No 2, pp. 155–174.
Callery, D. (2001). *Through the Body: A Practical Guide to Physical Theatre.* London: Nick Hern Books.
Case, S. E. (1988). *Feminism and Theatre.* London: Macmillan.
Connell, R. W. (1983). *Which Way Is Up?* Sydney: Allen and Unwin.
Connell, R. W. (1995). *Masculinities.* Sydney: Allen and Unwin.
Connell, R. W. (1999). Sex in the World. In Epstein, D., & Sears, J. T. (Eds.). *A Dangerous Knowing: Sexuality, Pedagogy and Popular Culture.* London: Cassell.
Crothers, L. (2007). *Globalization & American Popular Culture.* Lanham: Rowman & Littlefield.
Davies, B. (1989). *Frogs and Snails and Feminist Tales: Preschool Children and Gender.* Sydney: Allen and Unwin.
Davies, B. (1993a). *The Learning of Gender in the First Years of School: Questions of Violence and Social Justice.* (Keynote Address). The 5th Australia and New Zealand conference on the first years of school, Perth.
Davies, B. (1993b). *Shards of Glass.* St Leonards: Allen and Unwin.

Davies, B. (1997). Constructing and Deconstructing Masculinities through Critical Literacy. *Gender and Education*. Vol 9, No 1, pp. 9–30.

Davies, B. (2006). Subjectification: The Relevance of Butler's Analysis for Education. *British Journal of Sociology of Education*. Vol 27, No 4, pp. 425–438.

Dempster, E. (1988). Let's Watch a Little How She Dances. In Sheridan, S. (Ed.). *Grafts: Feminist Cultural Criticism*. London: Verso.

DePalma, R., & Atkinson, E. (2008). *Invisible Boundaries: Addressing Sexualities Equality in Children's Worlds*. Stoke on Trent: Trentham.

Drama Australia. (2005). *Drama Equity and Diversity Guidelines*. [Retrieved 12/12/09 from http://www.dramaaustralia.org.au/documents/Equity%20and%20 Diversity-.pdf]

Ducat, S.J. (2004). *Wimp Factor: Gender Gaps, Holy Wars, and the Politics of Anxious Masculinity*. Boston: Beacon Press.

Epstein, D., & Johnson, R. (2008). Walking the Talk: Young People Making Identities. In DePalma, R., & Atkinson, E. (Eds.). *Invisible Boundaries: Addressing Sexualities Equality in Children's Worlds*. Stoke on Trent: Trentham.

Erskine, S. (2005). The Dancing Mind. *All in the Mind* with Natashia Mitchell, aired Saturday, 19 March 2005, ABC Science, Radio National, Australia. [Retrieved 15/01/10 from http://www.abc.net.au/radionational/programs/allinthemind/the-dancing-mind/3442236#transcript]

Fanon, F. (2008). *Black Skin, White Masks*. New York: Grove Press.

Feldenkrais Method. (2008). *The Feldenkrais Method*. [Retrieved 02/11/08 from http://www.feldenkraismethod.ca]

Fierstein, H. (2002). *The Sissy Duckling*. New York: Simon & Schuster Books for Young Readers.

Fisher, J., & Shay, A. (2009). *When Men Dance: Choreographing Masculinity across Borders*. New York: Oxford University Press.

Flanagan, O.J. (1982). Freud: Masculinity, Femininity and the Philosophy of Mind. In Vetterling-Braggin, M. (Ed.). *Femininity, Masculinity and Androgyny*. Totowa, NJ: Rowan & Allanheld.

Foster, S.L. (1996). The Ballerina's Phallic Pointe. In Foster, S.L. (Ed.). *Corporealities. Dancing Knowledge, Culture and Power*. New York: Routledge.

Foster, S.L. (1998). Choreographies of Gender. *Signs: Journal of Women in Culture & Society*. Vol 24, No 1, pp. 1–33.

Foster, S.L. (2001). Closets Full of Dances: Modern Dance's Performance of Masculinity and Sexuality. In Desmond, J.C. (Ed.). *Dancing Desires: Choreographing Sexualities On and Off the Stage*. Madison: University of Wisconsin Press.

Foucault, M. (1977). *Discipline and Punish: The Birth of the Prison*. London: Peregrine.

Francis, B. (2010). Re/Theorising Gender: Female Masculinity and Male Femininity in the Classroom. *Gender and Education*. Vol 22, No 5, pp. 477–490.

Frank, B. (1993). Straight/Strait Jackets for Masculinity: Educating for 'Real' Men. *Atlantis: A Women's Studies Journal*. Vol 18, Nos 1–2, pp. 47–59.

Freire, P. (1990). *Pedagogy of the Oppressed*. New York: Continuum.

Fuchs, S. (2001). *Against Essentialism: A Theory of Culture and Society*. Cambridge: Harvard University Press.

Gard, M. (2001). Dancing around the 'Problem' of Boys and Dance. *Discourse: Studies in the Cultural Politics of Education*. Vol 22, No 2, pp. 212–225.

Gard, M. (2003a). Being Someone Else: Using Dance in Anti-oppressive Teaching. *Educational Review*. Vol 55, No 2, pp. 211–223.

Gard, M. (2003b). Moving and Belonging: Dance, Sport and Sexuality. *Sex Education*. Vol 3, No 2, pp. 105–118.

Gard, M. (2004). Movement, Art and Culture: Problem-Solving and Critical Inquiry in Dance. In Wright, J., Macdonald, D., & Burrows, L. (Eds.). *Critical Inquiry and Problem-Solving in Physical Education*. London: Routledge.

Gard, M. (2006). *Men Who Dance: Aesthetics, Athletics, & the Art of Masculinity.* New York: Peter Lang.
Gere, D. (2001). Effeminate Gestures: Choreographer Joe Goode and the Heroism of Effeminacy. In Desmond, J.C. (Ed.). *Dancing Desires: Choreographing Sexualities On and Off the Stage.* Madison: University of Wisconsin Press.
Goffman, E. (1959). *The Presentation of Self in Everyday Life.* New York: Anchor.
Goffman, E. (1997). The Arrangement between the Sexes. *Theory and Society.* Vol 4, No 3, pp. 301–331.
Gorely, T., Holroyd, R., & Kirk, D. (2003). Muscularity, the Habitus and the Social Construction of Gender: Towards a Gender-Related Physical Education. *British Journal of Sociology of Education.* Vol 24, No 4, pp. 429–448.
Grady, S. (2000). *Drama and Diversity: A Pluralistic Perspective for Educational Drama.* Portsmouth: Heinemann.
Graham, M. (1991). *Blood Memory.* London: Macmillan.
Greer, G. (2003). *The Boy.* London: Thames & Hudson.
Grosz, E. (1994). *Volatile Bodies.* London: Allen and Unwin.
Guillaumin, C. (1993). The Constructed Body. In Ehrenreich, J., & Burroughs, C.B. (Eds.). *Reading the Social Body.* Iowa: University of Iowa Press.
Halberstam, J. (1998). *Female Masculinity.* Durham: Duke University Press.
Hall, E.T. (1959). *The Silent Language.* New York: Anchor N.Y.
Hall, E.T. (1977). *Beyond Culture.* New York: Anchor N.Y.
Higgins, D.J., King, R.M., & Witthaus, D.E. (2002). *Pride and Prejudice: A Program for Secondary Students.* Victoria: Deakin University.
Hill, L. (2007). *The Cambridge Introduction to Jacques Derrida.* New York: Cambridge University Press.
Hillier, L., Jones, T., Monagle, M., Overton, N., Gahan, L., Blackman, J., & Mitchell, A. (2010). *Writing Themselves In 3: The Third National Study on the Sexual Health and Wellbeing of Same Sex Attracted and Gender Questioning Young People.* (Monograph series no. 78). Victoria: La Trobe University.
Hillier, L., Turner, A., & Mitchell, A. (2005). *Writing Themselves In Again: 6 Years On. The 2nd National Report on the Sexuality, Health & Well-Being of Same Sex Attracted Young People in Australia.* Victoria: Australian Research Centre in Sex, Health & Society (ARCSHS), La Trobe University.
hooks, b. (1994). *Teaching to Transgress.* New York: Routledge.
hooks, b. (1996). *Reel to Real.* London: Routledge.
hooks, b. (2001). Men: Comrades in Struggle. In Kimmel, M.S., & Messner, M.A. (Eds.). *Men's Lives.* Boston: Allyn and Bacon.
Jackson, C. (2002). 'Laddishness' as a Self-Worth Protection Strategy. *Gender and Education.* Vol 14, No 1, pp. 37–51.
Jenkins, R. (2002). *Pierre Bourdieu.* London: Routledge.
Johnson, K.L., Gill, S., & Reichman, V. (2007). Swagger, Sway and Sexuality: Judging Sexual Orientation from Body Motion and Morphology. *Journal of Personality and Social Psychology.* Vol 93, No 3, pp. 321–334.
Jones, C. (2003). Lesbian and Gay Cinema. In Neimes, J. (Ed.). *An Introduction to Film Studies* (third edition). New York: Routledge.
Kamler, B. (1993). *The Construction and Reconstruction of Gender in Classroom Discourse: Disciplining the Student Body.* (Paper). National Council of Teachers of English (83rd annual convention), Pennsylvania.
Kamler, B., Maclean, R., Reid, J., & Simpson, A. (1994). *Shaping Up Nicely: The Formation of Schoolgirls and Schoolboys in the First Month of School. A Report to the Gender Equity and Curriculum Reform Project Department of Employment, Education and Training (DEET).* Canberra: Deakin University.
Kehily, M. (2001). Bodies in School: Young Men, Embodiment, and Heterosexual Masculinities. *Men and Masculinities.* Vol 4, No 2, pp. 173–185.

Kehily, J. (2002). *Sexuality, Gender and Schooling: Shifting Agendas in Social Learning*. London: Routledge.
Kirby, S., & Hay, I. (1997). (Hetero)Sexing Space: Gay Men and 'Straight' Space in Adelaide, South Australia. *The Professional Geographer.* Vol 49, No 3, pp. 295–305.
Kolb, A. (2009). Nijinsky's Images of Homosexuality. *Journal of European Studies.* Vol 39, No 2, pp. 147–171.
Kosofsky Sedgwick, E. (1994). *Tendencies.* London: Routledge.
Kroeger, B. (2003). *Passing: When People Can't Be Who They Are.* New York: Public Affairs.
Lanzieri, N., & Hildebrandt, T. (2011). Using Hegemonic Masculinity to Explain Gay Male Attraction to Muscular and Athletic Men. *Journal of Homosexuality.* Vol. 58, No. 2, pp. 275–293.
Lecoq, J. (2002). *The Moving Body: Teaching Creative Theatre.* New York: Routledge.
Lingard, B., Martino, W., & Mills, M. (2009). *Boys and Schooling: Beyond Structural Reform.* Basingstoke: Palgrave Macmillan.
Linne, R. (2003). Alternative Textualities: Media Culture and the Proto-queer. *Qualitative Studies in Education.* Vol 16, No 5, pp. 669–689.
Mac an Ghaill, M. (1994). *The Making of Men: Masculinities, Sexualities and Schooling.* Buckingham: Open University Press.
Mac an Ghaill, M., & Haywood, C. (2007). *Gender, Culture and Society: Contemporary Femininities and Masculinities.* London: Macmillan.
Martino, W., & Mellor, B. (1995). *Gendered Fictions.* Cottesloe: Chalkface Press.
Martino, W., & Pallotta-Chiarolli, M. (2001). Gender Performativity and Normalizing Practices. In Haynes, F., & McKenna, T. (Eds.). *Unseen Genders: Beyond the Binaries.* New York: Peter Lang.
Martino, W., & Pallotta-Chiarolli, M. (2003). *So What's a Boy? Addressing Issues of Masculinity and Schooling.* Maidenhead: Open University Press.
Martino, W., & Pallotta-Chiarolli, M. (2005). *Being Normal Is the Only Way to Be.* Sydney: University of New South Wales Press.
Mauss, M. (1979). *Sociology and Psychology: Essays.* London: Routledge.
McCaw, D. (2011). *The Laban Sourcebook.* London: Routledge.
McCormack, M. (2012). *The Declining Significance of Homophobia: How Teenage Boys Are Redefining Masculinity and Heterosexuality.* Oxford: Oxford University Press.
McDonald, J. (2006). Playful Transgressions: Male Drama Teachers in Elite Boys' School. In Kiernander, A., Bollen, J., & Parr, B. (Eds.). *What's a Man Gotta Do? Masculinities in Performance.* Armidale, NSW: University of New England.
McKechnie, S. (2002). Movement as Metaphor: The Construction of Meaning in the Choreographic Art. In Stevens, C., Burnham, D., McPherson, G., Schubert, E., & Renwick, J. (Eds.). *Proceedings of the 7th International Conference on Music Perception & Cognition.* Sydney: University of New South Wales.
McKenna, T. (2001). Enactments of Difference. In Haynes, F., & McKenna, T. (Eds.). *Unseen Genders: Beyond the Binaries.* New York: Peter Lang.
McNay, L. (2004). Agency and Experience: Gender as a Lived Relation. In Adkins, L., & Skeggs, B. (Eds.). *Feminism after Bourdieu.* Malden, MA: Blackwell.
McRobbie, A. (2009). *The Aftermath of Feminism.* Thousand Oaks: Sage.
Mellor, B., Patterson, A., & O'Neill, M. (1991). *Reading Fictions.* Cottesloe: Chalkface Press.
Memmi, A. (1967). *The Colonizer and the Colonized.* Boston: Beacon.
Migdalek, J. (2002). Performing English: The Classroom as Rehearsal Space. *Prospect: An Australian Journal of TESOL.* Vol 17, No 2, pp. 53–61.
Migdalek, J. (2009). Masculine Moves: The Measure of a Man. *N J Drama Australia Journal.* Vol 32, No 1, pp. 45–54.

Monro, S. (2005). *Gender Politics*. London: Pluto.
Munsch, R. (1980). *The Paper Bag Princess*. Toronto: Annick Press.
Nayak, A., & Kehily, M.J. (1996). Playing It Straight: Masculinities, Homophobias and Schooling. *Journal of Gender Studies*. Vol 5, No 2, pp. 211–230.
Neimes, J. (2003). Gender and Film. In Neimes, J. (Ed.). *An Introduction to Film Studies* (third edition). New York: Routledge.
Nixon, S. (1996). *Hard Looks: Masculinities, Spectatorship and Contemporary Consumption*. New York: St Martins Press.
O'Connell, M. (2012). Don't Act, Don't Tell: Discrimination Based on Gender Non-conformity in the Entertainment Industry and the Clinical Setting. *Journal of Gay & Lesbian Mental Health*. Vol 16, No 3, pp. 241–255.
Ollis, D. (2008). *Sexualities and Gender in the Classroom: Changing Teacher Practice*. Cologne: Lambert.
Paechter, C. (2003a). Learning Masculinities and Femininities: Power/Knowledge and Legitimate Peripheral Participation. *Women's Studies International Forum*. Vol 26, No 6, pp. 541–552.
Paechter, C. (2003b). Masculinities and Femininities as Communities of Practice. *Women's Studies International Forum*. Vol 26, No 1, pp. 69–77.
Paechter, C. (2006). Reconceptualizing the Gendered Body: Learning and Constructing Masculinities and Femininities in School. *Gender and Education*. Vol 18, No 2, pp. 121–135.
Paechter, C. (2007). *Being Boys, Being Girls: Learning Masculinities and Femininities*. Berkshire: Open University Press.
Pallotta-Chiarolli, M. (2004). Weaving Textual Tapestries. In Scarparo, S., & Wilson, R. (Eds.). *Across Genres, Generations and Borders*. Newark, NJ: Delaware Press.
Pallotta-Chiarolli, M. (2010). *Border Sexualities, Border Families in Schools*. Lanham: Rowman and Littlefield.
Pascoe, C.J. (2007). *Dude, You're a Fag: Masculinity and Sexuality in High School*. Berkeley: University of California Press.
Payne, M. (1993). *Reading Theory: An Introduction to Lacan, Derrida, and Kristeva*. Los Angeles: Oxford.
Payne, R. (2007). Str8acting. *Social Semiotics*. Vol 17, No 4, pp. 525–538.
Pease, B. (2010). *Undoing Privilege: Unlearned Advantage in a Divided World*. London: Zed Books.
Pickering, M. (2001). *Stereotyping: The Politics of Representation*. Hampshire: Palgrave.
Plummer, D. (1999). *One of the Boys: Masculinity, Homophobia and Modern Manhood*. New York: Harrington Park Press.
Pratt, M. (1991). *Rebellion: Essays 1980–1991*. New York: Firebrand.
Pronger, B. (1990). Gay Jocks: A Phenomenology of Gay Men in Athletics. In Messner, M.A., & Sabo, D.F. (Eds.). *Sport, Men, and the Gender Order: Critical Feminist Perspectives*. Champaign, IL: Human Kinetics Books.
Renew, S. (1996). Acting Like a Girl: Lesbian Challenges to Constructions of Gender and Schooling. In Laskey, L., & Beavis, C. (Eds.). *Schooling & Sexualities: Teaching for a Positive Sexuality*. Victoria: Deakin University.
Renold, E. (2003). 'If You Don't Kiss Me, You're Dumped': Boys, Boyfriends and Heterosexualised Masculinities in the Primary School. *Educational Review*. Vol 55, No 2, pp. 179–194.
Renold, E. (2005). *Girls, Boys and Junior Sexualities*. London: Routledge Falmer.
Rich, A. (1987). *Blood, Bread and Poetry: Selected Prose 1979–1985*. London: Virago Press.
Risner, D. (2007). Rehearsing Masculinity: Challenging the 'Boy Code' in Dance Education. *Research in Dance Education*. Vol 8, No 2, pp. 139–153.

Rogers, L. (1999). *Sexing the Brain.* London: Weidenfeld & Nicolson.
Rubin, G. (1975). The Traffic in Women: Notes on the 'Political Economy of Sex'. In Reiter, R.R. (Ed.). *Toward an Anthropology of Women.* New York: Monthly Review Press.
Russo, V. (1981). *The Celluloid Closet: Homosexuality in the Movies.* New York: Harper & Row.
Said, E.W. (2003). *Orientalism.* London: Penguin.
Sallis, R. (2004). *Masculinities and Drama.* (Master's Thesis). Melbourne: University of Melbourne.
Savigliano, M. (1995). *Tango and the Political Economy of Passion.* Boulder, CO: Westview.
Saxton, J., & Miller, C. (2009). Opening Pandora's Box: The Ethics of Practice in Multicultural Communities. *N J Drama Australia Journal.* Vol 32, No 1, pp. 35–43.
Schirato, T., & Yell, S. (1996). *Communication and Cultural Literacy.* St Leonards, NSW: Allen and Unwin.
Schutz, A. (1944). The Stranger: An Essay in Social Psychology. *American Journal of Sociology.* Vol 49, No 6, pp. 499–507.
Sears, A., & Hollos, W.H. (2002). Actor Training in the Neutral Mask. In Zarrilli, P.B. (Ed.). *Acting (Re)Considered: A Theoretical and Practical Guide.* London: Routledge.
Shields, C. (2007). *Bakhtin Primer.* New York: Peter Lang.
Shilling, C. (2003). *The Body and Social Theory.* London: Sage.
Shilling, C. (2004). Educating Bodies: Schooling and the Constitution of Society. In Wright, J., Davies, B., Shilling, C., & Evans, J. (Eds.). *Body, Knowledge and Control: Studies in the Sociology of Physical Education.* London: Routledge.
Sinclair, C., Jeanneret, N., & O'Toole, J. (2009). *Education in the Arts: Teaching and Learning in the Contemporary Curriculum.* Victoria: Oxford University Press.
Sirin, S.R., McCreary, D.R., & Mahalik, J.R. (2004). Differential Reactions to Men and Women's Gender Role Transgressions: Perceptions of Social Status, Sexual Orientation, and Value Dissimilarity. *Journal of Men's Studies.* Vol 12, No 2, pp. 119–133.
Skattebol, J. (2006). Playing Boys: The Body, Identity and Belonging in the Early Years. *Gender and Education.* Vol 18, No 5, pp. 507–522.
Stoneley, P. (2007). *A Queer History of the Ballet.* London: Routledge.
Swain, J. (2004). The Resources and Strategies That 10–11-Year-Old Boys Use to Construct Masculinities in the School Setting. *British Educational Research Journal.* Vol 30, No 1, pp. 167–185.
Taylor, A., & Richardson, C. (2005). Queering Home Corner. *Contemporary Issues in Early Childhood.* Vol 6, No 2, pp. 163–173.
Threadgold, T. (1994). Performing Genre: Violence, the Making of Protected Subjects, and the Discourses of Critical Literacy and Radical Pedagogy. *Changing English.* Vol 1, No 1, pp. 2–31.
Threadgold, T. (2005). Performing Theories of Narrative: Theorising Narrative Performance. In Thornborrow, J., & Coates, J. (Eds.). *The Sociolinguistics of Narrative.* Amsterdam: John Benjamins.
Tierney, W.G. (1997a). *Academic Outlaws: Queer Theory and Cultural Studies in the Academy.* Thousand Oaks: Sage.
Tierney, W.G. (1997b). Border Guards: Ethnographic Fiction and Social Science. In Fine, M., Weis, L., Powell C.C., & Mun Wong, L. (Eds.). *Off White: Readings on Race, Power, and Society.* New York: Routledge.
Trinh, T. (1992). *Framer Framed.* New York: Routledge.
Turner, B. (1984). *The Body and Society.* Oxford, UK: Basil Blackwell.
Turner, B. (1992). *Regulating Bodies: Essays in Medical Sociology.* London: Routledge.

Valentine, J. (1994). *One Dad, Two Dads, Brown Dad, Blue Dads.* Los Angeles: Alyson.
Vicars, M. (2008). Memories of Homophobia in Childhood: Social Exclusion Is Not a Place Where One Chooses to Hang Out. In DePalma, R., & Atkinson, E. (Eds.). *Invisible Boundaries: Addressing Sexualities Equality in Children's Worlds.* Stoke on Trent: Trentham.
Victorian Department of Education and Early Childhood Development. (2004). *Catching On to Sexuality Education (Year 9 and 10 curriculum resource).* Victoria: Victorian Department of Education.
Viswanathan, G. (2004). *Power, Politics, and Culture: Interviews with Edward W. Said.* London: Bloomsbury.
Walliams, D. (2008). *The Boy in the Dress.* London: Harper Collins.
Wex, M. (1979). *Let's Take Back Our Space: Female and Male Body Language as a Result of Patriarchal Structures.* Munich: Frauenliteratur Verlag.
Witthaus, D. (2010). *Beyond "That's So Gay".* Melbourne: Hawker Brownlow Education.
Women's Health in the North & Reidy, C. (2011). *Pridentity: Inclusive Sexuality Education Resource Kit.* Thornbury: Women's Health in the North.
Young, I.M. (1990). *Throwing Like a Girl and Other Essays in Feminist Philosophy and Social Theory.* Indianapolis: Indiana University Press.
Zeig, S. (1985). The Actor as Activator: Deconstructing Gender through Gesture. *Women and Performance.* Vol 2, No 2, pp. 12–17.
Zizek, S. (1999). *The Sublime Object of Ideology.* London: Verso.

3 Frames of Investigation

PARTIAL PERSPECTIVES

I acknowledge that this book emerges from perspectives that are subjective, something that Laurel Richardson (1990) and William Tierney (1997a) contend is frequently at work in the collection, presentation, and interpretation of data. In order to make my subjectivity and personal connection to issues of gender embodiment visible, and not fall into third person omniscient voices that appear to erase subjectivity (see Trinh 1992, Tierney 1997b, Kerr & Nettelbeck 1998, Ellis & Bochner 2000), I choose to write much of this book in the first person. The autoethnographic approach I take is reflexive in that my inquiry focuses on myself as researcher in relation to institutional practices and fields in which I operate (Reed-Danahay 2009). A reflexive approach involves paying heed to the impact that my values, experiences, interests, commitments, and social identity have on my actions and understandings (Szarycz 2010). I am a Jewish, Australian, gay male who is a son, actor, dancer, educator, director, and choreographer, and I frequently refer to myself in these terms throughout this book. I should also draw attention to aspects of my positioning that I do not highlight. I am white, middle-class, middle-aged, and able-bodied, privileged and normative positions that I ordinarily, and unjustifiably, assume readers will take for granted (see Pease 2010). Yet these positions must also be taken into consideration as affecting and influencing my interpretations of and attitudes toward issues under discussion. For example, in reporting on my fieldwork, I refer to individual participants as male or female. These references are based on my observations of how these persons projected during fieldwork sessions via appearance, voice, and demeanor, and also on how they self-identified on response sheets. The issue of assignation of biological sex and gender identity is a sensitive one, and, in retrospect, I concede that my assumptions are grounded in, blinded by, and bound to dominant ideologies of gendernormativity.

MEANS OF EXPRESSION

Depending on context, some forms of language are more adequate than others (Trinh 1992). I embrace the notion that representing and making sense of one's data can be an artistic, interpretive endeavor (Richardson 1996, Denzin & Lincoln 2005, Leavy 2009) and incorporate expressive means of doing so. In finding the most effective ways to communicate and illustrate not only thoughts but also emotions, I include multiple forms of expression. I refer to these as vignettes. These include the written word (narrative, monologue, dialogue, theatrical script), illustration, and photography, as well as images from the media. All the vignettes are connected to my experiences and/or consciousness. I choose to present vignettes as artistic expression, as such forms of expression can be seen to resonate with readers more evocatively than conventional modes of academic expression (Knowles & Cole 2008, Leavy 2009).

The narrative vignettes that I have chosen to thread through the book center on experiences of embodiment and gender. Autobiographical narrative vignettes are informed by reflections on lived and embodied experiences from my own life as a child, son, student, actor, dancer, Australian citizen, educator, director, and choreographer, and these can be useful in illuminating the impact and effects of lived experiences on the individual. Fictitious narrative vignettes open up space for critique (see Kamler 2001) and fall under the banner of fictocriticism, which Stephen Muecke (2002) defines as inventions or stories through which philosophical arguments are made. Fictocriticism in forms such as prose, poetry, and dramatic scenarios can make meaning for the reader substantively clearer and emotionally more poignant than traditional modes of academic writing (Kilbourn 1999, see also Leavy 2009). I take the view that fictocriticism is a "space of possibility" (Schlunke & Brewster 2005, p. 394) and intend that the imagined experiences and events that emerge from my own consciousness will resonate with the reader on an emotional level while also progressing and substantiating the propositions that I put forward. My voice and gaze will shift back and forth between the perspectives of commentator, artist, and subject. Using multiple voices and means of expression will allow me to display multiple levels of consciousness, connecting the personal and the local to the cultural and political (Denzin & Lincoln 2000, Ellis & Bochner 2000).

The process of research can affect and change us as people and as researchers (Szarycz 2010). It can lead not only researchers but also fieldwork participants to new understandings around particular issues (Lincoln 1995, Gunzenhauser 2006). In such cases, the research itself can be understood as an act of intervention. I report on how discomforts triggered through the research process shifted and enhanced my own perspectives and understandings of gender and embodiment, as well as those of a number of fieldwork participants. Hopefully the contents of this book will do the same for its readers too.

REFERENCES

Denzin, N.K., & Lincoln, Y.S. (2000). *Handbook of Qualitative Research* (second edition). Thousand Oaks: Sage.

Denzin, N.K., & Lincoln, Y.S. (2005). *The Sage Handbook of Qualitative Research* (third edition). Thousand Oaks: Sage.

Ellis, C., & Bochner, A.P. (2000). Autoethnography, Personal Narrative, Reflexivity. In Denzin, N.K., & Lincoln, Y.S. (Eds.). *Handbook of Qualitative Research* (second edition). Thousand Oaks: Sage.

Gunzenhauser, M.G. (2006). A Moral Epistemology of Knowing Subjects: Theorizing a Relational Turn for Qualitative Research. *Qualitative Inquiry.* Vol 12, No 3, pp. 621–647.

Kamler, B. (2001). *Relocating the Personal: A Critical Writing Pedagogy.* New York: State University of New York Press.

Kerr, H., & Nettelbeck, A. (1998). *The Space Between: Australian Women Writing Fictocriticism.* Nedlands, WA: University of Western Australia Press.

Kilbourn, B. (1999). Fictional Theses. *Educational Researcher.* Vol 28, No 9, pp. 27–32.

Knowles, J.G., & Cole, A.L. (2008). *Handbook of the Arts in Qualitative Research.* Thousand Oaks: Sage.

Leavy, P. (2009). *Method Meets Art: Arts-Based Research Practice.* New York: Guilford Press.

Lincoln, Y.S. (1995). Emerging Criteria for Quality in Qualitative and Interpretive Research. *Qualitative Inquiry.* Vol 1, No 3, pp. 275–289.

Muecke, S. (2002). The Fall: Fictocritical Writing. In Walker, B. (Ed.). *The Writer's Reader.* Broadway: Halstead Press.

Pease, B. (2010). *Undoing Privilege: Unlearned Advantage in a Divided World.* London: Zed Books.

Reed-Danahay, D. (2009). Anthropologists, Education, and Autoethnography. *Reviews in Anthropology.* Vol 38, No 1, pp. 28–47.

Richardson, L. (1990). *Writing Strategies: Reaching Diverse Audiences, Qualitative Research Methods.* Thousand Oaks: Sage.

Richardson, L. (1996). Educational Birds. *Journal of Contemporary Ethnography.* Vol 25, No 1, pp. 6–15.

Schlunke, K., & Brewster, A. (2005). We Four: Fictocriticism Again. *Continuum.* Vol. 19, No 3, pp. 393–395.

Szarycz, G.S. (2010). *Research Realities in the Social Sciences: Negotiating Fieldwork Dilemmas.* New York: Cambria Press.

Tierney, W.G. (1997a). Border Guards: Ethnographic Fiction and Social Science. In Fine, M., Weis, L., Powell C.C., & Mun Wong, L. (Eds.). *Off White: Readings on Race, Power, and Society.* New York: Routledge.

Tierney, W.G. (1997b). Lost in Translation: Time and Voice in Qualitative Research. In Tierney W.G., & Lincoln Y. S. (Eds.). *Representation and the Text: Re-framing the Narrative Voice.* New York: State University of New York Press.

Trinh, T. (1992). *Framer Framed.* New York: Routledge.

4 Signification of the Body

READING SYMBOLS—READING BODIES

Please read the following word out loud: 'VIGNETTE'. It is very probable that you sounded the combination of those letters as VIN-YET. It is unlikely that in reading the word, you were mindful that the same combination of letters could also be sounded in a multitude of other phonetic ways such as *vij-net, vig-net-tee, vignyet, vignyetie, vin-et, vin-et-ie, vigh-net, vigh-netie, vigh-nyet,* or *vigh-nyetie.* You probably sounded and pronounced the word as you did because of what those letters placed in that learned combination signify to you. Even though that pronunciation is only one possible interpretation, it was taken for granted as being the right one in accordance with how you—and I—have come to automatically and unquestioningly use language.

It is your established and embedded cultural knowing that bestows on you the confidence with which you pronounced the word 'vignette'. However, the signification of those written characters in that combination is culturally specific. Although the same Roman letters are native to people from a variety of countries and regions, their pronunciation in certain combinations may differ greatly. Similarly, the cultural readings of human bodies embodying in certain ways may also signify differently to those of varying cultures or cultural backgrounds (Turner 1984, Burt 1995, Greer 2003, Paechter 2003a). How bodies and certain embodiments are read is, as for written characters, not a construction of nature but a construction of culture and time. Their signification is not necessarily universal.

When I see a swastika shape, my enculturation has me understand it by the meaning with which I associate it, being the Nazi regime. The lines and form of the symbol are rendered invisible by the workings of the Jewish and other cultures that have inscribed its meaning for me. The semiotics of the symbol as sinister and abhorrent are so powerful that they constrict how we use or repeat it within certain cultures, even though in other cultures the same symbol has traditionally signified 'well-being' (Heller 2008). Similarly, through repeated exposure, certain embodied performances take on meanings that align them as fitting to male or female biology. The semiotics of these embodied forms carry a weight that influences the way individuals within, or related to, that culture might replicate or endeavor *not* to replicate them.

Just as the swastika has become much more than simply a geometric form, so too have particular embodied forms of performance become much more than simply actions or poses that able-bodied persons of any biological sex are capable of producing. It is likely that certain bodies posed, reposed, or moving in certain ways will signify very specifically to us because of how we have culturally come to understand particular forms of embodied imagery. Bodies may signify as male, female, aggressive, friendly, timid, heterosexual, or homosexual, whether they are these things or not.

Pretty in Pink

Kim picks up the newborn swaddled in pink. She cuddles the infant softly and gently.

KIM: (cooing) Isn't she gorgeous!

Informed that the baby is a boy, Kim apologizes, then nuzzles her face into the baby's chest, and play-acts pummeling the baby's cheeks and nose with a clenched forefinger.

KIM: (growling like a bear) Hello fella. Grrrr!

Had the baby not been swaddled in pink, Kim would not have assumed that she should refer to the newborn as 'she'.

Nell and I watch her son, Ryan, playing with his elder sister, Gemma.

NELL: When Ryan was a baby, I thought, "Stuff it, I've got all these baby clothes from when Gemma was a baby. Why not use those?" You know, pink all-overs, pink bunny rugs. Well, the remarks I got: firstly, people would say things like *"Isn't she adorable! How old is she? What's her name?"* assuming he was a girl. And then, when I would tell them that he was a boy and his name was Ryan, I got responses like *"What are you doing to that poor kid? He's not going to know if he's Arthur or Martha."* This happened all the time. I started to feel really bad, like maybe I was an unfit mother. After a while I buckled under the pressure and tossed those pink things out.

Nell shakes her head and shrugs at me.

If Nell had dressed her baby *girl* in blue, would she have met with the same reaction and scrutiny as she did for dressing her baby boy in pink? Something in the fabric of mainstream Western society makes it more vital that a male not display feminine traits or characteristics. Yet why is it so vital to be marked as male or female from as soon as we are born? "The categorization of people as 'male' or 'female' permeates our society on every level, including our language, relationships, social institutions" (Monro 2005, p. 10). Just how uncomfortable society is about non-disclosure of a child's biological sex is evidenced in worldwide public protest over Canadian couple Kathy Witterick and David Stocker's decision not to divulge the biological sex of their newborn child, Storm.

Dominant branches of science tell us that the biological sex of an individual is determined through genitalia (Rogers 1999), yet we ordinarily identify individuals as males or females without seeing this part of their anatomy. The faces, sizes, and body shapes of infants and pre-pubescent children do not vary according to biological sex (Rogers 1999), so it is usually other symbols, such as how children are clothed, groomed, accessorized, and named, that indicate to us whether a child is male or female. These are social symbols—imposed by parents and carers—in the form of first names, haircuts, clothing (colors, fabrics, textiles, textures, designs, prints), adornments (ribbons, bracelets, watches), accessories (pencil cases, lunch boxes, backpacks), toys, and so on.

When I was a child, feminine styles of design and fashion were not common, nor deemed appropriate, for male bodies. For example, design motifs such as flowers and/or butterflies, fabrics such as chiffon and tulle, and accessories such as frills and ribbons consistently signified that which was of and for female bodies, not male. Connections between the feminine and female, and masculine and male, were so overwhelmingly common that they came to seem 'natural' to me.

The perceived sex of a child affects how they are responded to, handled, treated, enabled, and restrained (Young 1990, Rogers 1999, Paechter 2007). As a child, how I was named and clothed, and had my hair cut, signified to others that I was a boy. As such, it was with a certain set of gendered expectations that new teachers, adults, and other children met me. They assumed particular things about me that were common to their understanding and expectations of boys. The same set of gendered expectations derived via the names, clothing, and haircuts of other children and adults whom I came across dictated my expectations of who they were and what they might be like.

Just as clothing sections in department stores clearly display and define feminine designs, colors, and fabrics as being for females and not for males, so too do certain feminine and masculine embodied behaviors also come to be associated with female and not male biological sex. I recall being anxious about not necessarily fulfilling the criteria signified by my boy's name, clothing, or haircut. These anxieties hinged not only on the biological sex that these trappings signified me to be but also on how my body was regulated and self-regulated as a result of such signification.

Boy or Girl?

A new student, introduced as Jay, was brought in to join Len's preschool class. Jay wore a green T-shirt, blue track pants, and orange runners; was of average height; and had curly, mid-length brown hair. Len did not know whether Jay was a boy or a girl, and as the day progressed, the question of Jay's biological sex niggled at him. Where would he direct Jay when the student asked to be taken to the toilet? What would he say to Jay's mom or dad when they came to pick him/her up?

> *MOM/DAD:* How did Jay do today?
> *LEN:* Jay seemed to have a good day. Jay is well behaved. I think Jay is settling in well. In music, Jay demonstrated good coordination and rhythmic skills. Jay . . .

Eventually and ultimately, the English language demands the use of gendered pronouns (he, she, his, her) to define one as male or female.

What strategies can a teacher like Len use to discover whether a child like Jay is male or female:

- Have all students remove their clothing and determine Jay's biological sex by looking at Jay's genitalia?
- Ask Jay whether he is a boy or a girl?
- Separate the boys from the girls: "*I want all the boys to go to the activity corner and all the girls to gather around the arts and crafts table*"?
- Monitor how Jay is dressed? Watch out for anything frilly or pink, in which case it may be assumed that Jay is a girl?
- Observe Jay's interests? "*Hands up who likes Thomas the Tank engine. Hands up who likes Cinderella. Hands up who likes to play with dolls. Hands up who likes to play with cars. Hands up who wants to be a nurse when they grow up. Hands up who wants to be a firefighter when they grow up.*" Jay might be assumed to be a boy or a girl according to the stereotypical interests of other boys and girls.
- Observe what and how Jay plays? If Jay plays French skipping and if Jay is gentle, one might assume that Jay is a girl. If Jay plays rough-and-tumble, one might assume that Jay is a boy.

- Observe whether Jay plays predominantly with boys or girls? If Jay plays with boys one might assume that Jay is a boy. If Jay plays with girls one might assume that Jay is a girl.

How accurate or fair is each of these methods of deducing Jay's biological sex? How many of these strategies are based on stereotypes of females behaving in a feminine manner and displaying feminine interests and of males behaving in a masculine manner and displaying masculine interests? Ultimately, why does it matter whether Jay is a male or a female?

It is one thing for an infant's clothing or accessories to signify that the child is a boy or a girl, but situations exist where an infant's interests or embodied behavior leads us to make the same assumptions. It is problematic when a boy's or girl's interests or embodied behavior leads us to make assumptions about their gendernormativity and heteronormativity, causing us to view or treat them as being 'other'. My principal in Grade 2 spoke to my mother of concerns he had for me because my interests were more akin to those of the girls in my class than the boys (from an interview with my mother). He did not view such behavior as healthy or normal for a boy. That cues of femininity in males can have such potency from a young age signposts how oppressive social signifiers of biology and embodiment can be.

To this day I find it disturbing to have heard from several people that they *knew* that I was gay from when I was a child, especially as I was not fully aware myself of my sexual orientation until I was in my twenties. It amazes me that signals such as an individual's embodied behavior can be so defining as to lead to being classified and labeled in terms of sexual orientation (see Sirin et al. 2004, Johnson et al. 2007). This is especially concerning as being gay is perceived as subordinate (Connell 1995, Nayak & Kehily 1996, Paechter 2003a, Martino & Pallotta-Chiarolli 2005) and may lead to negative consequences or outcomes for subjects labeled as such. Embodied signification of who we are does not occur only in childhood nor just as an indication of biology. Examples of embodied signification that differentiate males and females in varying ways exist in the rituals of cultural, religious, and sporting traditions, be it through attire, physical positioning, and/or practice.

SOUND AND THE SIGNIFICATION OF GENDER AND EMBODIMENT

While tangibles such as adornment and grooming—in the form of clothes, accessories, and hairstyles—impact on how bodies signify, even intangibles such as sound and music have an effect on the signification of bodies and embodiment. How you *read* a segment of music will depend on your enculturation and the associations you make with certain melodies, sounds, and instrumentation. Music may be read and perceived differently according to meanings and associations related to human life assigned it by our cultures (McClary 1998, see also Leavy 2009). The extent to which you read a segment of music similarly to the way I do is likely to depend on commonalities in our enculturation.

Persons who live in Western cultures and are exposed to mass media—as I am—are likely to perceive feminine and masculine qualities in sounds similarly to how I myself do. The commonality of our readings of melody and music is dependent on commonalities in our enculturation. Even those who have never attended the ballet are likely to associate signature melodies from *Swan Lake* with images of femininity due to associated images that go hand in hand with these pieces of music as experienced through the mass media. In the West, we are very used to soft, flowing, gentle music being played alongside that which is female, poised, and graceful in movies, television dramas, and advertising. The 2010 *Lancôme* commercial in which actor Kate Winslet poses luxuriously and caresses her face and hair to the accompaniment of lilting harp and strings is a typical example. On the other hand, we are very used to strong and forceful music being played alongside that which is male, macho, and powerful. The 2010 *AussieBum Swimwear* commercial in which a muscular male jogs through the surf to the accompaniment of a rock beat accented by pounding steady drumming is a typical example. The semiotics of what kind of music matches the male body or the female body become so universal that they place composers in a bind. Consider the difference in briefs that a composer might receive for music to be featured in a beer advertisement targeting the drinking bodies of male clients as opposed to a beer advertisement targeting the drinking bodies of female clients.

Music is a cultural and social construction that by differentiating feminine versus masculine also serves to differentiate, by default, female and male. Musicologist Susan McClary (1998) contends that traditional and established musical codifications such as masculine and feminine cadence (driven and powerful versus soft and flowing) are invariably connected with male and female characterization, as evidenced in most dramatic musical utterances in which characters are inflected on the basis of gender. Musical sounds, as cultural constructions, have become so embedded and iconic that certain sounds come to be associated with the demure, the fragile, the dependent, and, by default, that which is 'female', in opposition to sounds that come to be associated with the powerful, the forceful, the dominant, and, by default, that which is 'male'.

If certain styles of music appear to fit certain products, such as beer, perfumes, lingerie, or fast cars, then it is reasonable to consider similar connections between music and certain embodiment as performed by particular biological bodies. For example, the pumping drive of Queen's *We Will Rock You* may well suggest the guzzling down of beer. However, it is more likely to suggest a male body gulping down beer than a female. This is due to our enculturation, and not because females are physiologically incapable of guzzling down a drink. Similarly, the sophisticated laid-back feel of Andre and Schwandt's *Dream a Little Dream of Me* is more likely to suggest a female body taking slow sips of a strawberry daiquiri than a male. Again, this is due to our enculturation toward the relationship between certain kinds of sounds and particular styles of embodiment performed by male or female bodies.

Mauss contends that "things we find natural have a historical origin" (1979, p. 116), claiming that the body techniques an individual takes on as normal are affected by external influences such as cinema. Taking this contention, it can be argued that exposure to music and other cultural constructions, such as design, that consistently connect that which is soft, lilting, and feminine to female bodies, and that which is strong, powerful, and masculine to male bodies, leads us to subconsciously internalize such connections and eventually serves to make them seem natural; deviations from these then seem marked, if not ludicrous. In short, our enculturation to connections between particular cultural constructions, such as music, and particular embodiment narrows the types of music and movement we deem to be appropriate for male or female bodies.

CULTURAL CONTEXTS

The following vignettes demonstrate that the same embodiment on a male or female body can signal and signify differently according to the cultural setting and context.

When we were children we received a photograph of our sixteen-year-old female cousin who lived in Israel and had been studying ballet for many years. The photograph showed our cousin in a classical ballet tutu, on her toes with arms overhead. Her underarms were unshaven. The sight of the classic ballerina with underarm hair greatly amused my sister and me. It was something that in Australian mainstream culture we had never seen before. We found the image hilarious.

The image of the quintessential ballerina is so much a part of Western enculturation that the image—whether to our liking or not—is not an unusual one to witness, be it on television, in advertising, and/or on billboards. The classic image of the ballerina in mainstream Western circles is always female, slender, white, and demure, without underarm hair. Breaches of any of these norms stand out as marked or remarkable ("We found the image hilarious"). Our reaction to the underarm hair of our

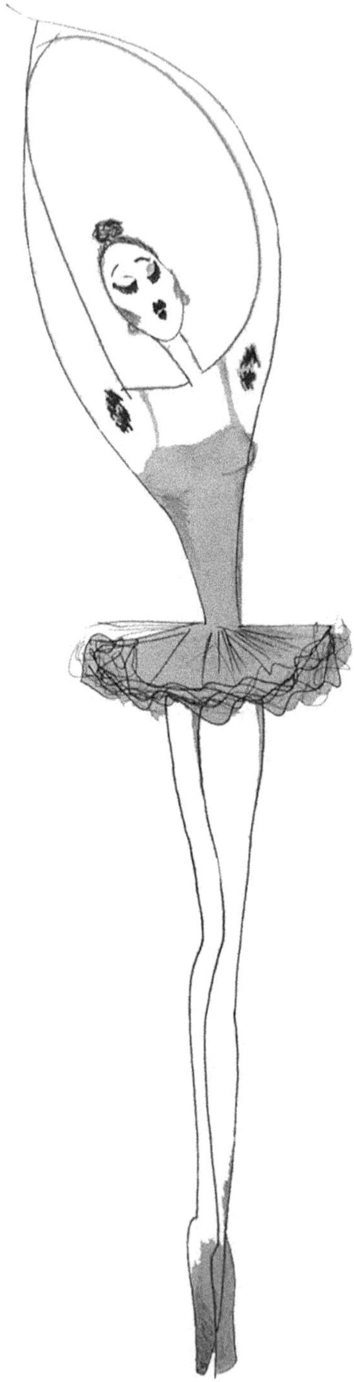

Figure 4.1 Ballerina with underarm hair. Artwork by Jack Migdalek.

I had just arrived in Japan, along with around 3,500 other Australians, New Zealanders, Canadians, Brits, and Americans who were on an exchange teaching program. It was stiflingly hot. We thousands were seated for a rather lengthy orientation briefing in an enormous auditorium, while on stage were Japanese officials—predominantly men—from various departments of the Ministry of Education: all cleanly shaven, all with neatly cropped and combed hair, all in conservative black, navy, or gray suits, shoes, and neck-ties. The hall was stuffy and still.

One be-suited Japanese man seated on the stage reached into his suit jacket and withdrew what looked at first to be a pen. With a flick of the wrist the object snapped open, and the man was fanning himself with the paper fan that had materialized. I was totally startled and amused, as were many of the other Westerners around me. We shared stifled titters of laughter. As the proceedings progressed, several of the other be-suited men on stage also revealed and flicked open fans to relieve themselves from the heat.

We just looked on, hot and fan-less, as the thin air stagnated around us.

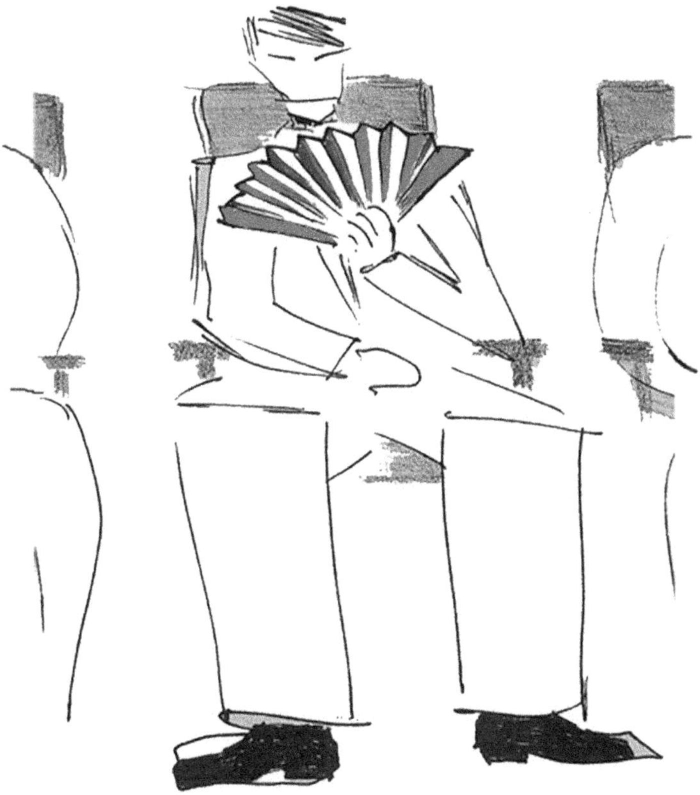

Figure 4.2 Hot. Artwork by Jack Migdalek.

ballerina cousin was not merely due to the difference between her body and the bodies of ballerinas to which our eyes were accustomed but to our perception and categorization of that difference as amusing, ludicrous, and strange.

The ways in which we are enculturated will necessarily inform how we see and read that which we are exposed to. Where an action is foreign to our culture and our enculturation, then it is likely to stand out. Our reaction to such marked performance will depend on our culture's regard for that which is different. In the case of what we are enculturated to define as a feminine action performed by a male (see Figure 4.2), the titters from across the assembled audience of Westerners indicate a discomfort with this embodied combination. Referring to Zizek's (1999) master-signifier theory, the feminine action that we found amusing was attributed meaning because of how it related to our understanding of *masculine* action as performed by a male. In my case, I was startled, amused, surprised, and confused, each a reflection of how I was positioned by the discourses and ideologies that had shaped me to date: startled at the incongruity of the action I had seen, amused because of what I saw as a glaring mismatch between the action performed and the biological sex of performer, surprised because I had never seen a man who was not in drag perform this action, and confused because for me the semiotics of a feminine action performed by a male signified homosexuality.

It may be that effeminate embodiment on a male signifies homosexuality (Gard 2001, Gere 2001, Martino & Pallotta-Chiarolli 2001), but such signification is culture specific. Where fanning one's face with a paper fan may be regarded as effeminate in one culture, it may not be regarded in the same manner in another. For the Japanese men it was a functional and normative action that held no comic or remarkable connotations.

My reactions to the Japanese men fanning themselves hinged on my enculturation. To my mind, and in my experience to date, the action of fanning oneself had been a languid action, something only for the soft or delicate, a feminine, coy act or possibly a flirting or seductive act as seen performed in the mass media. It makes sense that an action that is foreign to us comes to be marked as different, but why is it that differences become hierarchical with some acts of difference simply accepted as different, while others stand out as comic, ludicrous, deviant, or strange? This is relevant to ways in which taste (Bourdieu 1990) causes us to view, value, and perform embodied activity in particular ways, to be investigated in the next chapter.

During my six years in Japan, I frequently found myself double-taking and giggling at practices that were foreign to me: seeing men using paper fans (we saw this as an effeminate practice), seeing people who had colds wearing white face masks (we joked that they were surgeons), seeing people drink soup directly from a bowl (we used spoons). These practices were a source of amusement only in that they were different from those I had been brought up with. On reflection, these practices make good sense: fanning oneself to cool down, wearing a face mask so as not to spread germs, ingesting soup directly from the receptacle it is served in. However, being foreign to me, they signified as strange (and humorous), in contrast to oriental/exotic practices that were not so foreign to me, such as eating with chopsticks. Where an embodied performance of gender is perceived to be different, it may evoke responses ranging from amusement to abhorrence. In the case of children, these responses are likely to depend on the influences of carers, siblings, and/or peers, as suggested in the following vignette.

Lunch hour at a public restaurant. Seated at tables 1–5 are children with their parents/carers (see Figure 4.3). A young man is sitting alone at a table for two. His friend, another male, arrives to join him. They kiss.

Male to male kisses are part and parcel of the day to day embodied cultural practices of the family at table 5, yet not so for those at tables 1–4. The way in which children might glare at, stare at, giggle about, or not even notice a male to male kiss in a restaurant may hinge on the perceived perspectives of their carers, peers, or siblings. Our perspectives are shaped and affected by the discourses and cultures we come from. How aware are we of the power of our carers and cultures in forming our attitudes and taste (likes, dislikes, prejudices)? McRobbie (2009) cautions that we should not overlook the relationship between culture and subjectivity and the ways in which socially constructed notions, such as what is attractive, come to feel as though they are our own rather than externally imposed.

An embodied performance such as a kiss or an embrace can signify differently according to the enculturation of the individuals who view the act. It can also signify differently according to the biological sex of those engaged in the act. Within contemporary mainstream Western culture, a non-sexual kiss or embrace between a male and a female or between two females signifies differently from a non-sexual kiss or embrace between two males. Non-sexual kisses between or involving females seem to be regarded as unremarkable behavior within mainstream Western cultures. Similar differentiation in attitudes toward pornography also exists whereby girl on girl pornography for straight men is generally accepted as being titillating while boy on boy pornography for straight women is not (Pallotta-Chiarolli 2010). Where certain behaviors, such as a non-sexual kiss between two males, are consistently viewed in an aversive or comic light across a dominant cultural group, individuals inclined to perform such embodied practices in public settings are likely to develop a heightened degree of self-consciousness (see Foucault 1977, 1981). To this day I am very self-conscious of how my kissing or being kissed by another male will be received in public contexts and settings that I do not know to be accepting of such practices.

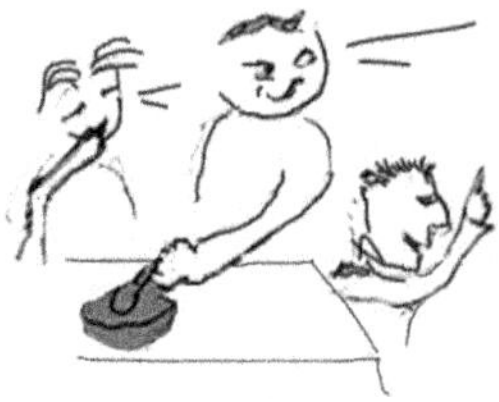

At table 1:
THE MALE TO MALE KISS AS A JOKE
Carer at table 1: "*Ugh!* Get a load of that! Now where do you suppose they left their handbags today?"

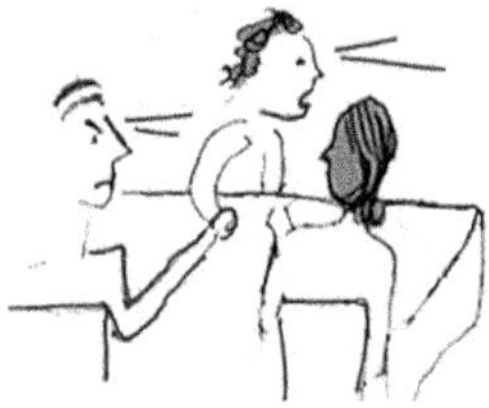

At table 2:
THE MALE TO MALE KISS AS AN ABOMINATION
Carer at table 2: "*Disgraceful!* Finish your meal children, we're leaving."

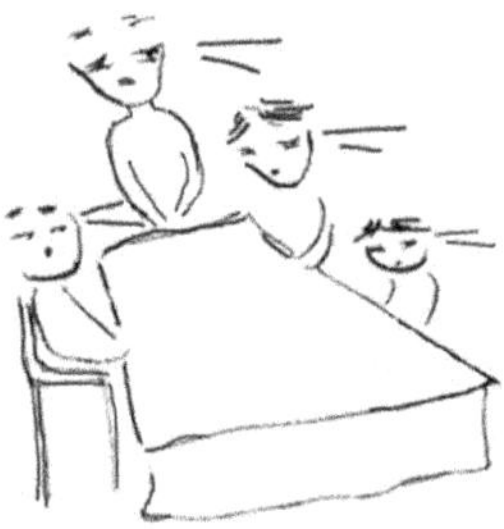

At table 3:
THE MALE TO MALE KISS AS THAT WHICH SHOULD NOT BE ACKNOWLEDGED
Carer at table 3: (to children who are staring at the men) "Don't look."

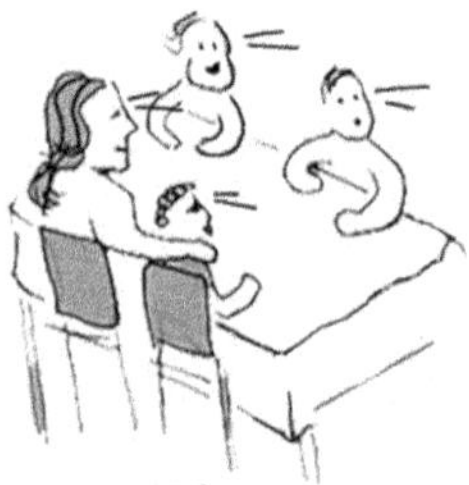

At table 4:
THE MALE TO MALE KISS AS AN ACT OF LOVE TO BE AFFIRMED
Carer A: "See those two guys there. They obviously care for one another very much, perhaps in a platonic way, or even in a way that your mom and dad love one another."
Carer B: "That's right, kids. Kissing is a way of showing affection to others, and something we should all do, regardless of our sex or sexuality."
Carer A: "In other words, kiss those you love."

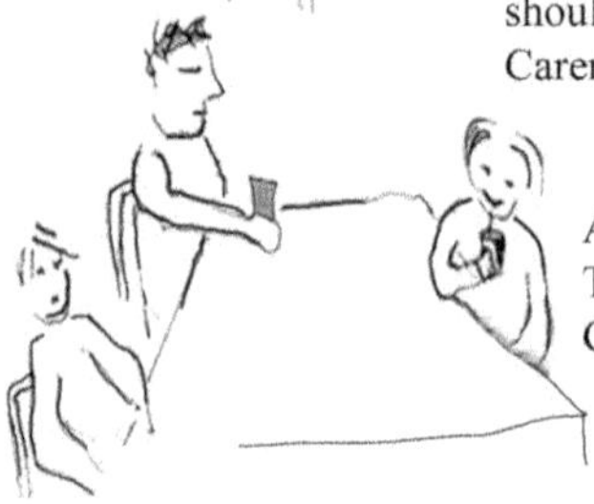

At table 5:
THE MALE TO MALE KISS AS ORDINARY
Carer at table 5: "Pass the sauce Alfredo."

Figure 4.3 Diners. Artwork by Jack Migdalek.

Pouted Lips

The following vignettes investigate the powerful means by which the engagement of facial muscles, as though about to kiss or blow out a candle, signifies differently according to the biological sex and culture of the performer.

The Look

We face ourselves in the mirrors lining the wall. Form-fitting fine woven fabrics stretch across and around our sweaty, toned bodies. Kenneth leads us through a new routine—setting, directing, defining, and refining our moves. We subject ourselves to his scrutiny. We trust his expertise, his eye. I'm still new and considered to be a promising young dancer, I am told. We come to Kenneth's classes in order to have him watch and teach our bodies, in the hope that he might recognize in us what it takes to do his moves 'on air'. He's the country's top commercial television choreographer.

We go through the motions with the music and then without it, in large groups, in small groups, a blur of pastel and primary colored leg-warmers, headbands, leotards, tights, jazz shoes. Yes, it is the 1980s! The girl in front of me helps me with a step I've not mastered. I'm grateful for her help. "You're welcome", she smiles (poor thing—I know she'll never make it: too fleshy). We work with our own 2D images in the mirrors, trying to embody and master the moves Kenneth talks us through. He demonstrates and corrects a phrase of movement on Natalie's lithe form, her concentration absolutely committed to the move and how it appears on her body in the mirror. Anorexic Meryn hardly matches Natalie's extension as she mirrors the correction earnestly. Kenneth barely acknowledges her. Along with Meryn, we strive to naturalize Kenneth's moves on our own bodies in the same way that Barbara, Darlene, and Rachelle (his top dancers) seem to have done. "God, if only I could dance like that."

An Epidemic

"OK kids, let's take it in groups of 6." Barbara, Darlene, Rachelle, and several others go first. We watch, scrutinize, and admire their forms, their finesse, their attitude, in the knowledge that these are the dancers always on the top rung of the dance work that's going, that they've got what it takes. From watching and admiring, and admiring and watching, the likes of 'in-work' Darlene, Rachelle, and Barbara, we attempt to duplicate, imitate, replicate.

I swear that when Kenneth taught us routines he said nothing about what to do with our lips. Nevertheless, over time, lip by lip, like an epidemic we acquire that expression, 'the look' (even we new students). Their lips, our lips, all lips pushed forward and pouting at our reflections, the promise of a kiss, the proffering of self. Like an infection (or affectation) setting in, we contract 'the face'. And why not? It's on the faces of the dancers that Kenneth uses consistently, the dancers we so look up to. We're the dancers who want work. We take on the look. It makes sense.

Kinesthetic Misdemeanor

I started dancing relatively late. It was empowering to realize that I possessed control over my body as I literally watched it transform and develop into a beautiful, finely tuned, aesthetic instrument. I watched myself becoming stronger and more flexible. I watched as my body became toned and pencil thin, secure in the knowledge that if I didn't eat two hours prior to class, I had no stomach at all. Routines became easier to pick up, and Kenneth sometimes even remembered my name! I sensed that I was close to getting professional work as a dancer. The proof was there in the mirrors. My body in motion had begun to match the bodies of the pros. Darlene was my #1 model of perfection. She was the best dancer in the class, and always on television in variety shows, rock videos, commercials. I was beginning to dance like Darlene. I was beginning to look like Darlene. Kinesthetically I knew I'd captured her dance style and demeanor. When I danced, I felt fantastic, like I really had what it took. I did have what it took!

I eventually came to realize, as my focus on my mirror image went from body to body and face to face, that the essence of Darlene that I had so successfully embodied worked differently on me. How embarrassed I felt when I finally saw my mirror reflection as it might have appeared to television-viewing Joe Public. The lip infection I had contracted did not serve me in the same way as it did Darlene, Rachelle, and the others. My focus shifted from the likes of Darlene to the less gifted Robert and Stephan. With some effort I exorcised the infection, substituting a straight-lipped cool, detached, occasionally aggressive, occasionally sardonic expression in its place. Having laid to rest what I'd taken to be the essential dancer in me, I learned a new essential way of dancing; my dream came true; I became a professional dancer, balls and all.

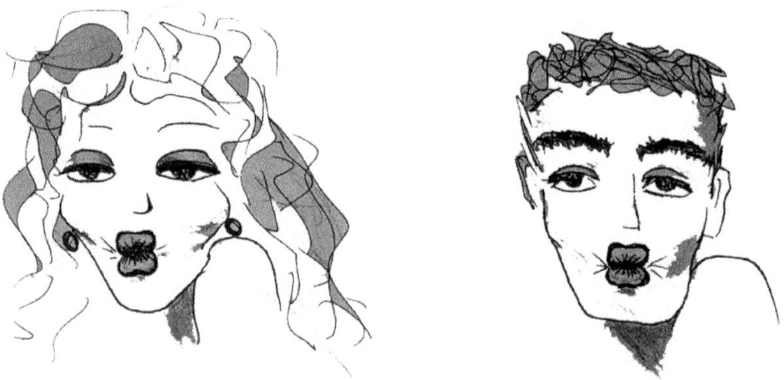

Figure 4.4 Pout. Artwork by Jack Migdalek.

For me, during the 1980s, the embodiment of pouted lips figured in and across many aspects of pop-culture and the mass media. Embodying and reading the look signified a disturbing confusion of multiple meanings. I saw and still see pouted lips on female dancers and models in advertising and commercial dance, and even on females in settings such as dance clubs. To me, the pout is an expression I did not and do not see on men except when adopted in parody of women, or when feigning preciousness such as in the television personas of Mr. Humphries in *Are You Being Served* (BBC), Jack in *Will and Grace* (NBC), Mark St. James in *Ugly Betty* (ABC), and Simon and Kylie in *Beautiful People* (BBC).

Males and females come to a very strong sense of being male or female at a very young age (Connell 1983, 1995, 2000, Plummer 1999, Rogers 1999, Kimmel & Messner 2001, Kehily 2002, Renold 2003, Shilling 2003, Swain 2004, 2005, Davies 2006, Paechter 2007, DePalma & Atkinson 2008) largely due to socialization that emphasizes the differences between the sexes. Unlike the fictional male dancer in the preceding narrative, I, as a male dancer in dance classes, identified with and became attuned to modeling myself on the male dancers in classes. This was despite the fact that there were usually far more females in classes than males. Whereas the fictionalized character in the story above took some time to realize that taking on the same embodied facial expression as the females in the dance class would not serve him well as a male choreographic subject, I realized this very early in my dance training, which began in my late teens. If nothing else, it was clear to me that there were no models of 'in-work' male dancers who embodied the facial expression adopted by so many 'in-work' female dancers. The physical capital—and poverty—attached to certain models of femininity and masculinity will be investigated in the next chapter.

Having lived in Japan from 1991 to 1997, I was amazed to find that the 'pouted-lips' look was a face worn publicly by males in that country. I saw it on the faces of Japanese principals, lecturers, and teachers in education institutions where I worked, as well as characters in Japanese television dramas. The expression manifested itself predominantly on the faces of Japanese male white-collar workers and signified being deep in contemplation or in the processes of decision making.

Due to globalization via mass media, the pouted-lips look, as seen on female models in advertising, female dancers in performance, and female actors in seductive scenes, has become prevalent across many countries. I wonder if there is a confusion of meaning in a country like Japan when the pouted-lips look is familiar both as a face of seduction via female faces in the mass media and as a face of concentration via the faces of Japanese males in the process of decision making. Or, as a result of multiple meanings, will Japanese men change—or have they changed—how they physically express being deep in contemplation? I wonder—as a result of the multiple meanings that pouted lips seem to hold—how Japanese wives and lovers might read or misread the look as it manifests on their businessmen partners in the throes of making love.

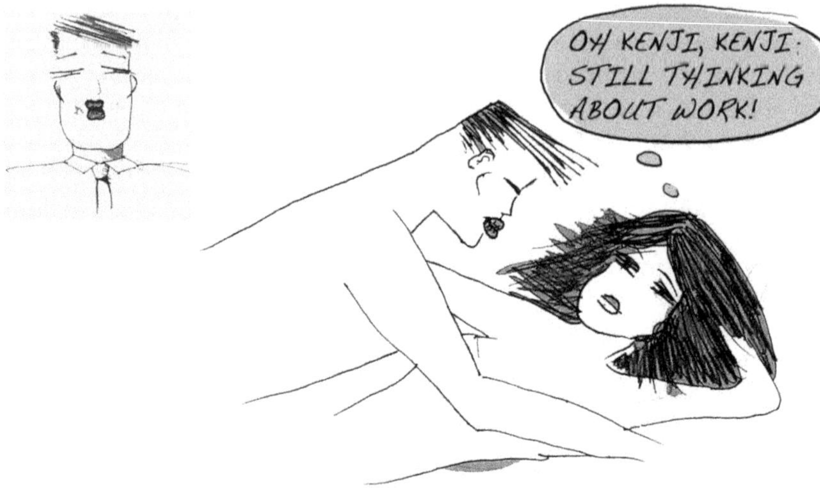

Figure 4.5 Kenji's pout. Artwork by Jack Migdalek.

The same embodiment can signal and signify differently according to biological sex and according to the cultural and temporal context.

POSE, REPOSE, ACTION

The pictured individuals in Figure 4.6 (overleaf) stand with the weight resting on one leg, the other leg bent at the knee. Able-bodied males and females are equally capable of performing this pose (known in the visual arts as contrapposto), yet within mainstream Western contexts it is a pose that one does not ordinarily see on the bodies of males.

Most people in contemporary mainstream Western contexts would see the contrapposto pose as feminine, and given that feminine embodiment on a male signifies homosexuality (see Pronger 1990, Gard 2001, Gere 2001, Martino & Pallotta-Chiarolli 2001), they would see it as homosexual when performed by a male body. Such conceptions are social. As mentioned previously, postures struck by men that may be considered soft or feminine were not associated with homosexuality until the 1900s (Wex 1979, Burt 2001, see also Greer 2003). Indeed, contrapposto poses such as those of Hermes (in the fourth-century iconic sculpture of *Hermes and Dionysos* by Praxitele) and Napoleon (as depicted in *Napoleon in His Study in the Tuilleries Palace* by Jacques Louis David in 1812) were seen to project as noble and heroic, and not as homosexual. Clearly, a change in how the pose signifies has occurred.

Although it can be argued that pressures still exist on how women should acceptably embody (including how they might walk, chew, or drink)

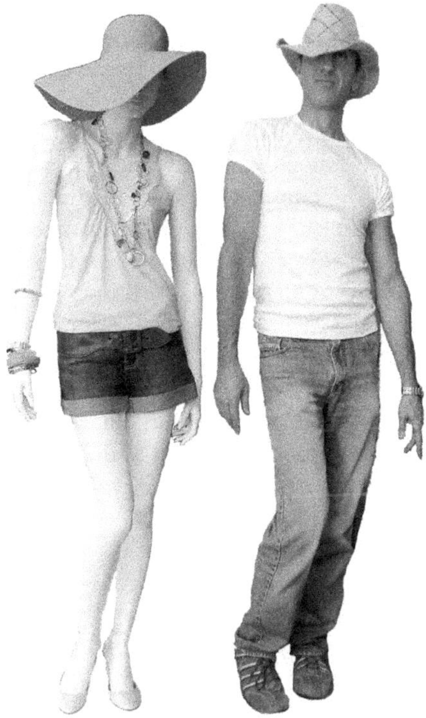

Figure 4.6 Contrapposto 1. Photograph by Esther Erlich.

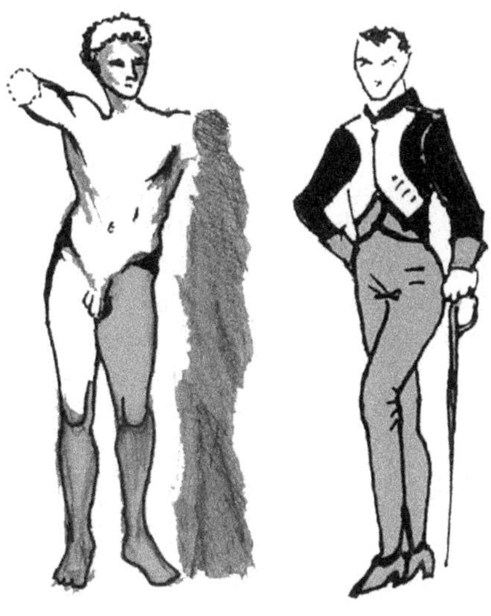

Figure 4.7 Contrapposto 2. Artwork by Jack Migdalek.

in contemporary mainstream Western societies, in recent times there has been a marked broadening in embodied behaviors that are socially acceptable for a female body to perform. Where broad straddle-legged poses on women may be socially acceptable in contemporary—and ancient—times within many cultural settings, such postures struck by women were not so distantly considered to be socially improper and for the most part as proffering sex (Wex 1979). The feminist movement can be credited with having improved the scope of what has come to be considered acceptable embodiment for women. The demarcation of the boundaries of what is deemed inappropriate for women's bodies to perform in contemporary mainstream society is not as clear-cut as what is deemed inappropriate for men. Males in contemporary mainstream Western cultures—who had more flexibility in how they could embody in past times—are now more restricted in the range or options of embodiment that they might assume. It is as if master-signifiers (Zizek 1999) of masculine embodiment on males cast a light over embodiment on males that is not masculine.

As yet, neither queer movements nor male movements have achieved much in destabilizing traditional codings and categories of what it is for a male to be gay or effeminate within wider society (Nixon 1996, see also Mac an Ghaill & Haywood 2007). The same can be claimed regarding the stability of what is choreographically acceptable embodiment for straight males in contemporary Western society. In theory, what is regarded as metrosexual behavior (behavior by a heterosexual male that is stereotypically regarded as homosexual) may herald a broadening of acceptable embodiment for males. However, in such cases the heterosexuality of the metrosexual is frequently at the forefront, serving to blatantly eliminate any misconception that the male in question might be homosexual (see Dunbar 2000, Mac an Ghaill 2007). Having proven his 'normal' credentials the metrosexual is thus allowed to '*play*' at being 'not normal'. On the whole the consequences for males whose embodiment is feminine continue to place such males at risk (Courtenay 2000, Paechter 2003b, Martino & Pallotta-Chiarolli 2005).

In this chapter, I have focused on the differential signification of male and female bodies. It must also be acknowledged that the way physical embodiment projects can vary according to more than just the biological sex of the performer. The same pose may project differently on a body that is thin, fat, short, tall, aged, hairy, freckled, scarred, pale, or dark. The person whose embodiment does not fit the norm tends to be defined by those very qualities as one who is 'other'.

REFERENCES

Bourdieu, P. (1990). *The Logic of Practice.* Oxford: Polity Press.

Burt, R. (1995). *The Male Dancer: Bodies, Spectacle, Sexualities.* London: Routledge.

Burt, R. (2001). Dissolving in Pleasure: The Threat of the Queer Male Dancing Body. In Desmond, J. C. (Ed.). *Dancing Desires: Choreographing Sexualities On and Off the Stage*. Madison: University of Wisconsin Press.

Connell, R. W. (1983). *Which Way Is Up?* Sydney: Allen and Unwin.

Connell, R. W. (1995). *Masculinities*. Sydney: Allen and Unwin.

Connell, R. W. (2000). *The Men and the Boys*. St Leonards, NSW: Allen and Unwin.

Courtenay, W. H. (2000). Constructions of Masculinity and Their Influence on Men's Well-Being: A Theory of Gender and Health. *Social Science & Medicine*. Vol 50, No 10, pp. 1385–1401.

Davies, B. (2006). Subjectification: The Relevance of Butler's Analysis for Education. *British Journal of Sociology of Education*. Vol 27, No 4, pp. 425–438.

DePalma, R., & Atkinson, E. (2008). *Invisible Boundaries: Addressing Sexualities Equality in Children's Worlds*. Stoke on Trent: Trentham.

Dunbar, M. (2000). Dennis Rodman: Do You Feel Feminine Yet? Black Masculinity, Gender Transgression, and Reproductive Rebellion on MTV. In McKay, J., Messner, M. A., & Sabo, D. (Eds.). *Masculinities, Gender Relations, and Sport*. Thousand Oaks: Sage.

Foucault, M. (1977). *Discipline and Punish: The Birth of the Prison*. London: Peregrine.

Foucault, M. (1981). *The History of Sexuality. Volume One, An Introduction*. London: Penguin.

Gard, M. (2001). Dancing around the 'Problem' of Boys and Dance. *Discourse: Studies in the Cultural Politics of Education*. Vol 22, No 2, pp. 212–225.

Gere, D. (2001). Effeminate Gestures: Choreographer Joe Goode and the Heroism of Effeminacy. In Desmond, J. C. (Ed.). *Dancing Desires: Choreographing Sexualities On and Off the Stage*. Madison: University of Wisconsin Press.

Greer, G. (2003). *The Boy*. London: Thames & Hudson.

Heller, S. (2008). *The Swastika. Symbol beyond Redemption*. New York: Allworth Press.

Johnson, K. L., Gill, S., & Reichman, V. (2007). Swagger, Sway and Sexuality: Judging Sexual Orientation from Body Motion and Morphology. *Journal of Personality and Social Psychology*. Vol 93, No 3, pp. 321–334.

Kehily, J. (2002). *Sexuality, Gender and Schooling: Shifting Agendas in Social Learning*. London: Routledge.

Kimmel, M. S., & Messner, M. A. (2001). *Men's Lives*. Boston: Allyn and Bacon.

Leavy, P. (2009). *Method Meets Art: Arts-Based Research Practice*. New York: Guilford Press.

Mac an Ghaill, M., & Haywood, C. (2007). *Gender, Culture and Society: Contemporary Femininities and Masculinities*. London: Macmillan.

Martino, W., & Pallotta-Chiarolli, M. (2001). Gender Performativity and Normalizing Practices. In Haynes, F., & McKenna, T. (Eds.). *Unseen Genders: Beyond the Binaries*. New York: Peter Lang.

Martino, W., & Pallotta-Chiarolli, M. (2005). *Being Normal Is the Only Way to Be*. Sydney: University of New South Wales Press.

Mauss, M. (1979). *Sociology and Psychology: Essays*. London: Routledge.

McClary, S. (1998). *Feminine Endings: Music, Gender, and Sexuality*. Minneapolis, MN: University of Minnesota Press.

McRobbie, A. (2009). *The Aftermath of Feminism*. Thousand Oaks: Sage.

Monro, S. (2005). *Gender Politics*. London: Pluto.

Nayak, A., & Kehily, M. J. (1996). Playing It Straight: Masculinities, Homophobias and Schooling. *Journal of Gender Studies*. Vol 5, No 2, pp. 211–230.

Nixon, S. (1996). *Hard Looks. Masculinities, Spectatorship and Contemporary Consumption*. New York: St Martins Press.

Paechter, C. (2003a). Learning Masculinities and Femininities: Power/Knowledge and Legitimate Peripheral Participation. *Women's Studies International Forum.* Vol 26, No 6, pp. 541–552.

Paechter, C. (2003b). Masculinities and Femininities as Communities of Practice. *Women's Studies International Forum.* Vol 26, No 1, pp. 69–77.

Paechter, C. (2007). *Being Boys, Being Girls: Learning Masculinities and Femininities.* Berkshire: Open University Press.

Pallotta-Chiarolli, M. (2010). *Border Sexualities, Border Families in Schools.* Lanham: Rowman and Littlefield.

Plummer, D. (1999). *One of the Boys: Masculinity, Homophobia and Modern Manhood.* New York: Harrington Park Press.

Pronger, B. (1990). Gay Jocks: A Phenomenology of Gay Men in Athletics. In Messner, M.A., & Sabo, D.F. (Eds.). *Sport, Men, and the Gender Order: Critical Feminist Perspectives.* Champaign, IL: Human Kinetics Books.

Renold, E. (2003). 'If You Don't Kiss Me, You're Dumped': Boys, Boyfriends and Heterosexualised Masculinities in the Primary School. *Educational Review.* Vol 55, No 2, pp. 179–194.

Rogers, L. (1999). *Sexing the Brain.* London: Weidenfeld & Nicolson.

Shilling, C. (2003). *The Body and Social Theory.* London: Sage.

Sirin, S.R., McCreary, D.R., & Mahalik, J.R. (2004). Differential Reactions to Men and Women's Gender Role Transgressions: Perceptions of Social Status, Sexual Orientation, and Value Dissimilarity. *Journal of Men's Studies.* Vol 12, No 2, pp. 119–133.

Swain, J. (2004). The Resources and Strategies That 10–11-Year-Old Boys Use to Construct Masculinities in the School Setting. *British Educational Research Journal.* Vol 30, No 1, pp. 167–185.

Swain, J. (2005). Masculinities in Education. In Kimmel, M.S., Hearn, J., & Connell, R.W. (Eds.). *Handbook of Studies on Men and Masculinities.* London: Sage.

Turner, B. (1984). *The Body and Society.* Oxford: Basil Blackwell.

Wex, M. (1979). *Let's Take Back Our Space: Female and Male Body Language as a Result of Patriarchal Structures.* Munich: Frauenliteratur Verlag.

Young, I.M. (1990). *Throwing Like a Girl and Other Essays in Feminist Philosophy and Social Theory.* Indianapolis: Indiana University Press.

Zizek, S. (1999). *The Sublime Object of Ideology.* London: Verso.

5 Model Bodies

THE CULTIVATION OF TASTE

In this chapter I chart and comment on how embodied performances, as viewed in formal and everyday arenas, come to be valued or devalued as attractive, unattractive, desirable, undesirable, tasteful and aesthetic, or distasteful and un-aesthetic. As already stated, a learner's principal agent is a model used for imitation (Hall 1959).

The gendered ways in which male and female bodies themselves are repeatedly represented, projected, and idealized in the media impact on the social mindset toward embodied adherence to or transgression of heteronormativity. Consistent with this, they can also impact on how males and females approach certain physical tasks, making them likely to embody or aspire to embody in ways that seem to befit their biological sex.

The widespread gendered presentation and representation of embodied behavior that occur within media and public performance arenas of dance, drama, musicals, game shows, talk shows, and public sports events (as seen on the stage, screen, television, or sports sites) reinforce deep-seated gendernormative/heteronormative, dominant outlooks on what is appropriate or desirable embodiment for male and female bodies respectively. Norms of embodied masculinity and femininity come to represent physical and cultural capital (Bourdieu 1990, Shilling 2003). Inversely, deviations from embodied sex-specific norms of masculinity/femininity are marked as subordinate forms of masculinity/femininity and come to represent physical and cultural poverty. In this chapter I will contemplate the relationship between physical and cultural capital and poverty, as projected by bodies around me, and my own history and sense of personal physical capital and poverty.

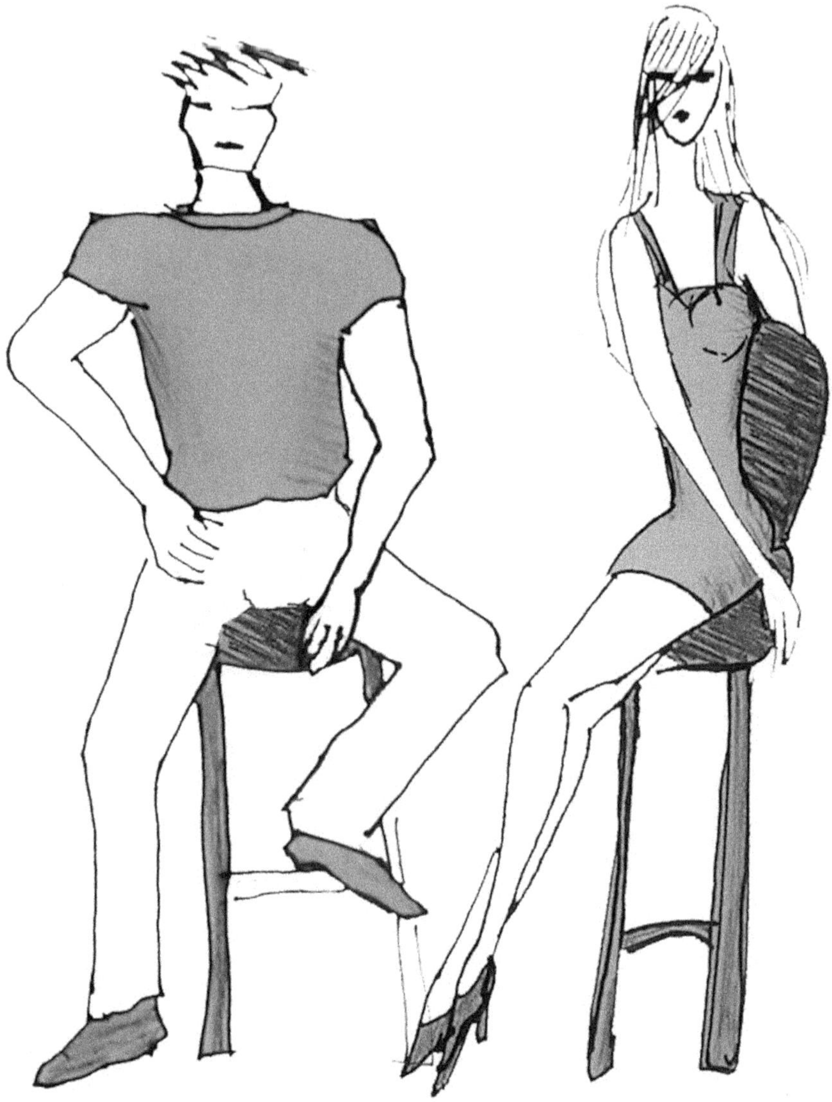

Figure 5.1 Model bodies. Artwork by Jack Migdalek.

BODIES IN MEDIA—BILLBOARDS, NEWSPAPERS, MAGAZINES

> The material the media supplies is not passively absorbed. Each of us actively appropriates this material to make sense of ourselves and our place in the social world.
>
> (Kirk 2002, p. 83)

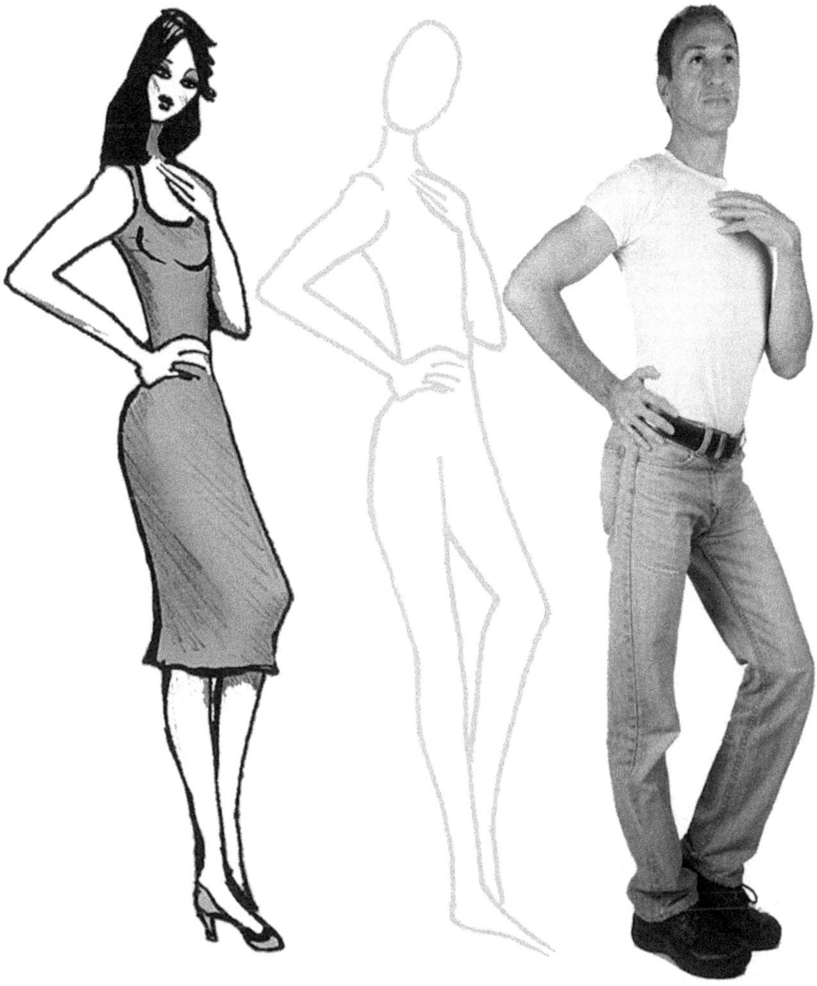

Figure 5.2 Embodiment/demeanor deemed acceptable and/or attractive on one body may not be so on another. Photograph by Rob Chiarolli (www.photosthattell.com). Artwork by Jack Migdalek.

Bodies posed in billboard, newspaper, and magazine advertisements for goods such as fashion items are frequently slim and attractive. Looking beyond these bodies as matter, I note a difference in the range of pose and repose that the male and female subjects of these advertisements strike. Although one may come across advertisements in which the bodies of male and female models are posed or reposed in strong or arguably 'masculine' poses, it is not so common in the mainstream to find advertisements in which male bodies are posed or reposed in languid, delicate, or arguably 'feminine' poses. Where they are posed in these ways it tends to be in advertising in magazines such as *DNA* (DNA publications), which markets to consumers who fit into categories such as queer or metrosexual, reinforcing links between such embodiment and the non-normative.

While it can be argued that there has been some accentuation of softness in the male as an object of the gaze in fashion advertising particularly, such imagery has had little impact on traditional gendernormative codes, perceptions, and practices of masculinity as taken up by males in lived culture (Nixon 1996, Mac an Ghaill & Haywood 2007). The gulf between what appears on a catwalk and what is accepted in the everyday was emphasized in the post-story comment of TV-journalist Tracy Grimshaw following a report on the feminine stylings of *femi-man* model Andre Pejic (Jean Paul Gaultier's muse), when she remarked, "Wonder how he'd go at the Broadmeadows pub" (*A Current Affair,* network 9, Australia, aired 29/03/11).

BODIES IN MEDIA—SPORTS ARENAS

Male and Female Bodies in Sports

How our bodies perform every day is influenced by the bodies we see in public arenas (Hall 1959, Kirk 2002). A public arena, where thousands of

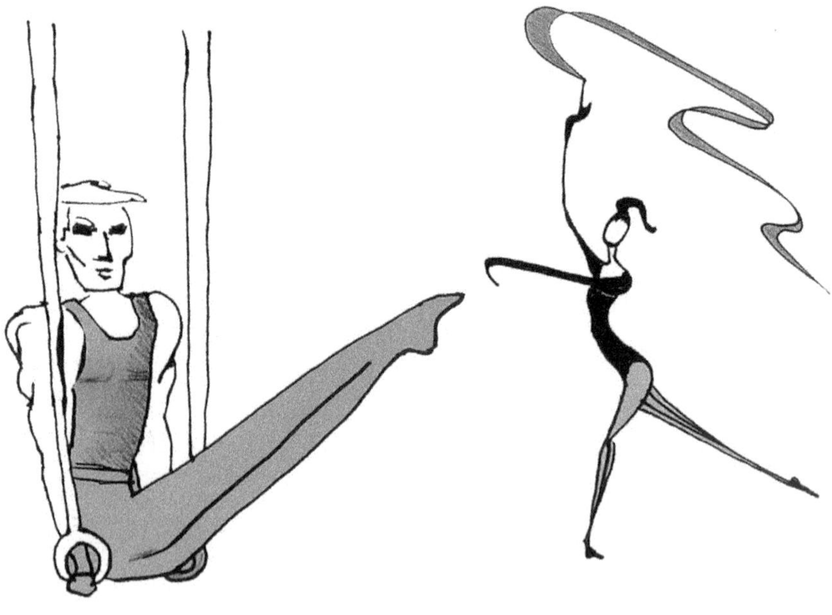

Figure 5.3 Men's sports—women's sports. Artwork by Jack Migdalek.

bodies were under international gaze, was the Commonwealth Games in Melbourne, Australia (March 2006). What we witness in such events is the continuation of unequal constructions of women's and men's bodies where patriarchy, hegemonic masculinity, and homophobia continue to dominate.

On the one hand, some equalizing change has occurred. Despite recurring references in the media to their attractiveness, more and more women's bodies are moving in ways that were previously the exclusive action domain of men. They are physically doing more with their bodies and taking more space than they were permitted to in the past (Young 1990). This is exhibited by their participation in sports and other activities previously considered inappropriate for women. Within some arenas sportswomen now do pole-vaulting, shooting, and weightlifting, as well as Australian rules football, soccer, boxing, and wrestling.

In current Olympic and Commonwealth Games, sportswomen are ineligible to compete in the rings or pommel horse events, just as sportsmen are ineligible to compete in rhythmic gymnastics, the beam, or synchronized swimming. (Although *mixed* pair synchronized swimming does exist, at the time of writing it is still not a category for the 2016 Olympic Games). The reasons for non-participation are probably very different. Given the access to and mastery of sports from which females were previously excluded, it is likely that in time women will also master the rings and pommel horse as muscles not previously tuned toward such action become developed. Why men do not do, perform, or compete in synchronized swimming and rhythmic gymnastics with ball and sash is a different matter altogether. I argue that the reasons males do not perform activities such as these are not connected to physical ability but to social perceptions and preconceptions of what motions are not suitably masculine. Certain forms of male embodied performance are valued above others (see Martino & Pallotta-Chiarolli 2001, Kirk 2002, Gorely et al. 2003). My concern is that deep-seated notions of differential embodiment being suited or becoming to male or female bodies are so deeply embedded that their gendered machinations rarely call our notice.

Synchronized swimming and rhythmic gymnastics are sports that males can physically master. However, notions of the feminine and the masculine are presented as so diametrically opposed that presuppositions of "binaried embodiment" prevail (Crowley 2004, p. 180), making crossover—especially from masculine to feminine—problematic. In a 2002 Uncle Toby's muesli bar television advertisement—featuring champion male swimmers Ian Thorpe, Grant Hackett, and Kieren Perkins—the notion that synchronized swimming was not a sport or arena suitable for men is reinforced. In the advertisement, the three elite male swimmers clown around with synchronized swimming moves. Ultimately, they toss in the towel on the sport because of how awkward and ludicrous they perceive themselves to be when moving in these ways. This is no wonder, given dominant masculinist attitudes that classify and dismiss the type of motion performed in synchronized swimming as feminine and girlie. The impact of male swimming heroes parodying such embodiment performed by male bodies further reinforces already existing rigid gendered roles.

Another example where the message that effeminate embodiment on sportsmen is not valued or welcome was evidenced in the commentary by veteran Canadian sportscasters Claude Mailhot and Alain Goldberg, and Australian commentators Eddie McGuire and Mick Molloy, who joked that because of his flamboyant skating and effeminate stylings, Winter Olympic ice-skater Johnny Weir should be competing in the *women's* competition, not the men's.

That certain sports are viewed as feminine and therefore suitable for female bodies to perform and not for male bodies to perform only reinforces the value or physical capital (Shilling 2003) of certain forms of male behavior above others, thus serving to sustain existing patriarchal ideologies of hegemonic masculinity. It can be argued that movements in men's gymnastics events are equally graceful to movements in rhythmic gymnastics and synchronized swimming. However, due to the sheer and obvious muscularity involved, men's gymnastics events tend to be seen as acceptably masculine. Indeed, there is a correlation between perceptions of masculinity and muscularity (Gorely et al. 2003).

I became aware at a young age of what type of motion was seen to be appropriate and desirable for males to embody. This occurred through exposure to representations of male bodies that were deemed to be successful: bodies—such as those of popular male sports icons—that took up space and moved forcefully, expansively, and powerfully. At the same time, I became aware of what type of motion was deemed to be *in*appropriate for males to embody. This occurred through exposure to representations of male bodies that were deemed to be comic, ludicrous, or homosexual. Examples of such bodies were those that were physically delicate, weak, fat, slight, and/or effeminate. These were the types of bodies that did not make sports teams. I disliked sports such as Australian rules football and chose, where possible, not to play. The social capital (Jenkins 2002 after Bourdieu) of the boy who participated in gentler recreational activity was valued very differently from those of the boys who played Australian rules football (see Renold 2005, Epstein & Johnson 2008, Lingard et al. 2009). The fact that my male body did not engage in rougher physical play left me feeling alienated from the majority of other boys, who did.

When I became a dancer, with a body that was necessarily a strong body possessed of power and stamina, I still found myself alienated from most other males because dance was regarded as an effeminate and suspect activity for a male body. It was in the guise of aerobics instructor that my fit and powerful body was less suspect. Exerting one's body to music in a gym setting where movement was obviously a demonstration of muscularity and arguably devoid of artistry proved to be more acceptable. Demonstrating that I could out-run, out-kick, out-last those whom I led through a fifty-minute aerobics routine awarded me respect and physical and social capital within mainstream circles that I would never achieve in dance.

Awards Ceremonies—Kisses

In the medal ceremonies of the 2006 Commonwealth Games held in Melbourne, Australia, male and female dignitaries and officials consistently shook hands with winning athletes. Occasionally there were also kisses between athletes and officials. It was not always clear who initiated the kisses, but that is not relevant. What is relevant is that within the Commonwealth Games' forum that involved males and females from seventy-one nations, this action was only practiced with female athletes and never male athletes. Why did kisses occur between males and females, and between females and females, in these medal ceremonies, but never between two males? Male to male kisses do occur between dignitaries and male athletes of some cultures, even in settings such as the Olympic Games. What is it about the Commonwealth culture that keeps the practice in check? In line with theories on colonialism and oppression (see Memmi 1967, Freire 1990, Said 2003, Fanon 2008), it can be argued that cultures where male to male kissing had been an acceptable expression of congratulation have been colonized to perform otherwise. Britain has subsumed the cultures of the countries and provinces that it took possession of, which have adapted to and taken on the British colonizer's gender inequitable 'kissing values and practices'—at least within contexts that are internationally viewed and scrutinized, particularly by Westerners, such as the Commonwealth Games.

Many practices are so ingrained in us that they become non-consciously performed and part of our habitus (Bourdieu 1990). Examples of this pertaining to embodiment would include actions such as nodding one's head when in agreement, clapping one's hands at the end of a speech, and standing on being introduced in a formal setting. These actions or habitus are

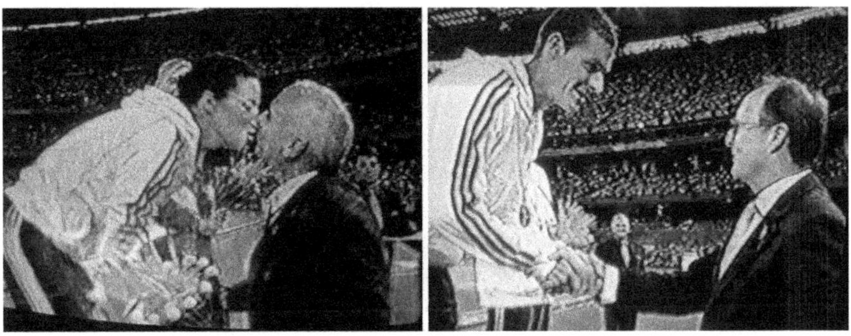

Figure 5.4 Medal ceremonies. Commonwealth Games coverage, Nine Network Australia 2006.

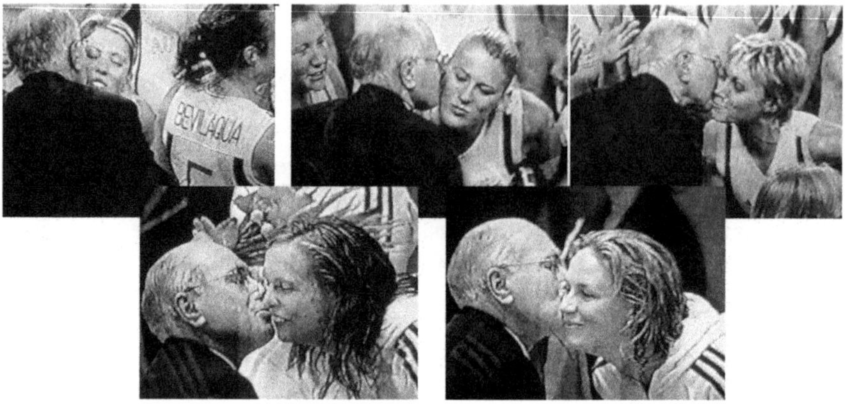

Figure 5.5 John Howard, Australia's prime minister (1996–2007), kissing female Commonwealth Games athletes, 2006. He only ever shook hands with male athletes. Commonwealth Games coverage, Nine Network Australia 2006.

performed without conscious thought. I argue that some body habitus—such as kissing a female athlete and not a male in Commonwealth Games award ceremonies—serve only to maintain patriarchal gender inequity.

> Gendered practices and images of the body exert an influence which does not remain at the level of consciousness or discourse. The ways in which we perceive, categorize and value women's and men's bodies are undoubtedly important in legitimising and reproducing social inequalities.
>
> (Shilling 2003, p. 98)

Where differences in practice according to the biological sex of the performer are invisible to us they are likely to legitimize gender inequities as natural. Performing actions that signify differently according to the biological sex of the performers involved can be seen as not merely symbolic but constitutive of gender inequalities.

If males and females should arguably have the same status in society, why do we position and allow ourselves to be positioned differently? Just what do public congratulatory kisses, such as those practiced in the Commonwealth Games, represent? Are they (1) sexual, (2) caring, or (3) merely congratulatory? If these kisses are sexual, is it not demeaning for a woman to be publicly subject to physical contact of a sexual and potentially unwelcome nature? If these kisses are signs of care and nurturing, is it not demeaning for a woman to be positioned or to allow herself to be in the position of one who is in need of care or protection—or, by the same token, why doesn't the male athlete also need care and nurturing? If these kisses are signs of warmth and congratulation, then why don't kisses take place between male officials and male athletes also? Why only where there are females involved?

Had a kiss been exchanged between a male official and male athlete during a medal ceremony it would have been noticed and noted very differently from kisses that occurred between males and females, or indeed kisses between two females. Although medal ceremony kisses were visible to the eye, the gendered make up of the practice remains largely *in*visible unless transgressed. What does this indicate about the cultures of the Commonwealth Games and Commonwealth nations and the differential positioning that women and men continue to inhabit? What does this indicate about the globalized colonial culture of Commonwealth nations within which specific colonized cultures have been subsumed? Where practices—such as those that differ according to biological sex—become habitual, their workings fade from consciousness, nor are they necessarily open to change (Bourdieu 1990, 2001).

Kisses or embraces can be associated with sexual action. They are part of sexual intimacy. Why is it that a male or female kissing or embracing a female in an award ceremony is generally accepted as non-sexual behavior? Yet were a male kissing or embracing a male it would be seen as something out of the ordinary, something concerning sexuality. Why is it that friendly body contact between males is more likely to be taken as a signifier of sexual interest or sexual orientation than friendly body contact involving females?

Post-event Embraces

We are often witness to emotional hugs between athletes and fellow athletes, friends, and coaches that follow sporting events. Unlike medal ceremonies, these performances of congratulation *appear* to be embodied practices that do not differentiate according to the biological sex of the performers. However, male to male embraces tend to be punctuated and enhanced by what I call '*biff-slap* punctuation' such as slaps to the back or punches to the chest. Embraces between males and females, or between two females, are more sustained and not so physically forceful. In what ways does friendly body contact between two males signify differently from friendly body contact between a male and a female, or between two females? What does '*biff-slap* punctuation' in a male to male embrace signify? How would the male to male embrace signify were the '*biff-slap* punctuation' to be absent? How can the difference in signification be explained?

Slaps, biffs, and punches punctuating a male to male embrace can be seen to legitimize an action between men that might otherwise be at risk of being read as sexual. The slaps and punches signify a denial of anything beyond mateship. The machinations of these actions are steeped in aggression, violence, and a form of muscularity that signals power and domination. I assert that this '*biff-slap*' mechanism is a reflex action connected to homophobic social conditioning that is performed to ensure that

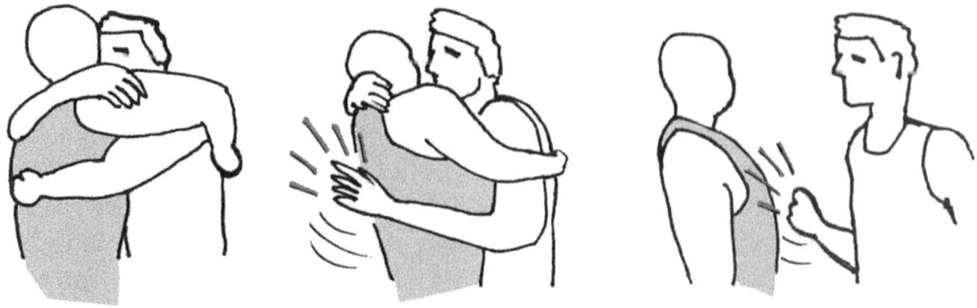

Figure 5.6 Biff-slap punctuation. Artwork by Jack Migdalek.

the sentiment of the moment is perceived as masculine and heterosexual. It is interesting to note that female to female embraces do not seem to be accented and marked by the same homophobic self-consciousness, nor are they read that way, despite the fact that these embraces tend to be sustained and gentler, making them more easily read as sensual and sexual than those between men.

What might these embodied sequences, these choreographic moments of men not touching men—unless accompanied by biffs and slaps, reinforce in society? That men's bodies are subject to regulations of hegemonic masculinity; that men who touch other men without the '*biff-slap*' mechanism are homosexual; that a man's social standing is in doubt if he is not perceived to be heterosexual; that same-sex kisses and embraces without force or a '*biff-slap*' mechanism are signifiers of softness, weakness, and feminine emotionality that render same-sex kissers who kiss without force or a '*biff-slap*' mechanism as soft, weak, and feminine; that individuals who perform same-sex kisses/embraces in this manner—usually women—are inferior/subordinate to heterosexual men?

It seems that patriarchal masculinist ideologies still have power over embodied behavior in spite of the impact of feminist, equal rights, queer, and other anti-discrimination movements that have effected disruptions in recent decades. The effects of embodied practices such as kisses—the meaning and reading of which vary according to the biological sex of performers—are not benign. They signify that women's and men's bodies are in the grip of a socially constructed paradigm where hegemonic masculinity continues to dominate.

Regarding my own body in the everyday, I too punctuate embraces with males in most public contexts with some form of back-slap, something that I do not incorporate in my embracing of females. The gendered machinations of my 'back-slap habitus' as applied to males and my 'gentle embrace habitus' as applied to females are so embedded and invisible that, as Bourdieu (1990) theorizes, these practices come to appear and feel nothing but 'natural'. My performing of this practice is informed and naturalized by a lifetime of witnessing limited models in mainstream media and public arenas of particular ways in which successful males (such as male sports stars and athletes) physically relate to one another (for example, the '*biff-slap*' mechanism) and of being wary of the consequences of what is signified when males physically relate to one another in 'other' ways that are commonly regarded as weak, feminine, homosexual, ludicrous, or deviant. The regulation of physical embodiment and the ways in which mainstream panopticonic scrutiny (Foucault 1977) follow me into non-mainstream, 'safe' settings will be discussed in subsequent chapters.

BODIES IN MEDIA—THE TELEVISION QUIZ SHOW

Temptation is a television quiz program adapted from an American television game show. Previously called *Sale of the Century,* the program has aired nationally in Australia (Nine Network) in a midweek, early evening timeslot on and off for over twenty years (it aired until the end of January 2009). Taking the definition of 'field' as being a socially constructed setting (Bourdieu 1990), *Temptation,* the television show, can be regarded as a field with which a large number of television viewers are familiar. The *Temptation* mainstream public arena as field is one that is gendernormative and heteronormative in nature. This is evident in the strict consistency of the differential choreography and embodied performances of the male and female cast and contestants who appear in all versions of the program.

The embodied congratulations that occur when contestants win the finals of *Temptation* is consistent with the gendered choreography of congratulations that occurred in Commonwealth sports arenas as discussed previously. Three generations of *Temptation* male hosts (Ed Phillips, Tony Barber, and Glenn Ridge) have shaken hands with male champions yet kissed female champions. Interestingly, generations of female hosts (Livinia Nixon, Alyce Platt, Barbara Rogers, Delvene Delaney, and Nicky Buckley) have kissed both male and female champions. It seems that in the *Temptation* quiz show culture, a female kissing a female signifies differently from a male kissing a male. I believe that whereas the impression of a kiss between females may be benign—and even pleasurable and sensual for male spectatorship (Pallotta-Chiarolli 2010)—a kiss between males in this setting may be perceived as a homosexual action, and so, due to dominant heteronormative views and the arguably low cultural capital of being perceived as homosexual (Connell 1995, Nayak & Kehily 1996, Paechter 2003, Martino & Pallotta-Chiarolli 2005), is an action to be avoided. Other television programs, including quiz shows, talk shows, and variety shows, follow the same unspoken rules. In television programs where male personalities embrace other male personalities or contestants, it is consistently forceful and punctuated by the '*biff-slap*' mechanism. Similar gendered choreography where males do not hug, kiss, or shake hands in a gentle manner—unless for comic effect—is evident on an abundance of other mainstream television programs. Where deviations occur they are marked as odd, comic, and sexual.

TV Quiz Show—Escorted Entrances

The *Temptation* mainstream public arena as field upholds its gendernormative and heteronormative ideological condition as evidenced through the strict gendered coupling and choreography of contestants with escorts at the start of each program. In each episode of *Temptation,* two new challengers enter and take their seats beside the current champion. The choreography for the entrance of the challengers is consistently as follows: female challengers are led to their seats on the arm of a male model; male challengers are led to their seats with a female model on their arm. In each case the arm of the female is placed over the proffered arm of the male. How do the workings of these specific permutations of male and female bodies mark what we see and feel to be 'normal' embodiment according to biological sex? Would the gendered make up of such choreography be noticeable should the usual biological sex-specific casting code be transgressed?

Even though the female model in the right-hand illustration is leading the male, her right arm is placed in a position of being led, her arm appearing to rest on the arm of the male. The man she is leading assumes a position of support, his arm proffered. This is consistent with the highly familiar, well-established (if not archaic) iconic choreography of brides and grooms,

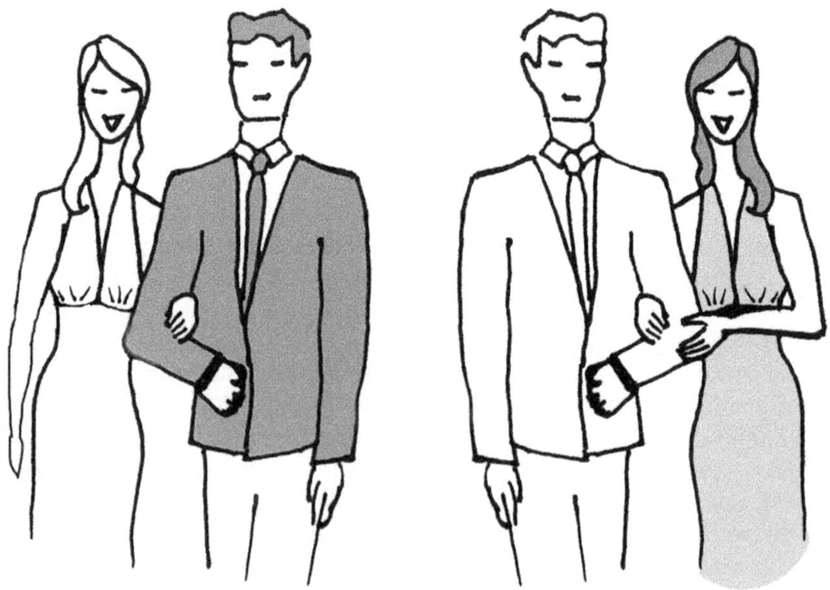

Figure 5.7 Escorted entrances. Artwork by Jack Migdalek.

Oscar Award candidates and their opposite-sex dates, debutantes with their boyfriends, and television and award show hosts with their opposite-sex co-hosts. In each case, regardless of who is leading whom, the physical positioning of arm in arm choreography is male with arm proffered, female with arm *resting* on male partner's proffered arm. The choreography itself is so normalized in our eyes that, regardless of who is leading whom, the male (arm proffered) is positioned as dominant, active, and supporting. This is in binary opposition to the woman (arm resting on male's), who is positioned as submissive, passive, supported, and led.

In *Temptation,* the choreography of a challenger making an entrance on the arm of an attractive model of the opposite biological sex draws very little attention to itself. Unless the escort is seen as a care-giver guiding one who is infirm and in need of assistance, the image within mainstream Western culture is one that ordinarily denotes the connection of a heterosexual couple, such as bride and groom. The iconic image of 'arm in arm male and female choreography' is highly familiar and well inscribed as normal and usual in the eyes of viewers who are products of cultures that repeatedly re-present this choreography.

I believe that being in or on the arm of a partner who projects as being of the *same* biological sex would be interpreted quite differently by mainstream Western society from being in or on the arm of a partner of the opposite biological sex. This less common image operates in direct contrast to what has come to be read as normal or familiar. Stigmas are attached to physical contact between persons of the same sex, especially males, even from a young age (Kehily 2001). Interestingly, I have found that members of cultural groups in which males may normally, comfortably link arms in many circumstances do not tend to do so in mainstream Australian general public contexts, or what Bourdieu might refer to as mainstream social fields (1990). To illustrate, I was recently at a public function attended by a mix of Italian-origin and Australian guests and was surprised that whereas Italian-origin males kissed and embraced females in attendance (both Italian-origin and Australian) they only shook hands with males (Italian-origin and Australian). My Italian-Australian friend confirmed that the same Italian-origin men would *definitely* embrace/kiss one another in other, solely Italian public settings. This editing of embodied behavior within certain Australian mainstream public contexts illustrates the force of mainstream hegemonic culture within Australia and the pressure it exerts on secondary cultures to conform.

In mainstream Western society, being on or in the arms of an attractive partner of the opposite sex can be seen as a form of what could be termed 'gender or sexual capital' that implies something of one's own cultural and social worth or value. Models on shows like *Temptation* are generally perceived as highly attractive, and so the impression of the choreography, connecting a contestant with such an object of desire, serves as a form of positive implication concerning the character, attractiveness, and desirability of the contestant. While in the present socio-cultural climate there is no sexual connotation about a connection between *Temptation* contestants and escort-models of the opposite sex, this might not be the case were the contestant and escort-model of the same sex.

In much the same way that many people feel good adorning their bodies with clothing and accessories that they know others find attractive (Swain 2004), the *Temptation* contestant may also feel good as a result of social, cultural, and sexual capital attached to being partnered by and connected with a physically attractive escort of the opposite biological sex, regardless of either person's sexual orientation and despite the fact that the escort is a relative stranger.

In the everyday we frequently hear people complimented on having beautiful or good-looking spouses or children. I recall as a teenager going out with a girl who was considered to be very physically attractive, and how terrific I felt when her physical attractiveness was commented on. It was as though my connection with her attractiveness in some way marked and elevated my cultural worth or capital. Inversely, being in or on the arms of someone not attractive or not of the opposite biological sex may signify the lowering of one's cultural capital and how one signifies to others. The manifestations of having an attractive partner of the same biological sex in or on one's arms may indicate a different level of cultural capital within heteronormative as opposed to non-heteronormative settings—such as gay and lesbian precincts, venues, and events. In my case I am highly conscious that what may serve as cultural capital in one field may serve as cultural poverty and potentially risky embodiment in others.

How might the *Temptation* challenger feel were they and their model escort of the same biological sex? In my own case, despite being homosexual, I know I would feel very conscious of how marked and noteworthy this performance would be within a mainstream public arena, and of the way in which it would be viewed/perceived by many. Anzaldua refers to tempering one's performance as a "survival tactic" resulting from a strong sense or awareness of when one is being stared at or thought about (1987, p. 39, see also Anzaldua 1990 on *making face/hacienda caras*). The sense of awareness Anzaldua refers to is field dependent and likely to be heightened in fields where this type of embodied performance is uncommon or in opposition to what Goffman (1959) and Bourdieu (1990) would refer to as dominant norms of embodied behavior.

The choreography of the *Temptation* quiz show is strictly heteronormative. Were I to be a contestant on *Temptation* I would be highly conscious of how my performance of entering as a male challenger would be reacted to should I make my entrance on the arm of a male escort. This panopticonic self-consciousness (Foucault 1977) is the result of years and years of exposure to, membership in, and practice of cultures that predominantly and consistently mark non-aggressive physical contact between males as that which is subordinate, deviant, comic, and worthy of distain or ridicule. So, even as a gay male who may be comfortable on the arm of another man in particular settings, I am also highly aware of how marked this same performance would be in mainstream contexts, fields, and settings in which patriarchal and sexist machinations of cultural capital are at play. For me to perform the choreography of entering a mainstream public field such as the *Temptation* quiz show on the arm of another man would be a political act, a deliberate and conscious breaking with convention in order to make a conspicuous statement for the attention and reaction of others. Although such an act may be admirable, it needs to be acknowledged that it may cause a high degree of anxiety and discomfort to the performer. Anzaldua (1987, 1990) speaks of persons caught between worlds adjusting their behavior as a method of survival, according to a sense of awareness of each world, in order not to stand out. These worlds can sometimes be as closely connected as two walls.

A gay male friend of mine, who is outspoken in his opposition to homophobic attitudes, appeared as a contestant on *Temptation* during 2006. He made a request to have the male model escort him to his seat. The request was laughed off and dismissed by producers of the show as something that was in no way possible. While traversing the physical space of the *Temptation* set on the arm of a male model would have been a physical possibility, the impossibility of traversing the psychological or emotional space involved in that proposition rendered physical transgression of the set gendered choreography inconceivable as well.

It is ironic to acknowledge how unproblematic it would be for me as a gay male to enter the *Temptation* mainstream public arena with a female model on my arm and to perform the iconic, stereotypical, recognizable, and commonly respected choreography of a heterosexual couple. The iconic image is so inscribed in my eyes due to years and years of exposure to public and private performances in which similar physical contact between males and females occurs, and is well regarded, that performing such choreography would not be uncomfortable in the least. This is in line with Goffman's (1959) theories of *virtual* performance informing what becomes *actual* performance. A lifetime of exposure to gendernormative/heteronormative performances—such as male with female arm in arm choreography—and perhaps conceiving of oneself performing the same (virtual performance) has equipped me to embody that choreography (actual performance) without feelings of discomfort or unfamiliarity.

Inversely, I recall the discomfort and self-consciousness I experienced the first times I danced with, embraced, kissed, or held hands with another male. I believe that despite my desire to perform those actions, my discomfort was largely due to having had barely any exposure to that kind of contact between males, in addition to an awareness of the negative perceptions that such actions would provoke in a great many contexts. The most prominent and consistent images that I viewed of non-violent physical contact between males were performed on the television screen by flamboyant and comic, two-dimensional persons of implicit but unspecified homosexual orientation, such as the character of Mr. Humphries in the British television comedy *Are You Being Served* (BBC 1972–1985). Even a benign character like Don on the 1970s Australian television series *Number 96* (Network Ten 1972–1977) was a deeply tortured individual, something I believe most young viewers would not aspire to become. That the character of Don was gay further signified connections between non-violent physical contact between males and homosexuality. The impact of male and female embodiment of actors' bodies on stage and film is discussed later in this chapter.

TV Quiz Show—Choreographic Impacts

While it may be argued that sex-specific choreographic practices in television shows like *Temptation* are benign, I wonder how these repeating, set, biological sex-specific embodied performances impact on different viewers. The gendernormative/heteronormative choreography of *Temptation,* with its absence of same-sex arm in arm entrances or male to male congratulatory embraces, reinforces the unfamiliarity of such practices for the viewer who is uncomfortable with gentle tactile physical contact between those of the same biological sex. This may also increase such individuals' social intolerance of such practices. Inversely, the gendernormative/heteronormative choreography of *Temptation* would make viewers who are comfortable with, or desirous of, gentle tactile physical contact with those of the same sex as themselves (male viewers especially) feel all the more alienated. Viewing embodiment that goes against their inclinations and desires is likely to emphasize a sense of social non-acceptance, isolation, and social pressure to conform.

In the current mainstream cultural climate, breaks with established norms of embodiment continue to be marked performances. Although same-sex couples who appeared on televised ballroom dancing shows such as Australia's Endemol Southern Star's *Strictly Dancing* were met with positive and approving feedback, their appearance was perceived as an oddity that was pointed out and remarked on in the press.

BODIES IN MEDIA—DANCING BODIES ON STAGE AND IN FILM

The Classical Ballet Heritage

The female classical ballet dancer has been positioned and choreographed to be dependent on the support of her male partner. Without him in the picture she could not balance, turn, or perform in the ways conventionally choreographed for her. The male classical ballet dancer, when not performing bravura or bombastic shows of strength and power, has been positioned

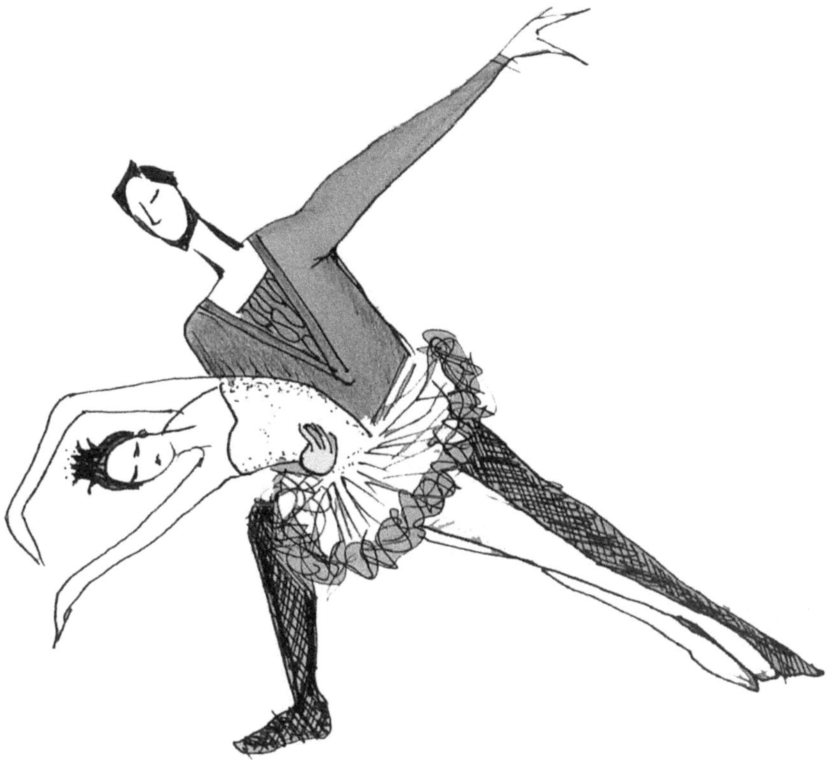

Figure 5.8 Pas de deux. Artwork by Jack Migdalek.

and choreographed to support and control the ballerina. Although many may regard the iconic image of the masculine, powerful male dancer and the feminine, delicate ballerina as archaic and fossilized, the gendered and patriarchal ideology behind the representations remains very much intact. The enduring legacy and structure of the classical ballet have seen the normalization of the male dancer as a figure of support and power, and of the female figure, no matter how powerful an athlete, as a decorative figure in a patriarchal construction: fragile, dependent, and in need of support and guidance (Dempster 1988, Foster 1996, Banes 1998, Gard 2006).

In 1661 what was a formalized dance practice of the court of Louis XIV became a codified performance art through the founding of the *Academie Royale de Danse*. The art form became widespread and popular throughout Europe. The fundamentals of the ballet were further refined in Russia and in time spread to countries throughout the world. This spread in popularity is remarkable considering that it occurred before high-speed travel and before mass communication modes such as film and television. Currently, ballet companies exist and operate throughout the world. Although new ballet works are produced, ballet companies continually reproduce and re-present ballet classics such as *The Nutcracker Suite, Swan Lake, Sleeping Beauty,* and *Giselle.* These classics continue to be performed with little variation in the basic choreography, music, or design of the original versions as choreographed by Marius Petipa for the Imperial Ballet in Russia (in 1892, 1895, 1890, and 1884 respectively). Even though ballet companies also produce modern ballet repertoire, the classics continue to be the most popular and marketable, as evidenced by how frequently they are restaged.

Contemporary dance forms may sometimes challenge and transgress the iconic norms of physical positioning for male and female bodies as established by the classical ballet. However, the number of people who subscribe to, attend performances of, or are familiar with contemporary dance is minute compared to the number who subscribe to, attend performances of, or are familiar with classic dance forms—such as conventional ballet, ballroom dance, and musical theatre—that toe the hegemonic gendered line (see Stoneley 2007).

Despite having the same foundation, the choreography of traditional classical ballet differs for males and females. In the classic pas de deux (duet dance between a male and female dancer), the female is frequently positioned in decorative ways that render her body dependent on the support of her male partner to assist or steady her turn or balance, to lift her, or to offer an arm for her to hold or catch on to. The ballerina, frequently in pointe shoes (ballet slippers that have a stiffened toe section), is able to balance for only short and arguably glorious moments of seeming weightlessness unless supported by someone. This support and physical guidance is ordinarily the province of the male ballet dancer.

Frequently, classical ballet storylines position the female character in roles that are fragile, delicate, vulnerable, and dependent on male heroes or villains (Dempster 1988, Foster 1998). This is not surprising considering the patriarchal times in which these ballets were originally created. Ironically, the physical demands for embodying these submissive roles require incredible strength and stamina from these female athletes (Dempster 1988). In some classical ballet storylines, female characters are agentic. Dance theorist Sally Banes (1998) argues that Aurora in *Sleeping Beauty* is very much an independent spirit who, in the famous *Rose Adagio,* dances with four suitors among whom she has the agency to choose. Nevertheless, when we look at the choreography of this iconic dance, the body of Aurora is repeatedly placed in positions of precarious balance where ultimately she must rely on and return to the physical support, guidance, and control of each of the suitors. This binary physical positioning of male and female dancers in the positions of supporter and supported is prevalent in a multitude of dance works. Even George Balanchine, who came to prominence in the 1930s and was known as a modern and innovative ballet choreographer, consistently placed female dancers in positions of physical dependence on their male partners. He spoke of the ballet as a purely female thing, "a garden of beautiful flowers [women], with man as the gardener" (*Dance Ballerina Dance,* BBC2 1998, originally quoted in *Life Magazine,* 11 June 1965). The woman is central, but only as cultivated and constructed by the patriarchal gardener/choreographer. This inequitable outlook positioning male and female in hierarchical, binary, and arguably unequal opposition continues to prevail despite some contemporary dance work that opposes it.

As a child, I never saw a classical ballet in the theatre. Even so, the form was highly familiar to me through ballet excerpts featured in television programs, movies, advertisements, ballet stills displayed in forms of paintings and photographs adorning walls in homes, ballet stills as branding on products such as cookies, and ballet motifs as printed and fashioned on bedspreads, female apparel, and jewelry. To my mainstreamed eyes, the configuration of a male dancer supporting a dependent female dancer was familiar and normal.

Modern Forms of Dance

Modern dance in the West was pioneered largely in the United States, where emerging choreographers such as Martha Graham, Doris Humphrey, Ruth St. Denis, and Ted Shawn broke with the ballet tradition and found new forms of dance expression. The iconoclastic pioneers of modern dance revolted against and challenged many of the established norms of the ballet form: they turned feet inward; they worked into the ground and not toward the heavens. Nevertheless, these choreographers continued to choreograph males as figures of strength who were positioned to project as powerful, physically athletic, and masculine (Burt 1995, Foulkes 2001). Reflective of times where softness in a male was deemed to be unattractive and might put the sexuality of a male in question, pioneering modern dance choreographers were deliberate in positioning and choreographing male dancers so as not to appear suspect of softness or homosexuality (Burt 1995, 2001, Foulkes 2001, Risner 2009). For example, in the case of Ted Shawn's all-male dance company (formed in 1933), the male dancers "never looked soft or flexible; they never curved. They never even touched except in those rare moments when the choreography stipulated that all bodies contribute to a common design" (Foster 2001, p. 168).

In contrast, choreographers who followed, such as Merce Cunningham in the 1950s and 1960s and Steve Paxton in the 1970s, consciously choreographed male and female bodies to perform in non-differential ways. Nevertheless, when it came to pas de deux (partner work), Cunningham still choreographed males and females according to classical protocols. For all Cunningham's "radical re-workings of choreography and movement, men usually still supported and lifted women in his pas de deux in quite traditional ways. Men did not partner men, nor did women lift or support women" (Banes 1998, 216, see also Burt 1995, Foster 2001). It has been said that Paxton's work, which had male and female bodies dancing truly equally, did so at the expense of dancers projecting as sexual or sexed beings at all (Foster 2001).

Even though the forms of dance and ways in which male and female bodies were displayed and presented were and are being challenged by modern dance forms, ingrained and established norms still exert control over the ways in which male bodies move. In commercial dance, male dancers continue to be choreographed to move with power and athleticism (see Fisher & Shay 2009, Risner 2009). Indeed, it was the vigor with which the male protagonist in *Billy Elliot* (Universal Pictures) danced that made the character's dance pursuits agreeable and appealing to the general public. For the most part, it is only in non-mainstream works, such as Australian choreographer Graeme Murphy's avant-garde *Air and Other Invisible Forces* (1999) and *Cut* (2006), and politically motivated repertoires of companies such as DV8 Physical Theatre, that male dancers might make sensual, non-aggressive physical contact with one another and/or dance in a decidedly soft and delicate manner. The exception here is works that are presented as parody. Parodic embodiment, which does sometimes achieve widespread mainstream exposure, is just as likely to reinscribe existing, limiting gender stereotypes as it is to challenge them (Butler 1990, 1993, Burt 1995). For a male dancer to dance in an effeminate manner in parody or imitation of a female is to a large degree a socially familiar and positively received occurrence, as can be seen in drag performances by the Trockaderos de Monte Carlo and musicals such as *La Cage Aux Folles* and *Priscilla, Queen of the Desert*. However, for a male dancer to dance in a feminine manner while not presenting as a comic or spectacle is not so socially familiar or palatable.

Enduring Gender Norms of Embodiment

Modern dance forms, even renowned ones, have not endured as the classical ballet has. How frequently do we see landmark or iconic modern or contemporary dance works such as Martha Graham's *Night Journey* (1947), Merce Cunningham's *Suite for Five* (1956), Steve Paxton's *Proxy* (1961), or Paul Taylor's *Aureole* (1962) remounted? Certainly these are not performed to the extent that the classics of the ballet are. Dance theorists Banes (1998), Foster (2001), and Burt (1995) speak about the gendered positioning of males and females in ballet, but it remains unclear why the classics of ballet endure.

For me the enduring problem of the classical ballet heritage is that its iconic emblems of masculinity and femininity have come to be perceived as fitting for male and female bodies respectively. The inherent gender inequities of these representations are compelling reinforcements of patriarchal ideologies. Iconic images of male and female dancing bodies projected through the ballet, as well as many modern forms of dance, exert an influence on the ways in which not only dancing bodies but also non-dancing bodies come to be perceived and appreciated. Females positioned as feminine figures in need or receipt of support, and males positioned as masculine figures of strength and support, become so habitual to the eye that they come to appear to be normalized states of being. Iconic and seemingly universal gendered images of male and female bodies in conventional (and even much contemporary) dance must have an impact on how individuals perceive what is an appropriate style of embodiment for male or female bodies; how individuals, who identify as male or female, perceive what is appropriate embodiment for their own male or female bodies; and the manner in which individuals come to embody their own male or female presenting bodies in the everyday.

Exposure to mainstream formal performance arenas in which the embodied choreography and positioning are consistently differential for male and female bodies serves to reinforce differential 'norms' of embodiment for male and female bodies as being natural, especially to individuals for whom such notions fit comfortably. By the same token, this exposure serves to reinforce any discomfort/anxiety on the part of those who may be inclined to embody differently from the norm of gendered representation to which they are exposed. Ultimately, it serves to restrict the ways in which males and females might otherwise embody in the everyday.

In my case, through exposure to dance as seen in advertising, billboards, still pictures on walls of homes, movies, television dramas, and variety programs, I became accustomed to impressions of males as strong, powerful, controlling figures and females as soft, delicate, decorative figures. I think this was the case for most urban Australians of my generation. Impressions of male or female dancing forms that did not fit this criteria were for the most part seen as comic or avant-garde. I recall the laughter that television stars such as Graham Kennedy evoked throughout the 1960s, 1970s, and 1980s, when on occasion he would prance around as program host on national television in an effeminate manner. When it came to my own embodiment, I understood well that soft or feminine movement was not considered manly or appropriate for a male. I did not enter the dance world until the age of eighteen, yet the exposure I had had to male bodies in dance and other formal performance arenas influenced my acceptance of masculine embodiment on a male as more attractive/aesthetic than feminine embodiment. Even at an early age, I came to understand from those around me that a male moving effeminately was unattractive, undesirable, and ludicrous. My inclination may have been toward feminine embodiment; however, I believe that my conceptions of the type of embodiment that was appropriate for men restricted how I might have otherwise operated. This will be charted in subsequent chapters.

Gendered Swans

Delicate, dainty female embodiment has become widely recognized and iconic as the conventional human representation and embodiment of swans. In standard versions of *Swan Lake* (originally choreographed by Marius Petipa in 1895) and *The Dying Swan* (originally choreographed by Michel Fokine in 1905) representations of these creatures are not only feminine but

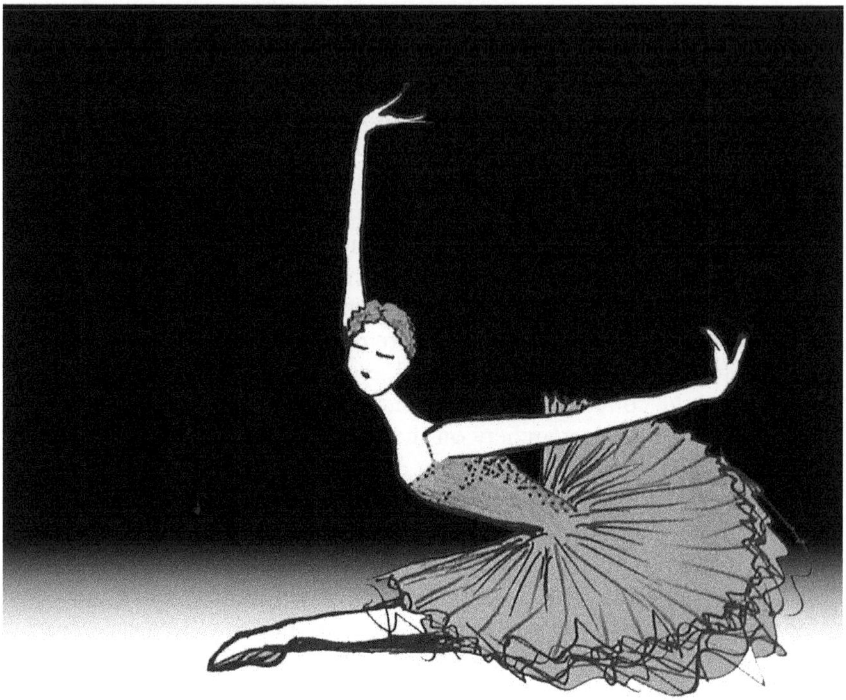

Figure 5.9 Classic ballerina. Artwork by Jack Migdalek.

also female. In mainstream Western circles a male body performing the same choreography is perceived and generally presented as an object of humor, as evidenced by male representations of these very poses and motions that occur in advertising, amateur performances, and professional dance troupes such as the Trockaderos de Monte Carlo.

When Matthew Bourne choreographed his version of *Swan Lake* (1996), he broke with conventional perceptions of human representation of swans as female by choreographing them as males. He also teased conventional gendered perceptions of swans as feminine by choreographing swans to move aggressively and powerfully (Foster 2001). However, as mentioned in Chapter 2, by choreographing his male swans to move in a masculine manner, Bourne too has remained bound by established aesthetic connections between gender and biology.

Aesthetics—Men Dancing like Men

> Dude, I'm here blowing my horn all the time about men dancing like men. What we have in front of us here is a real man, a bloke. Yeah, and

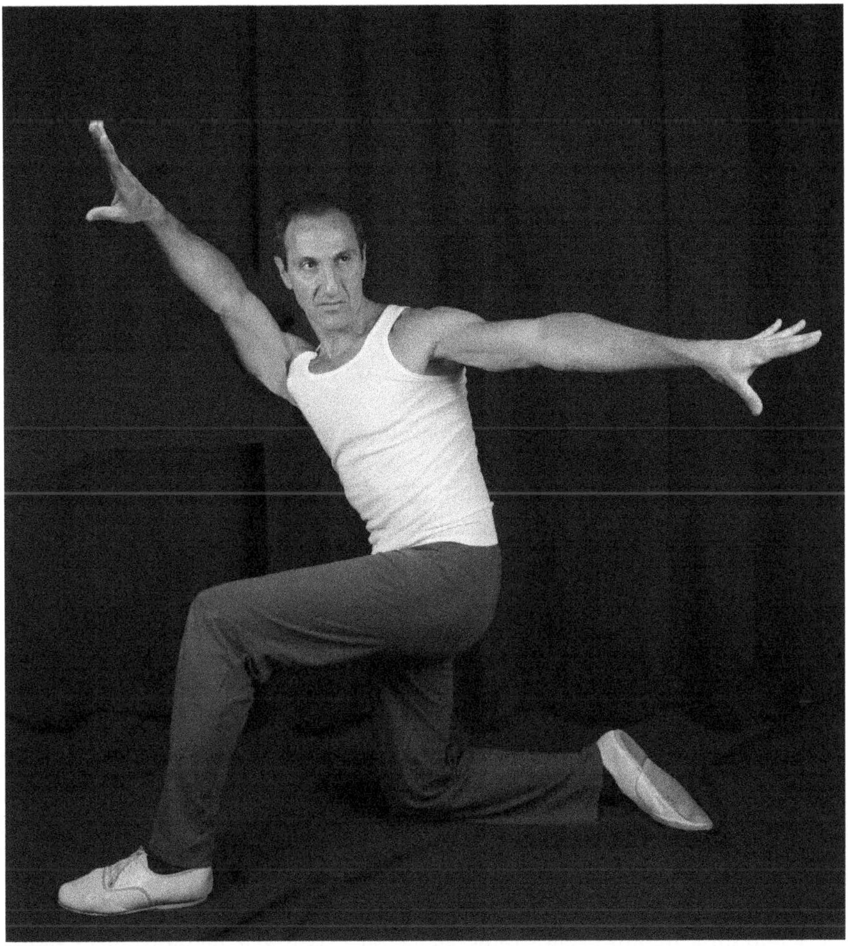

Figure 5.10 Dance like a man. Photograph by Rob Chiarolli (www.photosthattell.com).

> you danced like a bloke. It had a male energy, a male strength about it, you know it was like a real man dancing like a real man, and I love that. I'm a fan of that.
>
> (Jason Coleman—judge on *So You Think You Can Dance Australia*, Network 10, Episode 3, 2008—spoken to a male dancer auditioning to be in the competition)

If men who dance like men are *real* men, then the implication is that men who dance in other ways are not real men. How do we rank or value men who *dance* differently? How do we rank or value men who *move* differently?

So You Think You Can Dance Australia (produced by Fremantle Media) premiered in 2008 (the international television franchise of the program premiered in the United States in 2005) and attracted approximately 3,500 dancers, all competing to become Australia's most popular dancer of that year. The show enjoyed huge mainstream success and was the top-rating program in its timeslot from 2008 to 2010. (The show was revived in 2014.) Sentiments on men dancing like men, such as those above, surfaced frequently during the audition sessions for each series of the show. In the auditions, males who danced in a feminine manner were criticized as being "too girlie" and "too effeminate" and told to "really push the male" and "dance hard and strong like a man". This signaling of what is aesthetically attractive and unattractive was established by expert judges who narrowed down a diverse field of male dancers to ten males, who all danced, and were choreographed, week after week in a masculine manner. These dancers served as models—according to the expert judges—of how males should dance. Such commentary enforces for millions of viewers that males dancing in a strong or masculine manner are admirable and have a chance of success, as opposed to males dancing in an 'effeminate' or 'girlie' manner, who as a result will fail to make it to the finals. For the male dancer who moves in a feminine manner to succeed in the competition, he must adjust and move in a masculine manner. The implication is that off the dance floor too—in the everyday—masculine embodiment on a male is favored above feminine embodiment.

Despite rhetoric about multiple masculinities that promotes the notion that males should be able to display qualities such as femininity (Martino & Pallotta-Chiarolli 2001, Swain 2005, Paechter 2006), it is clear within the context of the *So You Think You Can Dance* culture that deep-rooted and established biases against males who embody in a feminine manner continue to be potent at this time. Negative perceptions regarding males who move in a feminine manner were reinscribed on a younger generation of dancers and audiences by both male and female judges on the program (all of whom were above the age of thirty) through the dismissal and degradation of males who did not dance in a masculine way. That female judges were also complicit in the denigration of the feminine when performed by males, but not when performed by females, is testimony to the power of patriarchy and to theories in which the oppressed take on the outlook of the oppressor (see Memmi 1967, Freire 1990), perhaps as a means of asserting authority within an existing system.

Although the judges have commended versatility and talked about the need to stand out in order to stay in the contest through advice like "be brave, be different", this advice was gender conditional and excluded standing out as a male dancer who moved in a dainty, delicate, or feminine style. In narrowing the field down to twenty male and female finalists, the judges on the program controlled the forms of male and female embodiment that were put forward to the general public as aesthetic, as *best*. The general public is likely to come to value and appreciate aesthetics of gendered embodiment that are put before them as being the best, week after week after week, not only in this public performance arena but far beyond. Exposure to consistently differential valorized modes of motion for male and female bodies is likely to impact on a viewer's own sense of what is appropriate or aesthetic for female bodies as opposed to male.

> I love your quirkiness and I love how different you are . . . but for me personally, I like boys to dance like boys.
>
> (Kelly Abbey, guest judge addressing male contestant Rhys on *So You Think You Can Dance,* aired 10/02/08)

During the 2008 auditions, Rhys, a male contestant who was runner-up in the competition, danced in a group-choreographed piece. He was seriously criticized by the judges for dancing the piece in a feminine manner. The message on aesthetics for heteronormative and gendernormative mainstream settings was made clear, and he learned early in the series that if he wanted to have a chance of success in the competition he had to adjust and dance in a masculine manner, which he consistently did from that point onward. In order to stay in the contest he had to comply with the gender aesthetics of the judges, regardless of how he might dance in queer or other settings. That said, aesthetic sensibilities in queer public settings also tend to be bound by conventions that favor masculine embodiment on figures that present as male (see Payne 2007 on the reverence in gay culture for the 'straight-acting' male; and Lanzieri & Hildebrandt 2011 on reverence in gay culture for heterosexual male idealizations of masculine embodiment). The imitating and replicating of dominant hierarchies and modes of embodiment in minority or disempowered groups may occur as a means of advancing one's self and gaining social capital and power (Kroeger 2003, see also Memmi 1967, Freire 1990, Said 2003, Fanon 2008). However, it may also occur as an effect of pervasive and continuing exposure to valorized representations of male and female modes of behavior presented in mainstream arenas (Schirato & Yell 1996).

Embodiment and Sexuality

Linked to notions of what kind of embodiment is desirable and aesthetic for a male is the implied connection between style of movement and sexuality. This is made blatantly clear in the following quote from *So You Think You Can Dance,* spoken by British judge Bonnie Lythgoe. She comments, in surprise, to a male dancer whose biography listed that he held the title of 'Mr. Gay Australia': "You're not what I expected. Well, on here it says 'Mr Gay Australia' . . . so you came on the floor, and I was O-Oh, Mr Gay is going to dance like very effeminate" (episode aired in Melbourne, 06/02/08).

The dancer in question danced in a strong and masculine manner and informed Bonnie, "I always try to dance as strong as I can. I really feel passionate about men dancing like men", to which she replied in a praising tone, "You *did* dance like a man". The expectation was that a gay male would move and dance in a feminine manner. Not all gay men embody in a feminine manner, and I imagine that the judge in question was well aware of this. Nevertheless, clichéd expectations that effeminacy in a male signifies homosexuality continue to prevail and endure (Gard 2001, Gere 2001, Martino & Pallotta-Chiarolli 2001, 2005), reinforcing and perpetuating their own truth. Males who dance in a feminine manner are not wanted on the *So You Think You Can Dance* stage—even if they are homosexual—as evidenced in Bonnie's comments to another male dancer:

> I don't care if you mince off the stage. I don't care if you mince up there [pointing toward the theatre exit. Then indicating the stage floor]. What I do want is that masculinity.
>
> (episode aired in Melbourne, 10/02/08)

Whereas feminine embodiment in a male was devalued on *So You Think You Can Dance* and linked with homosexuality, parallel inferences about female dancers were not evident. There was no suggestion that a woman dancing strongly was un-aesthetic, unattractive, or linked with homosexuality, indicating also that it is acceptable for a woman to be 'like a man'. It is as if trying to be, dance like, act like, or imitate those who hold power is an understandable and worthy endeavor.

The fact that, on the *So You Think You Can Dance* stage, feminine embodiment in a male is discouraged at the same time that the male who moves in a feminine manner is assumed to be homosexual implies a devaluation of both. The fact that a UK judge (who had also been a judge on the US series) brands feminine embodiment on a male in the same way Australian judges do indicates that the mindset that brands feminine embodiment on a male as undesirable, un-aesthetic, and homosexual may be commonly potent in the Western world. Indeed, the Australian judges on the program can be regarded as colonized subjects of British and American influences that have shaped and directed their dance and aesthetic sensibilities.

BODIES IN MEDIA—ACTING BODIES ON STAGE AND IN FILM

There are parallels between the signification of male and female forms dancing in particular ways and the signification of male and female forms acting in particular ways, as represented in dramas, comedies, and musicals seen on television, in cinema, and in the theatre.

Casting: Overwhelmingly, the casting and direction of male heterosexual characters involve masculine embodiment; the casting and direction of male

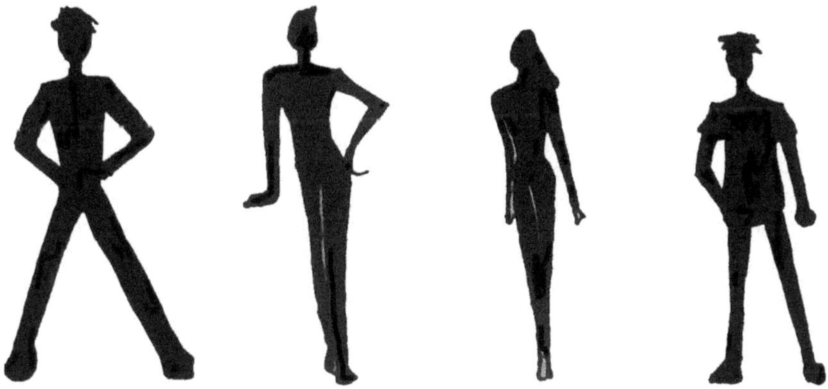

Figure 5.11 Stereotypes. Artwork by Jack Migdalek.

homosexual characters involve feminine embodiment; the casting and direction of female heterosexual characters involve feminine embodiment; and the casting and direction of female homosexual characters involve masculine embodiment.

How might these common embodied representations impact on the ways in which audiences regard and perceive males who move in masculine ways, males who move in feminine ways, females who move in feminine ways, and females who move in masculine ways? Where customary and familiar codes of representation such as those above are transgressed, viewers are likely to be amused or confused, despite the fact that in the real world there do exist and have existed gay males who move in masculine ways, heterosexual males who move—or are inclined to move—in feminine ways, gay females who move in feminine ways, and heterosexual females who move—or are inclined to move—in masculine ways.

There is a potent correlation between masculine embodiment and feminine embodiment on male and female actors and particular readings of character. Mainstream film producers and casting directors with whom I have become acquainted inform me that when casting for actors, they ordinarily narrow the field by laying photographic (embodied) images of actors before them and eliminating those who they consider do not suit the characters or roles being cast. This elimination is contingent on embodied forms, demonstrating that there are perceived links between character and embodied type.

Usual embodied representations of masculine males and feminine females as heterosexual characters in mainstream dramatized performance operate in binary opposition to representations of feminine males and masculine females as homosexual characters. These embodied representations are so potent and naturalized that viewers are likely to be amused, anxious, confused, or shocked where such codes of representation are transgressed

(Cohan & Hark 1993). For example, a major talking point concerning the 2005 movie *Brokeback Mountain* (Focus Features) was that neither male protagonist looked nor embodied in a feminine manner, even though their characters were homosexual. The movie was considered remarkable for the very reason that the masculine embodiment of the two gay protagonists disturbed familiar and common codes.

Russo (1981), hooks (1996), and Buchbinder (2004), when theorizing on the depiction of feminine and masculine characters in drama, comedy, and musicals, refer to the representation of character in regard to plot and storyline. Where a character like Annie in the musical *Annie Get Your Gun* moves and behaves in a masculine manner, she is a figure of interest because she does not fit neatly into her world. It is only when she adopts a feminine demeanor that she is able to find love and become complete. Similar storylines concerning gender non-conformity in theatre and film plots exist for characters such as Jane in *Calamity Jane,* Eliza in *My Fair Lady,* Kate in *The Taming of the Shrew,* Gracie Hart in *Miss Congeniality* (Warner Bros), and Tom in *Tea and Sympathy* (MGM), each of whom only reaches a happy conclusion when gender conformity occurs. Interestingly, feminine male characters' attempts toward gender conformity in drama, comedy, and musicals are more often than not doomed to fail, for example, the character of Albert in *La Cage Aux Folles* (Da Ma Produzione) and *The Birdcage* (United Artists) as well as characters such as Howard Brackett in *In and Out* (Paramount), Justin in *Ugly Betty* (ABC, Season 2, episodes 3 and 4), and Kurt in *Glee* (20th Century Fox Television, Season 1, episodes 3 and 4).

The embodiment of male and female bodies moving in masculine and feminine manners is a potent communicator of character and sexual orientation distinct from and even prior to the spoken text, story, or plot. Impressions of character are made through forms of stance, pose, repose, gait, and action, prior to dialogue or the unfolding of the plot or storyline. Where the stance and posture of a male are masculine, and where the stance and posture of a female are feminine, these images immediately project as normal. Where the stance and posture of a female are masculine, and where the stance and posture of a male are feminine, these individuals project in ways that are immediately viewed as suspect, comic, ludicrous, deviant, and/or subordinate.

How might universal representations of male and female bodies moving in masculine and feminine manners respectively impact on and affect gay males who move in masculine ways and gay females who move in feminine ways? Typical representations of males and females in dramas, comedies, and musicals are likely to imply to gay males who move in masculine ways and gay females who move in feminine ways that they will not ordinarily be perceived to be gay. Given that being perceived to be homosexual can marginalize an individual (Connell 1995, 2000, Nayak & Kehily 1996, Plummer 1999, Martino & Pallotta-Chiarolli 2001,

McKenna 2001), being a homosexual who is perceived to be straight may be a social advantage that makes it easier to advance and get by (Kroeger 2003). At the same time, where embodied semiotics of sexual orientation are rigidly held, there are likely to be contexts in which a gay individual may find it frustrating to have his/her sexuality signal as heterosexual, especially where that individual wants others to know his/her sexual orientation. In such cases it may be possible to consciously adopt or affect perceived gay behaviors, including styles of embodiment, in order to let other queers know that he is one of them (Pronger 1990). Thus, the choreography of the self can be about culturally 'fitting in' to subcultures in order to 'belong'.

How might universal representations of male and female bodies moving in masculine and feminine manners, respectively, impact on and affect heterosexual males and heterosexual females who move, or are inclined to move, in feminine and masculine ways, respectively? Typical representations of males and females in dramas, comedies, and musicals are likely to imply to heterosexual males who move, or are inclined to move, in feminine ways and heterosexual females who move, or are inclined to move, in masculine ways that they will be perceived as gay. Given that this is not always a positive thing—as reflected in an abundance of gay characters in dramas, comedies, and musicals who are clichéd comic, deviant characters who frequently come to lonely if not miserable ends (Russo 1981, Jones 2003)—anxiety over projecting as gay may cause acute self-policing in an effort not to project as gay. It concerns me that, in contrast to master-signifiers (Zizek 1999) of embodied heterosexual orientation, feminine embodiment on a male and masculine embodiment on a female have come to signify as homosexual orientation. Therefore, many females and, more particularly, males (gay, bisexual, straight, and even those unaware of their sexual orientation), endeavor *not* to project in such ways, despite being physiologically capable of doing so (see Kirby & Hay 1997). It is unreasonable to make assumptions about the sexual orientation of an individual based on that person's physical demeanor. Yet this even occurs to pre-pubescent subjects who may still be unsure of their sexual orientation (Renold 2005, Davies 2006, DePalma & Atkinson 2008).

Representations of males in dramas, comedies, and musicals led me to perceive at a young age that feminine embodiment on a male was undesirable and connected with homosexuality. I believe that representations that demeaned, subordinated, and trivialized feminine and gay males stalled my realization and acceptance of my sexuality as a gay male (see Allen & Oleson 1999). In my case, constant self-policing of my embodiment—in order not to project as gay—caused me a good degree of anxiety. The toll exacted as a result will be taken up in the next chapter.

Embodied representations of male and female characters that I saw projected in drama, comedies, and musicals, in films, in the theatre, and on television, greatly affected the ways in which I came to perceive embodied performance in the everyday. I viewed the female who stood with legs straddled and hands on hips differently from the man who stood in the same way: her as butch, aggressive, power-hungry; him as powerful, self-confident, assertive. I viewed the male who stood with feet together, hands crossed in front of his pelvis, head tilted to the side differently from the female who stood in the same manner: him as effeminate, posh, peculiar, fussy; her as feminine, modest, demure.

The norms—and *ab*-norms—of male embodiment projected in dramas, comedies, and musicals affected how I myself would embody in the everyday. I identified as a male and wished to project, as did the males in those movies and shows, as successful and worthy of respect. Desiring to be perceived in ways that harmonized with these positive role models, I endeavored to take on embodied forms that aligned with those representations. More to the point, I became acutely conscious of how *not* to embody if I wanted to achieve respect and acceptance. I became conscious that I should not stand with my hands crossed before my pelvis, not sit with my feet together, not stand with my hips cocked to one side, not walk in a feminine manner, not cross my legs.

DISCRIMINATORY PERCEPTIONS

Bodies are cast, directed, and choreographed in mainstream performance arts arenas such as theatre, film, and television in gendered ways that lend themselves to discriminatory perceptions. Male characters who embody in a feminine manner—such as Jack in *Will and Grace* (NBC), Stanford in *Sex and the City* (HBO), Niles in *Frasier* (NBC), Alan in *Two and a Half Men* (Chuck Lorre Productions), Kurt in *Glee* (Fox), Simon and Kylie in *Beautiful People* (BBC), and Cameron in *Modern Family* (20th Century Fox Television)—are perceived as objects of humor or pathos and as homosexual or homosexually inclined (see Crothers 2007). Male characters who embody in a masculine manner—such as Elliot in *Law and Order: SVU* (NBC), John McClane in *Die Hard* (Fox), Al Bundy in *Married with Children* (Columbia TriStar), Dalziel in *Dalziel and Pascoe* (BBC), Big in *Sex and the City* (HBO), Luke in *Gilmore Girls* (Warner Bros), Jeff in *Rules of Engagement* (CBS), and Doug Heffernan in *King of Queens* (CBS)—are perceived to be sturdy, stalwart, and unarguably heterosexual. The dramatic plots in these programs are reflective of heteronormative discourses that trivialize and marginalize effeminate and/or homosexual males through stereotypical, one-dimensional depictions—usually comic or deviant (Russo 1981, Butler 1993, Jones 2003, Neimes 2003). Limited readings of feminine embodiment on a male on screen or on stage serve to reinforce the gendered status quo, leaving little discursive space for alternative readings. Similarly, female characters who embody in a masculine manner—such as Coach Beiste and Sue Sylvester in *Glee* (Fox), Rosario in *Will and Grace* (NBC), and Berta in

Two and a Half Men (Warner)—are generally perceived as being oddball, lesbian, or sexually suspect.

There is a spillover from the abovementioned readings of character to acceptance and respect afforded to homosexual public figures who project themselves in particular ways. It may be argued that homosexuality is now accepted within contemporary mainstream cultural contexts. It may be that prominent public figures are non-problematically acknowledged as being homosexual. However, masculine embodiment on the homosexual male is more acceptable than softer feminine embodiment. For example, when he was in office (1996–2012), the embodiment of Senator Bob Brown, an openly gay Australian political leader, was akin to that of most male politicians. He had a direct gait and what appeared to be a strong handshake. I wonder whether he would have been as easily accepted/respected if his embodiment had been feminine. It can be argued that physical deportment should have nothing to do with one's position or station, yet corporeal projection does seem to affect how one is perceived (McWilliam 1997). Indeed, former New Zealand prime minister Helen Clark, who identifies as heterosexual, was subject to a degree of conjecture regarding her sexuality and biology. Her grooming and deportment, as well as her deep voice, did not sit comfortably with critics as being suitably feminine. Although notions of multiple masculinities and femininities may have had some impact on broadening the ways males and females may acceptably talk, respond, and feel, there is little sign of a broadening of the ways males and females may acceptably embody without being categorized in ways that marginalize and alienate. In short, hegemonic heteronormative constructions of masculinity/femininity promote a hierarchy of 'acceptable' forms of homosexuality, which gay men/women may arguably internalize and perform, or resist and transgress, depending on their desire to conform to or resist regulatory social forces. Options of resistance, compliance, and negotiation will be taken up in Chapter 7.

Overwhelming representations of males and females on stage and on screen whose embodiment is masculine and feminine respectively may impact negatively on the well-being of the individual who may not be inclined to perform according to dominant norms of sex-specific gender behavior. Such individuals are made to feel socially alienated and misfit. Embodied femininity and masculinity on the bodies of males and females as seen in media such as television, cinema, and the theatre, impacted on the ways in which I came to choreograph and endeavored to perform my own body, both in the everyday and as an aspiring performance artist. Embodied representations of males and females in the media also impacted on how I came (as director and choreographer) to cast and position the bodies of others. These developments will be investigated in Chapter 7.

Male and female bodies in the media are still positioned, performed, and choreographed in very unequal ways, as evidenced by the ways each tend *not* to be positioned, performed, and/or choreographed. Although bodies are visible to us, the machinations of what they perform, how they are choreographed, and how normative forms of choreography and performance can privilege them (see Pease 2010), are frequently invisible as practice and as such are not understood to be reflective of deep-seated patriarchal ideologies. This invisibility is part of a forceful cycle that is not easily opposed, exposed, or deconstructed.

In Chapter 2 I spoke of aesthetic ideals of masculinity and femininity as cultural constructions that may vary from culture to culture. However, the emergence in contemporary times of global access to mass media is seeing a globalization of ways of regarding and perceiving the world around us (Connell 1999, see also Crothers 2007, Mac an Ghaill & Haywood 2007) and likewise the globalization of particular valorized gendered representations of bodies. Through their very universality, the globalization of aesthetic ideals of masculinity and femininity for male and female bodies fortifies certain embodied behavior as being natural and not cultural constructions.

REFERENCES

Allen, D.J., & Oleson, T. (1999). Shame and Internalized Homophobia in Gay Men. *Journal of Homosexuality.* Vol 37, No 3, pp. 33–42.

Anzaldua, G. (1987). *Borderlands, La Frontera: The New Mestiza.* San Francisco: Spinsters/Aunt Lute.

Anzaldua, G. (1990). *Making Face, Making Soul: Creative and Critical Perspectives by Women of Color.* San Francisco: Aunt Lute.

Banes, S. (1998). *Dancing Women. Female Bodies on Stage.* New York: Routledge.

Bourdieu, P. (1990). *The Logic of Practice.* Oxford: Polity Press.

Bourdieu, P. (2001). *Masculine Domination.* Cambridge: Polity Press.

Buchbinder, D. (2004). *The Sign of the Dancing Men: Negotiations of Masculinity in Film Musicals.* (Conference Presentation). Masculinities: Gender, Art and Popular Culture Symposium, The University of Melbourne. [Retrieved 4/4/06 from www.art-museum.unimelb.edu.au/events_transcripts]

Burt, R. (1995). *The Male Dancer: Bodies, Spectacle, Sexualities.* London: Routledge.

Burt, R. (2001). Dissolving in Pleasure: The Threat of the Queer Male Dancing Body. In Desmond, J.C. (Ed.). *Dancing Desires: Choreographing Sexualities On and Off the Stage.* Madison: University of Wisconsin Press.

Butler, J. (1990). *Gender Trouble: Feminism and the Subversion of Identity.* New York: Routledge.

Butler, J. (1993). *Bodies That Matter.* New York: Routledge.

Cohan, S., & Hark, I.R. (1993). *Screening the Male: Exploring Masculinities in Hollywood Cinema.* London: Routledge.

Connell, R.W. (1995). *Masculinities.* Sydney: Allen and Unwin.

Connell, R.W. (1999). Sex in the World. In Epstein, D., & Sears, J.T. (Eds.). *A Dangerous Knowing: Sexuality, Pedagogy and Popular Culture.* London: Cassell.

Connell, R.W. (2000). *The Men and the Boys.* St Leonards, NSW: Allen and Unwin.

Crothers, L. (2007). *Globalization & American Popular Culture.* Lanham: Rowman & Littlefield.

Crowley, V. (2004). Perverse Hybridisations: Queering Postcolonial Pedagogies. In Hickling-Hudson, A., Matthews, J., & Woods, A. (Eds.). *Disrupting Preconceptions: Postcolonialism and Education.* Flaxton: Post Pressed.

Dance Ballerina Dance. (1998). BBC2 documentary, directed by Jill Marshall. Paladin Pictures.
Davies, B. (2006). Subjectification: The Relevance of Butler's Analysis for Education. *British Journal of Sociology of Education.* Vol 27, No 4, pp. 425–438.
Dempster, E. (1988). Let's Watch a Little How She Dances. In Sheridan, S. (Ed.). *Grafts: Feminist Cultural Criticism.* London: Verso.
DePalma, R., & Atkinson, E. (2008). *Invisible Boundaries: Addressing Sexualities Equality in Children's Worlds.* Stoke on Trent: Trentham.
Epstein, D., & Johnson, R. (2008). Walking the Talk: Young People Making Identities. In DePalma, R., & Atkinson, E. (Eds.). *Invisible Boundaries: Addressing Sexualities Equality in Children's Worlds.* Stoke on Trent: Trentham.
Fanon, F. (2008). *Black Skin, White Masks.* New York: Grove Press.
Fisher, J., & Shay, A. (2009). *When Men Dance: Choreographing Masculinity across Borders.* New York: Oxford University Press.
Foster, S.L. (1996). The Ballerina's Phallic Pointe. In Foster, S.L. (Ed.). *Corporealities: Dancing Knowledge, Culture and Power.* New York: Routledge.
Foster, S.L. (1998). Choreographies of Gender. *Signs: Journal of Women in Culture & Society.* Vol 24, No 1, pp. 1–33.
Foster, S.L. (2001). Closets Full of Dances: Modern Dance's Performance of Masculinity and Sexuality. In Desmond, J.C. (Ed.). *Dancing Desires: Choreographing Sexualities On and Off the Stage.* Madison: University of Wisconsin Press.
Foucault, M. (1977). *Discipline and Punish: The Birth of the Prison.* London: Peregrine.
Foulkes, J.L. (2001). Dance Is for American Men: Ted Shawn and the Intersection of Gender, Sexuality and Nationalism in the 1930s. In Desmond, J.C. (Ed.). *Dancing Desires: Choreographing Sexualities On and Off the Stage.* Madison: University of Wisconsin Press.
Freire, P. (1990). *Pedagogy of the Oppressed.* New York: Continuum.
Gard, M. (2001). Dancing around the 'Problem' of Boys and Dance. *Discourse: Studies in the Cultural Politics of Education.* Vol 22, No 2, pp. 212–225.
Gard, M. (2006). *Men Who Dance: Aesthetics, Athletics, & the Art of Masculinity.* New York: Peter Lang.
Gere, D. (2001). Effeminate Gestures: Choreographer Joe Goode and the Heroism of Effeminacy. In Desmond, J.C. (Ed.). *Dancing Desires: Choreographing Sexualities On and Off the Stage.* Madison: University of Wisconsin Press.
Goffman, E. (1959). *The Presentation of Self in Everyday Life.* New York: Anchor.
Gorely, T., Holroyd, R., & Kirk, D. (2003). Muscularity, the Habitus and the Social Construction of Gender: Towards a Gender-Related Physical Education. *British Journal of Sociology of Education.* Vol 24, No 4, pp. 429–448.
Hall, E.T. (1959). *The Silent Language.* New York: Anchor N.Y.
hooks, b. (1996). *Reel to Real.* London: Routledge.
Jenkins, R. (2002). *Pierre Bourdieu.* London: Routledge.
Jones, C. (2003). Lesbian and Gay Cinema. In Neimes, J. (Ed.). *An Introduction to Film Studies* (third edition). New York: Routledge.
Kehily, M. (2001). Bodies in School: Young Men, Embodiment, and Heterosexual Masculinities. *Men and Masculinities.* Vol 4, No 2, pp. 173–185.
Kirby, S., & Hay, I. (1997). (Hetero)Sexing Space: Gay Men and 'Straight' Space in Adelaide, South Australia. *The Professional Geographer.* Vol 49, No 3, pp. 295–305.
Kirk, D. (2002). The Social Construction of the Body in Physical Education and Sport. In Laker, A. (Ed.). *The Sociology of Sport and Physical Education.* London: RoutledgeFalmer.
Kroeger, B. (2003). *Passing: When People Can't Be Who They Are.* New York: Public Affairs.

Lanzieri, N., & Hildebrandt, T. (2011). Using Hegemonic Masculinity to Explain Gay Male Attraction to Muscular and Athletic Men. *Journal of Homosexuality*. Vol. 58, No 2, pp. 275–293.

Lingard, B., Martino, W., & Mills, M. (2009). *Boys and Schooling: Beyond Structural Reform*. Basingstoke: Palgrave Macmillan.

Mac an Ghaill, M., & Haywood, C. (2007). *Gender, Culture and Society: Contemporary Femininities and Masculinities*. London: Macmillan.

Martino, W., & Pallotta-Chiarolli, M. (2001). Gender Performativity and Normalizing Practices. In Haynes, F., & McKenna, T. (Eds.). *Unseen Genders: Beyond the Binaries*. New York: Peter Lang.

Martino, W., & Pallotta-Chiarolli, M. (2005). *Being Normal Is the Only Way to Be*. Sydney: University of New South Wales Press.

McKenna, T. (2001). Enactments of Difference. In Haynes, F., & McKenna, T. (Eds.). *Unseen Genders: Beyond the Binaries*. New York: Peter Lang.

McWilliam, E. (1997). Performing between the Posts: Authority, Posture and Contemporary Feminist Scholarship. In Tierney, W.G., & Lincoln, Y.S. (Eds.). *Representation and the Text: Re-framing the Narrative Voice*. New York: State University of New York Press.

Memmi, A. (1967). *The Colonizer and the Colonized*. Boston: Beacon.

Nayak, A., & Kehily, M.J. (1996). Playing It Straight: Masculinities, Homophobias and Schooling. *Journal of Gender Studies*. Vol 5, No 2, pp. 211–230.

Neimes, J. (2003). Gender and Film. In Neimes, J. (Ed.). *An Introduction to Film Studies* (third edition). New York: Routledge.

Nixon, S. (1996). *Hard Looks: Masculinities, Spectatorship and Contemporary Consumption*. New York: St Martins Press.

Paechter, C. (2003). Learning Masculinities and Femininities: Power/Knowledge and Legitimate Peripheral Participation. *Women's Studies International Forum*. Vol 26, No 6, pp. 541–552.

Paechter, C. (2006). Reconceptualizing the Gendered Body: Learning and Constructing Masculinities and Femininities in School. *Gender and Education*. Vol 18, No 2, pp. 121–135.

Pallotta-Chiarolli, M. (2010). *Border Sexualities, Border Families in Schools*. Lanham: Rowman and Littlefield.

Payne, R. (2007). Str8acting. *Social Semiotics*. Vol 17, No 4, pp. 525–538.

Pease, B. (2010). *Undoing Privilege: Unlearned Advantage in a Divided World*. London: Zed Books.

Plummer, D. (1999). *One of the Boys: Masculinity, Homophobia and Modern Manhood*. New York: Harrington Park Press.

Pronger, B. (1990). Gay Jocks: A Phenomenology of Gay Men in Athletics. In Messner, M.A., & Sabo, D.F. (Eds.). *Sport, Men, and the Gender Order: Critical Feminist Perspectives*. Champaign, IL: Human Kinetics Books.

Renold, E. (2005). *Girls, Boys and Junior Sexualities*. London: Routledge Falmer.

Risner, D. (2009). What We Know about Boys Who Dance: The Limitations of Contemporary Masculinity in Dance Education. In Fisher, J., & Shay, A. (Eds.). *When Men Dance: Choreographing Masculinity across Borders*. New York: Oxford University Press.

Russo, V. (1981). *The Celluloid Closet: Homosexuality in the Movies*. New York: Harper & Row.

Said, E.W. (2003). *Orientalism*. London: Penguin.

Schirato, T., & Yell, S. (1996). *Communication and Cultural Literacy*. St Leonards, NSW: Allen and Unwin.

Shilling, C. (2003). *The Body and Social Theory*. London: Sage.

Stoneley, P. (2007). *A Queer History of the Ballet*. London: Routledge.

Swain, J. (2004). The Resources and Strategies That 10–11-Year-Old Boys Use to Construct Masculinities in the School Setting. *British Educational Research Journal*. Vol 30, No 1, pp. 167–185.
Swain, J. (2005). Masculinities in Education. In Kimmel, M. S., Hearn, J., & Connell, R. W. (Eds.). *Handbook of Studies on Men and Masculinities*. London: Sage.
Young, I. M. (1990). *Throwing Like a Girl and Other Essays in Feminist Philosophy and Social Theory*. Indianapolis: Indiana University Press.
Zizek, S. (1999). *The Sublime Object of Ideology*. London: Verso.

6 Embodiment and Regulation

Sex-specific prescriptions of desirable and undesirable masculinities and femininities can impact on how we come to *do* gender through our own bodies. The vignettes and investigation in this chapter focus on the regulation of the body as a socially positioned embodied subject. Charting memories of my childhood body as a subject of enculturation and regulation, I focus on external ascription relating to the delimitations placed on my embodiment as a male within specific cultural settings such as school. I also ponder self-ascription relating to regulation that I imposed on myself in attempting to fit desired gender identities. This investigation indicates the delicacy of the relationship between personal and social control of one's embodiment of gender. It also signposts the threat of alienation, ostracism, and marginalization for those who transgress and fail to embody gender according to ways in which they are socially regulated.

THE BODY AS BONSAI

Bonsai are trained
By pruning branches and roots
Pinching off unwanted growth
Wiring branches and trunk
In order that they grow to desired shape
Some suggest Bonsai culture is cruel
Stifling, smothering a plant's natural inclination
But given adequate water, air, light and nutrients
Properly maintained bonsai
Can live as long as any full size tree.

(Migdalek 2003, p. 2–3)

Where the bonsai plant may appear to be a normal tree, it is actually the product of regulation imposed on it that restricts its natural inclination. So,

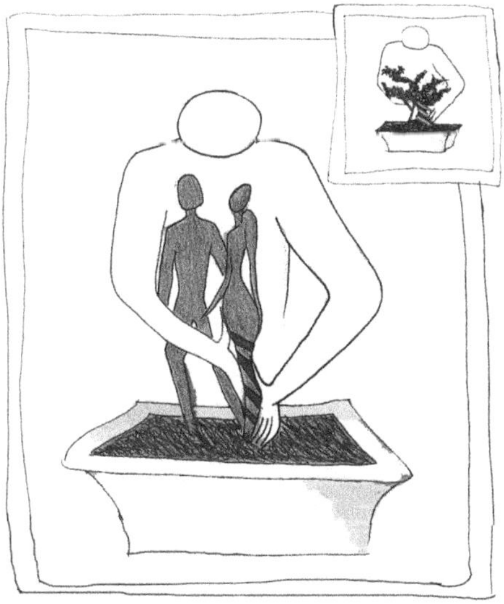

Figure 6.1 Bonsai. Artwork by Jack Migdalek.

too, the embodied behavior of males and females may to varying degrees be the product of regulation imposed on them—even those who appear to be 'natural'. The individual whose body is regulated against its inclination may be more vulnerable than it appears.

When children are not what parents, teachers, or society expect or desire, carers have a tendency to do what they can to have those individuals appear to fit in. Because of the social tendency to link feminine behavior in males and masculine behavior in females to homosexuality (Bartky 1990, J. Butler 1990, 1993, Mac an Ghaill 1994, Connell 1995, Plummer 1999, Green 2001, Martino & Pallotta-Chiarolli 2001b), and because being gay is frequently perceived to be subordinate (Connell 1995, Nayak & Kehily 1996, Paechter 2003b, Martino & Pallotta-Chiarolli 2005), there is an inclination, as stated in Chapter 2, to safeguard children's social acceptance by raising them in a manner that maximizes the possibility of a heterosexual gendernormative outcome (Kosofsky Sedgwick 1994). Embodying in what is deemed to be a heterosexual manner—which is masculine embodiment for males and feminine embodiment for females—is more socially acceptable and less likely to invite discrimination than embodying in other ways, regardless of what one's actual sexual orientation is. Where a carer is conscious of potential disadvantageous consequences for the charge whose embodied manner does not fit established embodied norms, the carer may endeavor to protect their charge from such consequences by whatever means they can.

REGULATING THE BODIES OF BOYS AND GIRLS

Where corporeal practices imposed on the bodies of children differ according to perceived biological sex, such practices can be seen to be gender inequitable and have the potential to cause a negative impact.

> A bow is pinned to the few strands of hair on the infant girl's head.
> She toddles around, exploring the world that seems so vast and full of curiosities.
> Whenever her head inclines forward, backward, or sideways
> the insecurely bound bow slips off her head.
> Each time this happens a big person's hand
> Stops her in her tracks and pins it ludicrously back in place
> Like an unwelcome magnet.
> The bow will stop falling off when the little girl learns to balance it there.
> That means no cartwheels, no forward rolls, no wrestling, no tumbling

The hair ribbon in the story above is more than just an accessory. It operates as a control mechanism akin to Pavlov's dog reinforcement behavior training (Kaplan 1966). If the ribbon is put back in place whenever it falls from her head, the girl will eventually learn what embodied action causes such corrective attentions to occur. She will also come to realize that if she stops actions that cause the ribbon to drop from her head (such as

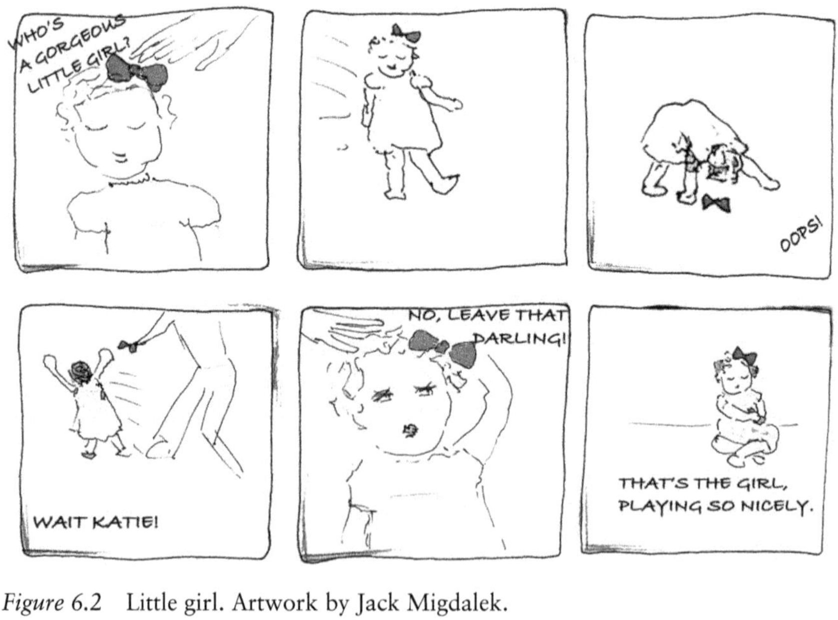

Figure 6.2 Little girl. Artwork by Jack Migdalek.

rough-and-tumble behavior), so too will the interruptive reapplications of said ribbon that continually stop her in her tracks be stopped. In a similar way, being dressed in skirts, or being adorned in clothing made from delicate, easily stained fiber, or with accessories such as fragile bracelets and necklaces, during childhood, in addition to being encouraged to participate only in particular activities and sports at school and elsewhere, is likely to condition an individual's embodied restraint (Young 1990, see also Paechter 2007). Given that we teach our young that it is rude, indecent, and improper to expose the genitals, it is those who are dressed in skirts who are inhibited and limited from cart-wheeling, inverting, or sitting straddle-legged (see Young 1990, Paechter 2007).

As children grow older, they face other forms of conditioning that establish a hierarchy of manners and embodied habits that signify differently according to whether they are male or female. Girls tend to get corrected for ways in which they walk, sit, and masticate, for which boys are not corrected. There are pressures on boys to embody in a masculine manner, and more specifically *not* to embody in a feminine manner, which, as discussed in Chapter 2, is more closely specified and penalized than are dominant configurations of femininity for girls (Paechter 2003a).

Males and females are subject to differential socialization from birth (Turner 1984, Connell 1995, Goffman 1997, Rogers 1999, Gorely et al. 2003, Shilling 2003, Paechter 2006). How they are handled, related to, and reacted to varies according to their biological sex. Frequently, this differential socialization involves physical regulation of the body. The bodies of infant boys tend to be jostled and subjected to rough play as opposed to the bodies of girls, which tend to be handled more gently. Differential handling and regulation of the bodies of infant boys and girls position notions of male and female as dissimilar to one another. It can be argued that "once a child is handled in a particular way, she or he will learn from or develop in accordance with that treatment" (Paechter 2007, p. 48). Where there are rigid differences in how male bodies and female bodies are regulated and socialized (controlled, handled, dressed, treated), deviations from such norms become marked. Where such deviations come to be seen as strange or ab-normal, this may impact on the self-image and confidence of boys or girls who become aware that their embodied inclinations do not align with gendernormative ways in which their bodies are coaxed, cajoled, and pressured to embody.

Differential regulation and perception of male and female bodies by influential adults and carers is likely to condition girls' and boys' embodiment, deportment, embodied disposition, and embodied restraint. As a child I came to restrain myself from pursuits and activities that were deemed to be feminine. I never questioned why as a boy I was clothed and groomed differently from how my sister was. I recall my sister skipping, playing hopscotch, and playing with hula hoops. Where I was inclined to also do these activities in my home environment, I was conscious that these activities were deemed to be girls' activities. I was conscious that a boy acting out such play preferences in public settings was not the same as doing so at home (see Paechter 2007). Being anxious about how I would be perceived and treated were I to act differently from other boys in public settings such as school, I censured myself accordingly. It was one thing to play Australian rules football badly and not join in rough play at school, but it became apparent to me that to join in *girls'* activities would be a confirmation of not being a regular boy (see Epstein et al. 2001, Renold 2005, Lingard et al. 2009). I was acutely self-conscious about how my body projected and feared that participating publicly in girls' activities would be received with teasing and disapproval.

I contend that within mainstream Western cultural settings, a boy or girl is likely to come to restrain himself or herself from pursuits and activities deemed to be feminine or masculine respectively: where one is physically positioned and conditioned to embody in certain ways; where one is made aware of binary differences between male and female; where one is made aware that certain activities and interests are deemed suitable exclusively for males or females; and where one becomes aware that deviations from norms of embodiment are regarded and treated as strange, misfit, ludicrous.

LOOKING OUT FOR THE YOUNG

Teachers, carers, and parents want the best for their charges. Achieving this may involve guiding and encouraging children to perform/embody in ways other than how they are inclined.

Setting: The Preschool Classroom

PREP TEACHER: Now boys and girls, we are going to prepare a performance for our moms and dads for the end of year concert. What I want you to do is to imagine an enormous and amazing garden. Each of us is going to become one of the things that live in the garden. Some of you might be flowers, and butterflies. Some of you might be insects and frogs . . . maybe dragonflies. Just imagine what you want to be.

(SOME TIME LATER): Alright boys and girls. Amanda, you want to be a . . .? Butterfly! And Jarrod . . .? A lizard! Great! And Steven . . .? A flower? Wow! Wouldn't you prefer to be one of the grasshoppers? Or a frog perhaps? No? OK. And do you think your mom would like to make you a flower costume for all those people to see you in at the concert? You sure you wouldn't prefer to be a beetle . . . or a dragonfly perhaps?

Why would the teacher in the episode above discourage Steven from taking on the role of a flower? Why would the teacher encourage boys in the concert to take on the roles of frogs or dragonflies as opposed to butterflies or flowers? The teacher is aware that flowers are considered to be feminine and therefore 'girlie', and as a result this would be likely to draw negative attention to young Steven should he take on that role; is conscious that cues of femininity in a male charge may not serve the child well in terms of social acceptance by his peers; regards a more masculine or non-feminine garden creature as more suitable for a boy; attempts to regulate Steven's embodiment in order to protect him from social marginalization; and is aware that gender non-conforming schoolboys and schoolgirls are at risk of being ridiculed, teased, and bullied (DePalma & Atkinson 2008, see also Mac an Ghaill 1994, Kehily 2002, Renold 2005, Lingard et al. 2009).

Carers (such as the teacher in the preceding vignette) who actively discourage their charges from transgressing gender norms of embodiment according to biological sex indicate how potent these norms are in defining or classifying children as normal boys or girls. The boy or girl who transgresses these 'norms' is likely to be marked as different, if not *ab*-normal. Reflecting on my work as a drama and dance educator of children, I unthinkingly never placed boys in situations that made feminine embodiment or characterization the only option or an attractive option for them to take up. I believe that in general we, as educators and parents, do not create opportunities for boys to publicly embody in feminine or delicate ways, in order to protect them from discrimination and marginalization that we know can occur in such cases. Why else would a teacher choose not to make such opportunities easily available to boys?

What might the consequences be for Steven in the above episode if the teacher had not discouraged him from being a flower? Steven might be teased by other students; Steven's parents, siblings, and/or grandparents might have apprehensions about Steven's role; Steven's parents might be unhappy about making a flower costume for Steven; audience members at the concert might notice or react to Steven's performance in derogatory or pitying ways. Is the experience of playing a flower likely to cause Steven to grow up to be effeminate? Will performing as a flower have an impact on Steven's as yet unacknowledged sexual orientation? These questions are pondered in the playscript *Sugarplum Fairies* in the Appendix.

EMBODIED INCLINATIONS

Knowledge of how one's embodiment may be perceived by others can have a panopticonic, regulatory effect on the ways in which an individual endeavors to project. In order to get ahead, it may be in one's interest to conform to dominant norms of embodied behavior (Kroeger 2003), even when it goes against one's performance inclination. Both conforming to and resisting dominant norms of embodied behavior when such norms go against one's inclination can have negative consequences: individuals who live life performing against their inclination in order to conform may lose something of a sense of self (Anzaldua 1990, Kroeger 2003) and a sense of how they might otherwise desire to or be inclined to perform; individuals who resist and transgress norms of embodied gender behavior may be subject to bullying and marginalization. Losing a sense of self as a result of the former may not be as fearsome as consequences such as being bullied, marginalized, and/or discriminated against as a result of the latter. However, the former may also result in feelings of alienation and low self-esteem that can have a profound effect on an individual's social and emotional well-being.

The photograph in the figure is of me at the age of ten. The occasion was my sister's twelfth birthday, a fancy dress party, held in our home, to which about ten of my sister's girlfriends were invited. My mother made me a butterfly costume that I had chosen from a book full of costume ideas.

What strikes me about this photograph is how effeminate my pose is: the bend of the front leg, the lifted heel of the foot, the elegant placement of the arms as wings, the slight tilt of the head. Drawing on interviews, memories, and photographs such as this one, I believe that I possessed some effeminate behavioral and embodied inclinations.

> You were delicate, you were dainty . . . You moved delicately . . . it did stand out, I remember, definitely . . . that delicate way you moved, and

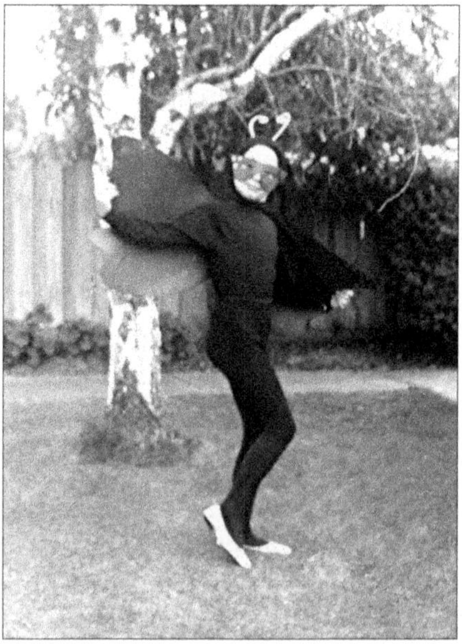

Figure 6.3 Fancy dress. Author's family photograph.

> that delicate way you were, which was so against what I guess men were meant to be like, or boys.
>
> (from interview with my cousin 2007)

I believe that this effeminate embodied disposition was part of what my natural gender inclination was meant to be. To me the photograph reflects a time when I was not self-conscious that my embodiment may have been effeminate. As I grew up, I became highly self-conscious about my embodiment, and a gulf occurred between my embodied inclination and how I predominantly came to embody. Basically, the uninhibited embodied inclination of that ten-year-old boy became lost. Was this occurrence part of growing up or a result of regulation? If regulation was part of losing that inclination—and I believe it was—then I may have unnecessarily lost a part of self that I experienced as feminine, which no longer manifests in embodied form.

Interestingly, my mother had no qualms about making me the requested butterfly costume. As a European immigrant, her cultural perspective was possibly different from that of mainstream Australian parents. As a new Australian, she may not have understood the potential consequences for the son who dressed and embodied as a butterfly in the same homophobic way that Australian parents might. That said, she acknowledged that she might have felt differently about the costume were it to have been for a school event as opposed to one held at home and with friends.

As I grew up I became conscious that a male embodying in a feminine manner was likely to be labeled as 'gay' or 'sissy'. The tone with which others spoke of or referred to sissies and gays led me to know that for a boy or man to behave as a 'girl' was a negative. Through exposure to representations of males in the media, I learned ways of being in the world that were sanctioned and others that were punishable (Linne 2003). I feared that were I to resist convention and embody in a feminine manner (as I was inclined), I would have to face consequences such as being bullied, marginalized, ostracized, and discriminated against. Fear of being perceived to be gay or sissy served to condition me to comply with convention and resist feminine embodied inclination, especially in public contexts such as school. The consequences of this were that I was not bullied or ostracized, but I experienced feelings of social isolation and a consciousness that there was something wrong with me.

> You became reclusive . . . You became more quiet and shy.
>
> (from interview with my mother 2007)

REGULATION AND CORRECTION OF THE YOUNG BODY

My male body was, and is, capable of performing in a feminine manner. However, the "astonishing gap between what bodies can do and what they 'choose' to do" (Gard 2003, p. 219) may be explained through investigation of our upbringing and enculturation. There were many practices in my upbringing as a male body that were different from those imposed on female bodies. These occurred across numerous sites and institutions in which I was inducted as a son, student, and largely docile participant.

The primary school I attended regulated boys' bodies and girls' bodies in different ways: boys wore pants, and girls wore skirts; in the classrooms, boys were seated next to boys, and girls next to girls; boys and girls were given concurrent sports classes in which the girls' bodies were made to play softball and basketball while the boys' bodies were made to play cricket and Australian rules football; boys' bodies were taught to do woodwork; girls' bodies were taught to sew; for the annual school ball, boys and girls were taught different steps to perform. Going against these sex-specific embodied practices was an option that was made to be unattractive. For example, boys and girls were seated next to one another only as a form of punishment.

The physical school site itself also regulates boys' and girls' bodies differently (Davies 2000, Renold 2005). In primary school, morning assemblies were held in the quadrangle, where we lined up on white lines painted on the asphalt that split us into classes, the boys on the right, the girls on the left. The school, as an embodied site, regulated the bodies of boys to play on one side of the playground and those of girls to play on the other side. There were separate gates from the playground for boys and girls that led into a quadrangle. I do not recall being told that boys were not to play in certain spaces or enter certain gates, but, nevertheless, through never seeing the practice transgressed, a knowledge that boys and girls were not to deviate from these structures was understood. Without external policing I came, as a subject of panopticonic control (Foucault 1977), to self-regulate my behavior in this regard.

A tendency to regard feminine behavioral and embodied qualities on a male as that which is in need of regulation or correction is illustrated in the following interview extract, in which it is implied that the root of my feminine tendencies was biological and in need of correction.

> Mr. W, your headmaster in primary school—I think grade 1 or 2, once came to me when I came to pick you up and said to me that you were—I think he said something about you being a bit, playing, always playing with the girls and being a bit effeminate, and he suggested that you have your testicles checked in case they're not—descended or something.
>
> (from interview with my mother 2007)

Implicit in the principal advising my mother to have me checked by a medical doctor is the assumption that feminine qualities or behaviors in a boy were problematic and not natural or healthy, and were something that could, and should, be remedied. The principal's line of thought was that a physiological problem or abnormality would explain why I played with girls and behaved in an effeminate manner. I am unsure why the principal found it so important to regulate me to behave like other boys, nor why he connected effeminacy in a young male with the physiological condition of undescended testicles. My mother, whose concerns were aroused by the principal, complied with his advice and had my body checked by a doctor, who told her that I was all right. Once she knew that I was physically healthy, my mother did not pursue the matter any further.

> I didn't sort of try to change you in any way but other people did. Like, for instance, Dad wanted you to play soccer, and even Nanna tried to give you boys' toys to play with.
>
> (from interview with my mother 2007)

At the time, I knew neither anything of what had been suggested to my mother by the principal, nor that there were worries for my normality. At the time, I was not yet acutely aware that my behavior and interests were not deemed appropriate for a boy. That my tendencies were disturbing to the principal is both alarming and touching. I am alarmed that my behavior, which was not disruptive or antisocial, was regarded as unnatural and in need of correction. At the same time, I am touched that perhaps his motives may have been that he foresaw that it would not be in my social interests to continue to behave in an effeminate manner. As I reflect back on how withdrawn and introverted I became as I grew older, it seems that the principal had reason to be concerned for my social well-being. My social withdrawal was prompted by a growing consciousness of not being like other boys.

> It was very obvious to me that you changed, because as a little boy you were very sociable—and always seeking company, and then you became more quiet and shy . . . You may have realized that you were different to other boys, I'm not sure. Maybe—you felt like an outsider perhaps . . . I think you were a little bit depressed. You were often in your own company. You didn't want to be in others' company much.
>
> (from interview with my mother 2007)

This was in contrast to my behavior and disposition before this period, which my mother described as:

> You were really cute . . . Everybody was always drawn to you because you were so friendly and outgoing and lively and sweet.

What the principal saw as problematic could have been dealt with in two ways: work on changing the little boy in order to protect him from being singled out, marginalized, or oppressed as a result of his effeminate tendencies; or work on combating the social mindset that is oppressive of difference by trying to influence a school culture's acceptance of difference, diversity, and that which may seem to be 'other'. Although I do not think many principals today would advise that an effeminate male student be given a medical check up, I think that there is still a mindset that finds effeminate behavior in males to be of concern. Contemporary school cultures promote ideas of diversity and acceptance, and the fighting of bullying (see Department of Education and Early Childhood Development Victoria 2008, 2014). However, boys and girls whose gendered behavior and interests are not aligned to those of other boys and girls respectively continue to feel pressured to regulate and conform to gendered norms of embodiment and behavior (Plummer 1999, Robinson et al. 2002, Martino & Pallotta-Chiarolli 2005). Where regulation and self-regulation are oppressive, they are bound to affect the social and emotional well-being of such individuals.

While my skipping, playing hopscotch, and wearing a butterfly costume were accepted by my parents in the home, my parents actively fostered and promoted gendernormative roles for my sister and myself. Where my sister was encouraged to help with the cooking, I was encouraged to help with fix-it jobs inside and outside the house. My sister was sent to ballet classes, while I was taken to soccer training. For my parents, these were natural activities to have us both do. Even though I was quite taken by the idea of dance, I never asked to be taken to ballet class, probably as a result of having come to understand that it was not an appropriate activity or interest for boys, but one for girls. It became clear to me that boys and girls not only were dressed differently but were also supposed to pursue different activities. Mine was a docile body (Foucault 1977) that adhered to how I was regulated. I remember disliking soccer, and also being bad at it. But I did not voice my aversion to playing, as I did not want to disappoint my father, who had been a keen soccer player himself. I understood that soccer was something appropriate for boys to do, and I was aware of my father's desire for his son to follow in his footsteps. It was only after some time, when my father asked how I felt about the weekly sessions, that I came clean and was able to stop going.

As a youngster I recall kissing and being kissed by many of the adult males and females in my life. From around the age of twelve, kisses were no longer generally practiced with my father and uncles but did continue with my mother and aunties. I am not certain whether it was my father and uncles who stopped kissing me, or whether I stopped kissing them. However, the situation worked differently with my sister, for whom the practice of kisses with all adult family members continued. Our induction or apprenticeship into socially appropriate forms of greeting that differed according to biological sex matched the forms of socially appropriate greeting projected by male and female bodies in mainstream surroundings and in the media.

We were not a religious family but did attend an orthodox synagogue on Jewish holidays. In this physical space, too, males and females were physically segregated, usually with women in a balcony area overlooking the men's section where the service was held. Males had to wear prayer-shawls on their shoulders and skullcaps on their heads. Women were not to wear pants. Like other religions Judaism specifies certain roles and rituals for male bodies and others for females, enforcing the notion of male and female embodiment being in binary opposition.

My enculturation as an obedient son and student enforced embodied norms for males and females. That those around me did not look positively on transgressions of these norms influenced me to conform to what I came to understand as being appropriate embodiment. I came to understand deviation or transgression of gender norms as being naughty, if not wrong. I wanted approval, and I wanted to fit in. I sensed that there was a lot at stake for boys or girls should they transgress from the clear demarcations of what was appropriate physical activity for each. My panopticonic conscience (Foucault 1977) made me uncomfortable about embodying any feminine inclinations I may have had. In my docility I attempted to toe the line by participating in activities that were seen to suit boys. I was conscious that my fascination with theatre and dance was not a usual interest for boys, and so I underplayed this interest before my father, teachers, and classmates, who I thought would not be accepting of such pursuits and would not see them as fitting for a male.

Since my childhood, Australian society has changed considerably. In many schools, boys and girls have access to the same play areas and are not segregated in assemblies, made to sit separately, or made to dress differently. Nevertheless, it can be argued that the bodies of contemporary Australian boys and girls continue to be conditioned and segregated via the sports and physical activities deemed suitable for each (see Epstein et al. 2001, Gorely et al. 2003, Renold 2005) and the continued valuing of differential deportment for each (see Kamler et al. 1994 regarding teachers' differing notions of what sitting up *nicely* is for boys and girls).

My enculturation and the regulation of my embodiment positioned me away from the transgression of masculine forms of embodiment, or, in other words, I avoided embodying in a feminine manner. Yet a transition took place that went against how I was enculturated, in that I took up theatre and dance, occupations that in Western cultural circles are commonly perceived as effeminate (Burt 1995, 2001, Foster 2001, Foulkes 2001, Gard 2008). My transition to acting and dancing came about through my own agency and will be explained and explored in the following chapter. Suffice it to say that through a desire to act and dance, I found ways and strategies that made such practices justifiable and acceptable to myself, my family, and my peers. Ironically, within the mainstream theatre and dance settings that I entered, there were regulatory forces at work that also promoted and valorized masculine embodiment for the bodies of males.

THE PERFORMANCE ARTIST AS CHOREOGRAPHED SUBJECT

My male body was—and is—capable of performing in a feminine manner, yet it was hardly ever directed or choreographed to move in this way. As a male actor and dancer performing in commercial productions for mainstream audiences, I was coached to move powerfully and strongly, and to occupy a large amount of space. As mentioned in Chapter 5, I saw and understood that working male actors and dancers moved with these qualities. Indeed, it was through taking on these qualities in my acting and dancing that I became a working professional performer myself. As a professional dancer and actor, working predominantly in mainstream commercial musicals, film, and television, my male body was almost always choreographed and directed to move in masculine ways. That was how I had been conditioned to dance and act, and how I came to feel comfortable in presenting myself. Although getting work as a professional actor and dancer was contingent on talent, I believe that it was also contingent on not embodying in a feminine manner. I regulated my body not to embody in a feminine manner, not just when acting or dancing, but also when presenting at auditions.

In regard to dance, although there may have been variation in the styles of the choreographers and dance teachers who choreographed my male body, the choreography they produced on male dancers' bodies was ultimately athletic and masculine, involving expansive leaps, spins, widely straddled legs, arms with splayed fingers or clenched fists, and the lifting and controlling of female dancers' bodies. In contrast, these choreographers choreographed their female dancers to move more slinkily, often with softer lines and flexed wrists, something they rarely ever imposed on the bodies of their male dancers. Notions of the aesthetics of a male dancer moving in a masculine manner were reinforced by the male dancer models I aspired to, self-policed by an awareness of how soft, feminine dancing on a male body was perceived.

In order to obtain work, my body became used to moving in ways demanded by the commercial directors and choreographers with whom trained. Through a process of practice, moving in these ways became natural and also comfortable for my body to perform. And so, influenced by the ways in which my male body was choreographed and directed, I developed my 'male actor/dancer habitus', or 'body memory' (Erskine 2005), which not surprisingly informed how I myself cast, choreographed, and directed the bodies of others, to be investigated in Chapter 7.

Performing against one's habitus is a difficult and often uncomfortable experience. In the case of dance, I recall how difficult it was for a classically trained dancer friend to learn to dance in a jazz style, despite the desire to do so. When habitus is deeply ingrained through consistent and ongoing practice, it is not easy to alter (Bourdieu 1990, Shilling 2003). It is probably even more difficult to alter one's practices when one finds the alternatives to be distasteful. In my case, the 'male dance habitus' into which I was enculturated was so ingrained that to dance against it and dance in a feminine manner was an uncomfortable and distasteful experience, one steeped in internalized 'femiphobia' (Ducat 2004), where male femininity was taboo. The one time I was choreographed differently still disturbs me: I was working in a children's musical, and I was choreographed, along with five female dancers and another male dancer, as a flower. I recall vividly how I detested performing the sequence, which was wafting and delicate. I felt very self-conscious and would dance the steps in a vigorous and sharp manner at performances where the choreographer was not present.

HEAVY HANDED POLICING OF EMBODIMENT

It is not just parents, teachers, carers, directors, and choreographers who regulate our embodiment but also those whose motives are not so caring. I refer back to the opening episode of this book, in which two pedestrians were abused as "Poofs" by the occupants of a passing car. The event happened to my partner and me not long ago. The event stunned, shocked, scared, and upset me. Had the car stopped, I believe that the situation could have been an unsafe experience for us. Regardless of questions of what may have provoked the prejudice and abuse of the people in the car, I am concerned about the regulatory effects that the reality of this kind of incident has/can have on the embodied behavior of individuals. The experience, which I believe occurred as a result of something in my embodiment, tempers my embodied self-regulation. It is safer for me not to project as a 'poof'. It is safer for me to pass as straight.

The incident, which occurred relatively recently, has served as a personal memo that for my own well-being I continue to need to be vigilant about the way I behave in many contexts. The threat from not sizing up to dominant social norms of embodiment may be physical or social. The former involves the threat of being beaten up. The latter involves the threat of being marginalized, ostracized, or labeled. In my case, the threat has served and continues to serve as a panopticonic device (Foucault 1977) to regulate my embodied behavior so as not to stand out or be perceived as that which is 'other'.

'OTHER'

A segment that regularly featured on the U.S children's television program *Sesame Street* (Sesame Workshop, formerly CTW), titled *One of These Things*, consisted of the presentation of a set of four pictures from which one was to be eliminated as not fitting into the set. When the picture that 'did not belong' was singled out, it was crossed out of the set broadly and dramatically. For each of the illustrated sets (overleaf), which of the four pictures would be most likely singled out as misfitting?

The *One of These Things* segment no longer features in contemporary episodes of *Sesame Street,* probably because, when applied to people, the notion of picking out that which does not belong negates notions of social acceptance of difference. For all the contemporary jargon that condones the celebrating and embracing of diversity, pressures for individuals *not* to deviate from the norm or not be 'other' are still forceful. The mindset of singling

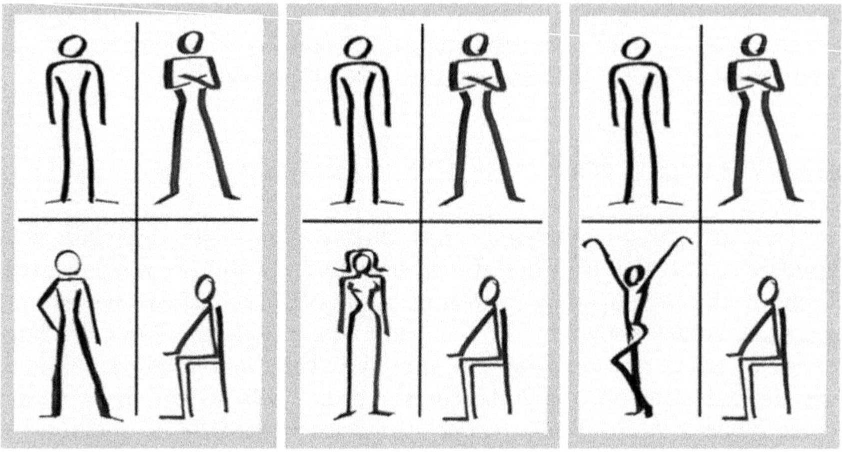

Figure 6.4 Odd one out. Artwork by Jack Migdalek.

out that which is different still prevails. I will refer to this as the 'Sesame Street mindset'. It is a mindset whereby, in contrast to master-signifiers, that which is different calls attention to itself (see Zizek 1999, R. Butler 2005). Where an action is foreign to our enculturation, it is likely to stand out as being different or other. Our reaction to such marked performance will depend on our culture's regard toward that which is different. In mainstream Western culture, that which is different is often marked as being ludicrous, comic, deviant, or pitiable, and not merely different.

The 'Sesame Street mindset' of finding that which is 'different from normal' to be amusing is established from an early age, as illustrated in the following scenario:

A carer sits with an infant who is drawing a picture.

CARER: What are you drawing?
INFANT: It's a garden and a house.
CARER: That's fantastic. What else are you going to put in the picture?
INFANT: Um, some trees.
CARER: Good idea. And what color are you going to make them?

Infant looks at his or her choice of colored pencils but does not respond.

CARER: (*playfully*) How about . . . purple?
INFANT: (*laughing*) No!
CARER: (*playfully*) Um . . . what about . . . blue?

INFANT: (*laughs*) No!
CARER: Mmmm. Yes, blue and purple are kind of stupid. What color then?
INFANT: Green!
CARER: That's excellent!

Both the Sesame Street segment and the scenario above make fun of picking out that which does not belong; make the thought of conceiving something that is 'other' as fitting into a ludicrous or comic notion; deny diversity within a category; situate that which is different as subordinate and worthy of opposition/ridicule; and regulate a mindset that positions that which is other as subordinate.

The scenario between the carer and the infant illustrates a situation in which an adult instills in a child a sense of humor toward that which is different or other. The suggestion is made that a tree painted purple or blue is absurd. This marking of that which is 'other' as being amusing or strange serves to situate that which is different in hierarchical binary opposition to that which is normal or correct (see Pickering 2001). Through the playful tone of the carer, the child is encouraged to see the notion of that which is different (the purple or blue tree) as not only comic but stupid. This kind of marking of difference can lead to negative attitudes toward that which is 'other than the norm' beyond the context of the previous narrative. Where this kind of marking of difference influences the ways that male and female embodiment is perceived, the effects of attitudes toward gendered embodiment that is *other* than normal may not be benign.

The theme that comes up again and again is that in mainstream Western settings, male and female bodies that are marked and draw attention for being different or 'other' tend, through not fitting the 'norm', to be regarded as any combination of curious, ludicrous, subordinate, revolting, obscene, depraved, and/or deviant. In being contrasted to a norm, they are not being simply regarded as different or other but as ab-normal. Being classified and marginalized in such ways can impact negatively on an individual's well-being (Plummer 1999, Swain 2004, Martino & Pallotta-Chiarolli 2005, Kimmel 2009). It is no wonder that individuals (or those who care for them) might endeavor to regulate their embodiment so as not to draw attention for being different or other.

I too am guilty of a 'Sesame Street mindset'. As a result of habitual and inequitable ways in which I had come to perceive the embodiment of gender, I am far more likely to do a double take or be amused on seeing a male whose gait is feminine, or a female whose gait is masculine, than a male whose gait is masculine or a female whose gait is feminine. Embodiment that I had habitually learned to find amusing or noteworthy is the result of my enculturation toward that which was 'different'—in binary opposition to what I was conditioned to regard as 'normal'.

CHOREOGRAPHIC PRESCRIPTION ACCORDING TO BIOLOGICAL SEX

To get by in social and cultural settings, one needs to have a feel for the field and the game (Bourdieu 1990). Knowing a field is to know the setting one is entering or proposing to enter, and knowing the rules of a game is to know the practices by which to engage or get by in that setting. Many fields (settings) and games (practices) involve embodiment or choreographic regulation (rules) to which an entrant's body must adhere in order to effectively enter or operate in them (Gee 2008). Deviating from these norms of embodiment will mark and marginalize an individual, and may inhibit participation in a field or game. For example, if I do not line up for service, it is unlikely that I will be served; if as a school student I do not put my hand up to speak, it is unlikely I will be called on to speak—just as if I speak without putting my hand up, I may be reprimanded.

Some choreographic practices on which effective participation in various fields and games is dependent are gendered in that they are performed and perceived differently according to the biological sex of a performer. For example, in the Western world a woman's handshake is not expected to be strong, whereas a man's is; in Japan, a man bows with hands toward the outside of his thighs, whereas a woman bows with hands toward the inside of her thighs. As already discussed, in most mainstream Western settings, males are expected to embody in ways that are not feminine, and females in ways that are not masculine, and deviating from these norms of embodiment can mark and marginalize an individual.

The choreographies to which we are expected to adhere physically are so clearly demarcated, and so solidly inscribed in relevant fields and contexts, that it rarely occurs to an individual to go against the choreography as prescribed or set. This is especially so where one desires to get by or operate within a field or game of a society or culture. I believe that operating as a subject of choreography and following the way other males and females perform is easier than operating differently from the norm and opposing what is set. Transgressing puts a lot at stake for the perpetrator and may lead to marginalization, abuse, ridicule, and exclusion. Stories verifying this abound (see Anzaldua 1987, 1990, hooks 1994, Martino & Pallotta-Chiarolli 2001a, Savin-Williams 2001, Kroeger 2003, Drummond 2005, Pascoe 2007). To transgress the pre-set and established choreography of a game is a more difficult path to take than to adhere to established norms.

As a choreographic subject of fields and settings into which I was born, I was inducted into cultures that idealized male embodiment in binary opposition to female embodiment. My body was subject to training that would not only maximize the possibility of matching prescribed masculine norms of embodiment for males but minimize the possibility of embodying in ways that were feminine. As mentioned earlier, I was taken to soccer as opposed to ballet training. On the subject of ballet classes my mother said:

> Well at the time it was sort of a girl's thing to do. Mostly girls went to ballet, and it didn't even occur to me to take you . . . You didn't sort of mention that you wanted to go, so it didn't occur to me at all. It was just what most girls did, and most mothers took their girls to ballet.

Even though my mother may not have feared that feminine embodiment on her son would result in him becoming a homosexual, she adhered to gendernormative conventions and never thought to have me learn to dance. I address how, when, and why I transgressed my enculturation and took up dance in the following chapter.

The impacts of how my body was regulated and enculturated in childhood have had a pervasive influence on my embodiment in adulthood. Like most individuals placed in and exposed to particular social and cultural settings or fields (Bourdieu 1990, Gee 2008), my body learned to play by the rules. My body was regulated as a docile subject (Foucault 1977) of the cultural settings into which it was born, so much so that the machinations of the ideologies by which I came to embody and which eventually became my embodied habitus—both in formal performance arenas and in the everyday—were beyond my awareness. Sets of options for embodiment that are given and taken up as representative of male, female, heterosexual, and homosexual are limiting and debilitating, especially for those who may be inclined to perform in contrast to those options. A lifetime of being regulated to comply with norms of embodiment along with an awareness of the consequences for transgressing these norms is what leads many individuals to conform to gendered norms of embodiment.

REFERENCES

Anzaldua, G. (1987). *Borderlands, La Frontera: The New Mestiza.* San Francisco: Spinsters/Aunt Lute.

Anzaldua, G. (1990). *Making Face, Making Soul: Creative and Critical Perspectives by Women of Color.* San Francisco: Aunt Lute.

Bartky, S. L. (1990). *Femininity and Domination: Studies in the Phenomenology of Oppression.* New York: Routledge.

Bourdieu, P. (1990). *The Logic of Practice.* Oxford: Polity Press.

Burt, R. (1995). *The Male Dancer: Bodies, Spectacle, Sexualities.* London: Routledge.

Burt, R. (2001). Dissolving in Pleasure: The Threat of the Queer Male Dancing Body. In Desmond, J. C. (Ed.). *Dancing Desires: Choreographing Sexualities On and Off the Stage.* Madison: University of Wisconsin Press.

Butler, J. (1990). *Gender Trouble: Feminism and the Subversion of Identity.* New York: Routledge.

Butler, J. (1993). *Bodies That Matter.* New York: Routledge.

Butler, R. (2005). *Slovoj Zizek: Live Theory.* London: Continuum.

Connell, R. W. (1995). *Masculinities.* Sydney: Allen and Unwin.

Davies, B. (2000). *(In)scribing Body/Landscape Relations.* Walnut Creek, CA: AltaMira Press.

DePalma, R., & Atkinson, E. (2008). *Invisible Boundaries: Addressing Sexualities Equality in Children's Worlds.* Stoke on Trent: Trentham.

Department of Education and Early Childhood Development Victoria. (2008). *Bullying.* [Retrieved 12/12/09 from http://www.education.vic.gov.au/school/parents/health/Pages/bully.aspx]

Department of Education and Early Childhood Development Victoria. (2014). *Unity through Diversity.* [Retrieved 07/30/14 from http://www.education.vic.gov.au/Documents/about/programs/cultures/unitydiversity.pdf]

Drummond, M. J. N. (2005). Listening to the Voices of Young Gay Men. *Men and Masculinities.* Vol 7, No 3, pp. 270–290.

Ducat, S. J. (2004). *Wimp Factor: Gender Gaps, Holy Wars, and the Politics of Anxious Masculinity.* Boston: Beacon Press.

Epstein, D., Kehily, M., Mac an Ghaill, M., & Redman, P. (2001). Making Masculinities and Femininities in School Playgrounds. *Men and Masculinities.* Vol 4, pp. 158–172.

Erskine, S. (2005). The Dancing Mind. *All in the Mind* with Natashia Mitchell, aired Saturday, 19 March 2005, ABC Science, Radio National, Australia. [Retrieved 15/01/10 from http://www.abc.net.au/rn/science/mind/stories/s1323547.htm]

Foster, S. L. (2001). Closets Full of Dances: Modern Dance's Performance of Masculinity and Sexuality. In Desmond, J. C. (Ed.). *Dancing Desires: Choreographing Sexualities On and Off the Stage.* Madison: University of Wisconsin Press.

Foucault, M. (1977). *Discipline and Punish: The Birth of the Prison.* London: Peregrine.

Foulkes, J. L. (2001). Dance Is for American Men: Ted Shawn and the Intersection of Gender, Sexuality and Nationalism in the 1930s. In Desmond, J. C. (Ed.). *Dancing Desires: Choreographing Sexualities On and Off the Stage.* Madison: University of Wisconsin Press.

Gard, M. (2003). Being Someone Else: Using Dance in Anti-oppressive Teaching. *Educational Review.* Vol 55, No. 2, pp. 211–223.

Gard, M. (2008) When a Boy's Gotta Dance: New Masculinities, Old Pleasures, *Sport, Education and Society.* Vol 12, No 2, pp. 181–193.

Gee, J. P. (2008). *Social Linguistics and Literacies: Ideology in Discourses.* London: Routledge.

Goffman, E. (1997). The Arrangement between the Sexes. *Theory and Society.* Vol 4, No 3, pp. 301–331.

Gorely, T., Holroyd, R., & Kirk, D. (2003). Muscularity, the Habitus and the Social Construction of Gender: Towards a Gender-Related Physical Education. *British Journal of Sociology of Education.* Vol 24, No 4, pp. 429–448.

Green, J. (2001). The Art and Nature of Gender. In Haynes, F., & McKenna, T. (Eds.). *Unseen Genders: Beyond the Binaries.* New York: Peter Lang.

hooks, b. (1994). *Teaching to Transgress.* New York: Routledge.

Kamler, B., Maclean, R., Reid, J., & Simpson, A. (1994). *Shaping Up Nicely: The Formation of Schoolgirls and Schoolboys in the First Month of School. A Report to the Gender Equity and Curriculum Reform Project Department of Employment, Education and Training (DEET).* Canberra: Deakin University.

Kaplan, M. (1966). *Essential Works of Pavlov.* New York: Bantam.

Kehily, J. (2002). *Sexuality, Gender and Schooling: Shifting Agendas in Social Learning.* London: Routledge.

Kimmel, M. (2009). Hostile High School Hallways. In Martino, W., Kehler, M. D., & Weaver-Hightower, M. (Eds.). *The Problem with Boys' Education.* Hoboken: Routledge.

Kosofsky Sedgwick, E. (1994). *Tendencies.* London: Routledge.

Kroeger, B. (2003). *Passing: When People Can't Be Who They Are.* New York: Public Affairs.

Lingard, B., Martino, W., & Mills, M. (2009). *Boys and Schooling: Beyond Structural Reform.* Basingstoke: Palgrave Macmillan.

Linne, R. (2003). Alternative Textualities: Media Culture and the Proto-Queer. *Qualitative Studies in Education*. Vol 16, No 5, pp. 669–689.
Mac an Ghaill, M. (1994). *The Making of Men: Masculinities, Sexualities and Schooling*. Buckingham: Open University Press.
Martino, W., & Pallotta-Chiarolli, M. (2001a). *Boys' Stuff*. Crows Nest: Allen and Unwin.
Martino, W., & Pallotta-Chiarolli, M. (2001b). Gender Performativity and Normalizing Practices. In Haynes, F., & McKenna, T. (Eds.). *Unseen Genders: Beyond the Binaries*. New York: Peter Lang.
Martino, W., & Pallotta-Chiarolli, M. (2005). *Being Normal Is the Only Way to Be*. Sydney: University of New South Wales Press.
Migdalek, J. (2003). *White Bred* (Theatre Piece). Melbourne: Chapel off Chapel.
Nayak, A., & Kehily, M.J. (1996). Playing It Straight: Masculinities, Homophobias and Schooling. *Journal of Gender Studies*. Vol 5, No 2, pp. 211–230.
Paechter, C. (2003a). Learning Masculinities and Femininities: Power/Knowledge and Legitimate Peripheral Participation. *Women's Studies International Forum*. Vol 26, No 6, pp. 541–552.
Paechter, C. (2003b). Masculinities and Femininities as Communities of Practice. *Women's Studies International Forum*. Vol 26, No 1, pp. 69–77.
Paechter, C. (2006). Reconceptualizing the Gendered Body: Learning and Constructing Masculinities and Femininities in School. *Gender and Education*. Vol 18, No 2, pp. 121–135.
Paechter, C. (2007). *Being Boys, Being Girls: Learning Masculinities and Femininities*. Berkshire: Open University Press.
Pascoe, C.J. (2007). *Dude, You're a Fag: Masculinity and Sexuality in High School*. Berkeley: University of California Press.
Pickering, M. (2001). *Stereotyping: The Politics of Representation*. Hampshire: Palgrave.
Plummer, D. (1999). *One of the Boys: Masculinity, Homophobia and Modern Manhood*. New York: Harrington Park Press.
Renold, E. (2005). *Girls, Boys and Junior Sexualities*. London: Routledge Falmer.
Robinson, H., Irwin, J., & Ferfolja, T. (2002). *From Here to Diversity: The Social Impact of Lesbian and Gay Issues in Education in Australia and New Zealand*. New York: Harrington Park Press.
Rogers, L. (1999). *Sexing the Brain*. London: Weidenfeld & Nicolson.
Savin-Williams, R.C. (2001). Memories of Same-Sex Attractions. In Kimmel, M.S., & Messner, M.A. (Eds.). *Men's Lives*. Boston: Allyn and Bacon.
Shilling, C. (2003). *The Body and Social Theory*. London: Sage.
Swain, J. (2004). The Resources and Strategies that 10–11-Year-Old Boys Use to Construct Masculinities in the School Setting. *British Educational Research Journal*. Vol 30, No 1, pp. 167–185.
Turner, B. (1984). *The Body and Society*. Oxford, UK: Basil Blackwell.
Young, I.M. (1990). *Throwing Like a Girl and Other Essays in Feminist Philosophy and Social Theory*. Indianapolis: Indiana University Press.
Zizek, S. (1999). *The Sublime Object of Ideology*. London: Verso.

7 Bodies Getting By

A QUESTION OF AGENCY

I now focus on the options that the individual not inclined to embody gender in socially prescribed ways may take in order to get by. While it can be argued that individuals have agency over their own behavior (Turner 1984, Connell 1995, Shilling 2003) and their own performances of self (Goffman 1959), I argue that even agency is conditioned to an extent by embedded (albeit invisible) ideological notions of gender that influence an individual's embodied habitus.

My body can be regarded as a choreographic *subject* affected by the ways in which it was socialized, regulated, and enculturated. At the same time, I have, and have always had, a degree of choreographic agency over my body. How I have operated and continue to operate as a choreographic *agent* is affected by ways of seeing and ways of doing that have come to feel right or wrong, appropriate or inappropriate, pleasurable or disagreeable. Where ways of seeing or doing become sedimented or fossilized, they are not easily upset or altered (Bourdieu 1990, Shilling 2003). The machinations of habitual states of mind and behavior—rendered invisible through not being conscious of them—delimit ways in which we not only *view* but also *do* embodiment.

In this chapter I chart and comment on my own experiences, socialization, and enculturation in regard to how I operated and continue to operate as an agent of my own actions. In addition to investigating my agency over my own embodiment and the ways in which I have 'gotten by', I will also investigate the ways in which I have operated as an agent over the embodiment of others as a director, choreographer, and teacher. While demonstrating that it felt both safe and comfortable to comply with mainstream norms of embodied performance of gender, I explore inequitable aspects of my own gender practices of which I was unaware.

SELF-REGULATION OF EMBODIED PERFORMANCE

As individuals we have the agency to perform the same choreography in different ways. I invite readers to consider the following piece of everyday 'coffee shop' choreography and ponder whether and why there are certain ways that you may *not* come to perform it.

> Step 1: How would you choose to stand? Are there ways that you would *not* choose to stand (feet together, wide apart, hip cocked, contrapposto, arms crossed, hand/s on thigh/s, hip/s, chest)? Why might any of these options be uncomfortable?

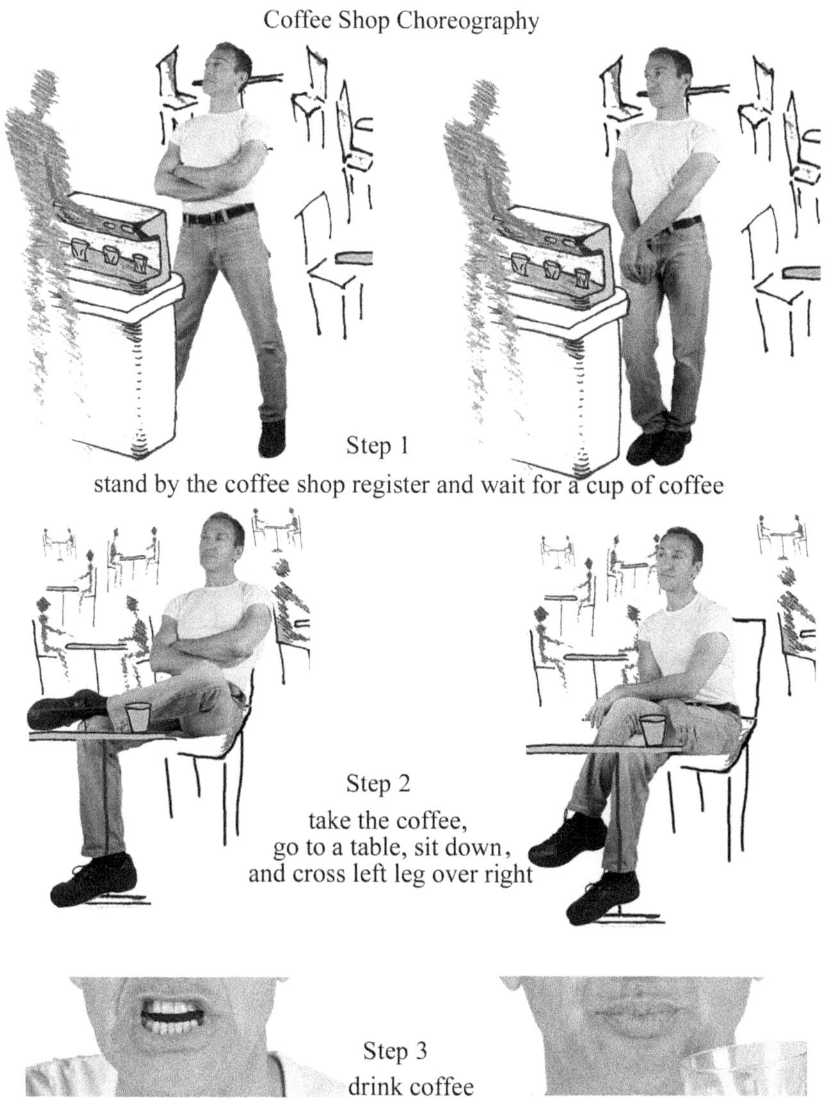

Figure 7.1 Coffee shop choreography. Photograph by Rob Chiarolli (www.photosthattell.com). Artwork by Jack Migdalek.

Step 2: How would you cross your left leg over the right? Are there ways you would *not* choose to cross your legs (knees neatly together, left foot broadly straddled over the right thigh)? Why/why not?

Step 3: In what ways would you sip and swallow? Are there ways in which you would *not* choose to drink (large/small mouthfuls, lips drawn together)? Why/why not?

I perform the 'coffee shop choreography' described above very frequently in my everyday life. While it is a performance that others might view, it is not a performance that I perform specifically for the attention of others. As far as I know, I do not perform the choreography in a feminine manner, despite having the agency to do so.

A theme that has repeatedly arisen in each chapter of this book is how the impact of choreography depends on the way it is performed. For example, it is not the *act* of ingesting coffee but the *manner* in which it is ingested that may make the performance come across as particularly masculine or feminine. The impression made by a performance that is masculine or feminine is also contingent on the biological sex of the performer. Sitting in a feminine manner signifies differently on a male body from the way it signifies on a female body.

Where a male or female is conscious that one's embodiment may draw negative attention, that person may choose to regulate his or her manner of performance in an attempt to go unnoticed. Where it may be physically comfortable to stand contrapposto in step #1 of the 'coffee shop choreography', I do not do so because I am conscious of negative ways in which males embodying in that manner in mainstream Western settings are perceived (see Plummer 1999, Martino & Pallotta-Chiarolli 2005). Choices made in the performance of choreography in the everyday, and the decisions made by directors, choreographers, and performers regarding how an action is to be performed on the stage, are likely to hinge on anticipation of how performances will be perceived. While performances on a stage are deliberately executed for the attention of an audience, there are performances in the everyday that, informed by external framing of how they might be perceived, are tempered so as *not* to draw attention. My self-consciousness about the attention I might draw should I perform the 'coffee shop choreography' in a feminine manner is the reason that I am deliberate about not performing it in that way.

OPTIONS AND STRATEGIES FOR GETTING BY

Using the example of embodying in mainstream everyday public settings, I consider my options as well as the costs and consequences of each, my options being to resist, to comply, or to negotiate. Through reflection on my own fears and experiences of transgressing social norms of gendered behavior, I argue that in the current climate, each of these options can be oppressive to the well-being of individuals whose inclination does not conform to norms of gendered behavior.

Resistance

In resisting, an individual would embody in ways that go against socially prescribed forms of embodiment for their biological sex. This may be done deliberately or unconsciously. As a male, were I to perform the 'coffee shop choreography' in a feminine manner it could be regarded as an act of resistance whereby my performance goes against norms of embodiment as prescribed within Western mainstream contexts. In my case, knowledge of negative outcomes suffered by males whose embodiment projects as feminine, such as verbal harassment or physical abuse, immediately comes to my mind. This knowledge comes from and is fueled by stories and incidents represented and presented in fiction, movies, television programs, and news reports, as well as hearsay from the experiences of friends.

Forms of resistance may be a means toward social change in favor of gender equity (J. Butler 1993, Connell 1995, Monro 2005). However, social change does not happen automatically, nor does it occur simply as a result of purely intellectual motivation (Shilling 2003). This implies that resistance against oppressive embodied gender norms should take a practical and embodied form. It may be that deliberately and courageously embodying in a feminine manner in mainstream public contexts will confront and challenge homophobic and gender conformist attitudes, leading to positive changes in the social mindset (Mac an Ghaill & Haywood 2007). I would like to be an agent toward social change by resisting mainstream norms and ceasing to police my body against the possibility of projecting feminine versions of myself. While I greatly admire those—such as queer activists—who have the courage to embody in resistance to mainstream norms, there are those like me who, on hearing and seeing the negativity that is dealt to those who do resist, are inclined to self-protect themselves from potential personal consequences. In other words, I fear consequences and repercussions should my performances of gender resist established norms of embodiment.

Compliance

As far as I am aware, my performances of the 'coffee shop' (and other everyday) choreography comply with norms of embodiment for males in mainstream Western cultures. Projecting this way makes me feel that I am unmarked and safe. Examining my own embodied behavior has made me conscious of how I regulate my embodiment in mainstream public settings. The way in which I stand, sit, and drink in various settings relates to my consciousness of my social and cultural location (Gee 2008). In settings where I am aware of potential non-acceptance and negative reactions, I self-regulate my embodiment in an attempt to ensure that as a male I do not stand out as a potential target of abuse, disapproval, alienation, or ridicule. If I find myself walking past a venue such as a mainstream public bar frequented predominantly by males, I am aware of making physical adjustments to my gait: I make my stride heavier; I hold my arms wider and further away from my body; I set my jaw and chin forward. "A sign for masculinity is a well-defined lower jaw" (Wex 1979, p. 9, see also Shilling 2003). Acting on panopticonic fear (Foucault 1977, Pallotta-Chiarolli 2010), I adjust my usual gait in this way in order to avoid the possibility of projecting as a feminine or homosexual male, which I have come to realize is a popular target of abuse. Knowledge of gay bashings and homophobic abuse can explain why males might actively avoid projecting as homosexual (Kirby & Hay 1997). It is ironic that displays other than sexual acts can define an individual's sexual orientation, when there are those whose performances of gender, be they consciously or unconsciously performed, contradict commonly understood modes of sexual expression. I find the use of reductionist definitions such as "homosexual behavior" (Taga 2005, p. 132, see also Kirby & Hay 1997, McKenna 2001) disheartening, especially when resorted to by queer theorists.

The threat of abuse, alienation, ostracism, or marginalization for those who fail to perform their gender in socially appropriate ways may cause acute consciousness of how one's body projects (J. Butler 1993, Shilling 2003). In contexts where I sense that projecting as anything but masculine may be unsafe for me, I try to pass (Kroeger 2003) so as not to be distinct from other males in that setting. As a male, I believe that I get by unharassed in public settings by not doing any of the following, despite having the agency and ability to do so: standing with legs close together and hips cocked, allowing my hips to sway from side to side when walking, sitting with one leg crossed closely and neatly over the other, pursing my lips, allowing my wrists to hang limply, gesticulating with limp wrists, drinking beverages in small sips, chewing food in small bites and with lips closed. Where individuals think they may be under surveillance and where they are aware of social consequences or penalties for behavior that is transgressive, it is likely that they will develop survival tactics, such as self-policing their behavior, in order to appear to fit in rather than stand out (Anzaldua 1990). Although I do not know how successfully I fit in, I am aware, in certain mainstream public settings, of consciously policing myself from embodying in ways that others might perceive to be feminine.

Continually complying in this way may impact on one's sense of self. Just as standing out will have consequences for the individual who embodies in ways that transgress social norms, so too will a lifetime of self-policing one's embodiment. Years spent editing out whole parts of oneself may cause depression, hostility, anxiety, and low self-esteem (Kroeger 2003). In my case, I believe that complying in this way was also, in a sense, empowering. It protected me from being singled out as sissy or effeminate and for the most part has made me feel safe.

Where an individual constructs or adopts masks, faces, personas, and identities as protective devices behind which to hide in order to avoid being singled out, rejected, oppressed, or marginalized for reasons of being different, this may be self-sabotaging in that an individual may lose a sense of self (Anzaldua 1987). Perpetually embodying gender in order to fit into valorized categories of male biology has had significant repercussions for my own sense of self. It has resulted in a dislocation from that part of my self that I experienced as feminine (discussed in the previous chapter) and the suffering of years of introversion and feelings of social isolation. Should males and females inclined to perform gender differently from prescribed norms wish to fit in, or not stand out, it may be to their social advantage to self-regulate and in effect colonize themselves (see Savigliano 1995). What concerns me is that through a lifetime of self-imposition of such control, the colonized individual—such as myself—may lose touch with their own inclinations, in my case embodied inclinations of femininity.

Relentless self-imposition of heteronormative embodied behavior must take a toll on an individual's embodied inclination. Indeed, I am so used to sitting, standing, walking, and gesticulating in certain safe ways that even when I know I can let my guard down, I continue for the most part to sit, stand, walk, and gesture in these ways, which are now my 'sitting, standing, walking, gesticulating habitus'. Where passing via embodied performance—such as masculine gait, deportment, and posture—becomes habitus, such non-consciously performed embodiment can impact and impede shifts or developments in how I may *desire* to project. Even if I desire to move (or allow myself to move) in a more feminine manner—as I believe I should be able to—feminine embodiment on my body feels foreign, odd, and uncomfortable.

Kroeger (2003) emphasizes that 'passing' can be a wondrous ability of being able to create and recreate the self, a way of achieving and fulfilling certain aspirations and advancement that hinge on social acceptance. She acknowledges that passing can be a means of avoiding conflict, danger, prejudice, discrimination, rejection, or undesirable outcomes (see also Anzaldua 1990, Butler 1990, Martino & Pallotta-Chiarolli 2001). My efforts to not project as feminine can be seen as trying to pass as masculine—and by default heterosexual—in order to avoid such conflict. My attempts at passing via my gait, stance, and physical disposition have not been a wondrous ability of being able to create and recreate the self but simply an effort not to be marked, not to stand out, to survive, be/feel safe, get by, and avoid undesirable outcomes.

Negotiation

In negotiating, an individual compromises in order to get along or get by. I regulate my body not to perform in a feminine manner in certain settings such as those that I sense may be potentially unsafe. This includes the majority of mainstream public contexts in which I find myself: a majority of streets, shops, restaurants, suburbs, schools, trains, and train stations. In these contexts I continue to be aware of negotiating my deportment to ensure that I do not project in a feminine manner. I am unaware of the same covert anxiety over my embodiment in settings that I regard to be safe, such as precincts, streets, and venues that are accepting of feminine embodiment on males. This knowledge occurs through witnessing transgressive embodiment on others within these settings that does not draw negative or aversive attention to the perpetrator. My sense in these settings is that I need not be anxious of the consequences should I project in feminine ways. Placing myself in 'safe' public settings makes it possible to let my guard down, meaning that I can temporarily drop vigilant self-policing of my embodiment of gender.

Where I operate differently according to context and setting I can be seen to be dwelling between or across borders (Anzaldua 1987, Pallotta-Chiarolli 2004), as described in Chapter 2. For me, negotiating how I embody between borders is a workable, though not always comfortable, situation. For example, being guarded about how or whether I kiss or embrace a platonic male friend differently according to setting/context can be strenuous and frustrating. While I might kiss and be kissed by platonic male friends in certain settings, there is a moment of contextual appraisal between us when we meet in other settings. During this moment we negotiate in a split second the form of greeting we will share: kiss, hug (with or without back-slap), smile, handshake, nod—all this in order to get by unharassed.

I am aware that it is possible to use my border-positioning to my advantage (Anzaldua 1987, Pallotta-Chiarolli 2004). However, I do not feel a sense of power or triumph when I pass unharassed as suitably masculine or heteronormative in mainstream public settings. I have had friends who, knowing of my research interests, comment that they had never found my gait, stance, or physical deportment to be feminine. To me, this indicated that I had successfully 'passed' (Kroeger 2003) as masculine. Although I was pleased to have passed, this was not helpful in coming to terms with feminine aspects of myself that I had so diligently suppressed for many years in many settings. I am so used to performing choreography such as the 'coffee shop choreography' in a particular non-feminine manner that even in settings in which alternative manners of performance feel acceptable and safe, my body is likely to perform according to what has become its usual 'non-feminine habitus'. I believe that that habitus has suppressed and overridden what may have been my feminine embodied inclination, an inclination that I am curious to explore, acknowledge, and reincorporate into the self, if that is still possible. Why I am unsure that this will be possible connects to embedded and repeating feelings of discomfort and distaste that I continue to experience on viewing males embodying in an effeminate manner, as well as continued experiences of self-consciousness and discomfort on performing feminine actions. Performing against my 'male embodied habitus' will be explored in the following chapter.

THEN AND NOW

Much of this chapter is based in and around my experiences and consciousness from when I was a boy growing up in the 1960s. I believe that despite some changes in social consciousness, the social pressures for a boy to fit in and get by are still forceful now, over forty years later. A participant in one of my fieldwork sessions expressed concerns for her twelve-year-old son, Allan, whose behavior and embodiment she defined as effeminate. Allan had initially not seemed to care what others thought of him. Here he can be seen to have resisted pressures to conform. However, it was reported that Allan had gradually became withdrawn and was self-conscious that he not project as effeminate.

> He's now much more aware of what he looks like . . . He was also very flamboyant . . . and now he's much quieter, and—he asks me how should I wear—does this look gay? So he's changing and—no matter what my husband and I do, it's the brothers "oh you're sitting like a girl" and it's his peers that he's really conscious of now, and he wasn't at all aware of before.

If an individual wants to fit in, he or she must conform or pass (Kroeger 2003) within the culture in which he or she must necessarily co-exist from day to day. Perhaps Allan had become conscious of what is at stake for the individual whose gendered embodied behavior is different from that of the majority of boys. In conforming he has chosen to comply with or negotiate normative male behavior in order to get by. What strikes me here is the desire not to project or be perceived as gay, even at this young age. My story and that of Allan are not dissimilar despite being almost forty years apart. As I grew older I also gave an increasing amount of credence to how I envisaged that others perceived me, and this led to endeavoring not to project as feminine, which—even before I was aware of social notions concerning homosexuality—I knew was not befitting of successful boys and men. As I became more aware that aspects of my embodiment were not in line with normative male behavior, my disposition faded from outgoing and confident to subdued and withdrawn. It seems that Allan is undergoing the same process, enforcing that in recent times too, effeminate embodiment on a male signifies homosexuality (Gard 2001, Gere 2001, Martino & Pallotta-Chiarolli 2001), and that being perceived to be gay continues to be an undesirable option.

SCAR-TISSUE

Despite my enculturation I think—and understand—that it is and should be fine for a male to embody in a feminine manner. However, when I see a male with a mincing gait or disposition, I often feel a sense of discomfort. I believe that this discomfort occurs because of a resurfacing of something of the way I used to think—and understand—that males should embody. I define this phenomenon as 'scar-tissue'. It is possible to parallel the scars of former perspectives that have been discarded to phantom sensations or scars left where something has been removed. At times, a phantom sensation of a previous condition can pervade or surface. So too, sometimes, something of discarded perspectives resurfaces.

I believe that scar-tissue is the forceful manifestation of discourses, ideologies, and experiences of an individual's past onto an individual's present. I define 'scar-tissue' as that which continues to affect the way we react to, read, or perceive things, even after our minds have altered or changed their ways of seeing, reading, or understanding. The concept of scar-tissue can be used to explain how being in certain embodied positions, or seeing certain embodied performances, may still feel or read as discomforting, despite one's

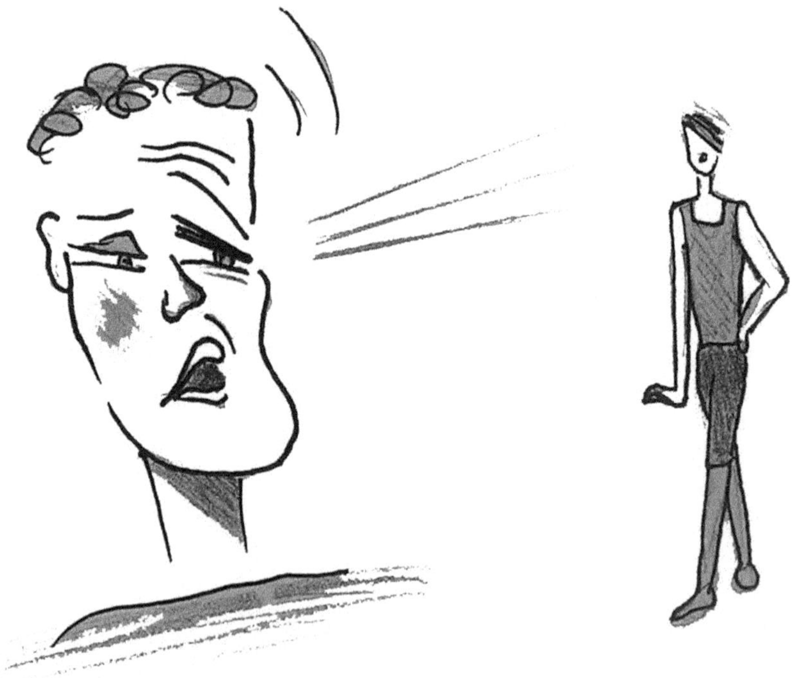

Figure 7.2 Double take. Artwork by Jack Migdalek.

current mindset or logic that may interpret or perceive such performances as acceptable. What follows is a contextualizing of scar-tissue with reference to Bourdieu's theories of habitus and taste in relation to how scar-tissue can impact on the perception and performance of gendered embodiment.

Scar-Tissue and Habitus

Bourdieu (1990) theorizes about habitus as non-consciously performed practices that manifest in forms of perception or physical action. These I will refer to as non-conscious ways of *seeing/perceiving* and non-conscious ways of *doing/performing*. An example of *seeing/perceiving* embodiment according to gendered habitus might be to perceive the graceful, dainty chewing of food with lips closed as being ladylike. An example of *doing/performing* embodiment according to gendered habitus might be for a male to walk with broad masculine strides.

That habitus is non-conscious implies that individuals do not have agency over it. Indeed, its very invisibility limits what one can say and see (Threadgold 1994). However, habitus can change, sometimes through osmosis, but also through individual agency or will (Schirato & Yell 1996). To illustrate, when I lived as a foreign resident in Japan, I came to control or hold back some aspects of my native habitus. It had been my habitus to wink at people in friendly interactive situations. It was brought to my attention that within the Japanese culture my wink was being construed as flirtatious. Aware of the tension between my habitual embodied behavior and how it was being interpreted, I attempted to revise my winking habitus, and in time succeeded. To affect change through agency or will is conditional on becoming conscious of one's habitus and having the desire or compulsion to affect change (Migdalek 2002). A *diagnosis* of the scar-tissue connected with revising gender-related habitual ways of seeing/perceiving and doing/performing follows.

1) revising habitual ways of *seeing/perceiving:*
   It is my habitus to cringe whenever I see the embodied performance of women boxing. I may become conscious of and question my habitus through coming to know that women can be physically strong and powerful. This may bring about a desire to revise or affect my 'seeing/perceiving women boxing habitus' in order to no longer cringe when I see women box.
2) revising habitual ways of *doing/performing:*
   It is my habitus to surrender my seat to women on public transport. I may become conscious of and question my habitus through coming to know that most women on public transport are capable of standing. This may bring about a desire to revise or affect my 'doing/performing standing for women on public transport habitus' and to no longer perform the action for able-bodied women.

Disposing of one form of habitus—be it a seeing/perceiving habitus or a doing/performing habitus—may result in a further non-conscious habitus: (1) habitus of being able to watch women boxing without cringing, and (2) habitus of not standing for women on public transport.

Scar-tissue comes into the equation where a discomfort or dis-ease is triggered that sees the resurfacing of old ways of perceiving or performing. This can occur even when one has come around to operating according to a revised or changed habitus. For example:

1) scar-tissue impacting on habitual ways of *seeing/perceiving:*
I may be used to the idea that women can and do perform the sport of boxing. However, years of 'knowing/perceiving' that it was not a women's sport will sometimes impact, in the form of scar-tissue, on my reaction to seeing women pursuing the activity in ways that watching males boxing does not. At such times it may strike me that the sport is 'unwomanly'.
2) scar-tissue impacting on habitual ways of *doing/performing:*
I may know that unless a woman is frail or weak, women are physically capable of standing on public transport. However, years of perceiving that males should stand for women continue to impact, in the form of scar-tissue, on my new habitus of not surrendering my seat to able-bodied females. At such times I will experience twinges of embodied discomfort when I do not stand up for a woman who does not have a seat.

Once one is fully acclimatized to a new or revised perception or practice, new habitual ways of viewing/doing may establish themselves and eventually become a new habitus. Although a change has occurred, I contend that the scar-tissue of how that practice used to be performed or perceived may pervade or surface from time to time. So pervasive are past memories and experiences that it is possible that scar-tissue will surface when triggered in certain ways. Threadgold (1994) claims that when a body is re-placed in postures, then thoughts, feelings, and states of mind associated with that posture are recalled. In this way, what is sometimes triggered when I find myself sitting with my legs neatly crossed in a way that I used to understand to be 'ladylike' is scar-tissue of what that practice used to mean. What is sometimes triggered when I see a male embodying in a feminine manner is scar-tissue of what that practice used to mean to me, in addition to my kinesthetic sense of how as a male I would feel performing or being perceived to perform that action.

Where we perform or perceive according to habitus it is ordinarily a non-conscious phenomenon and, as a result, not discomforting. However, where scar-tissue surfaces, one becomes conscious of and uncomfortable about what one is perceiving or embodying. While it may be possible for habitus to be consciously held back, revised, or modified (Schirato &

Yell 1996) it is not possible to affect, hold off, or override sensations of scar-tissue.

Scar-Tissue and Taste

Taste is the perception of that which is agreeable. It does not operate at the level of consciousness and is dependent on one's social location (Bourdieu 1990, Turner 1992, Shilling 2003). Taste directly impacts on the way we come to value, favor, or disfavor certain performances. In many cases these values and performances are gendered. My use of the term 'scar-tissue' relates to taste as regards the impact of habitual, ingrained, non-conscious ways of seeing or perceiving on my consciousness of embodiment, in and through my own body as well as the bodies of others. For example, the habitus I acquired through the cultures/fields in which I was raised did not include any gentle physical male to male contact (apart from situations of ill health and old age). In regard to taste, gentle physical male to male contact was painted in a negative light as something comic or deviant. The first time I witnessed men gently embrace I was not a comfortable observer. Despite my desire to do so, the first times I was embraced by another male were not comfortable experiences. This discomfort still resurfaces within certain settings. Despite change in one's mindset, one may still non-consciously slip back into ingrained, embedded, formerly habitual ways of perceiving.

Scar-tissue directly relates to one's past taste. Even though an individual's knowledge, mindset, or attitude may change, one's taste may not be so easily or instantly malleable. For example, even though my present mindset holds that it is fine for a male to embody in a feminine manner, my reaction when I see a male embodying in a dainty manner is that it is unattractive. This negative reaction is reflective of my taste as informed and developed according to my social and cultural location in my formative years. Much as I desire not to find such embodiment distasteful, and much as I can intellectualize that feminine embodiment on a male is just as aesthetic as masculine embodiment, sedimented taste is not easily altered.

The following instances, in which scar-tissue is triggered by embodied performances, illustrate how previous ways of seeing/perceiving continue to impact on and disrupt my current ways of seeing/perceiving: seeing a female with underarm hair continues to stand out differently to me than seeing a male with underarm hair despite knowing that underarm hair is part of the biology of both male and female bodies; seeing males dancing in a feminine and sultry manner continues to stand out differently to me than seeing females doing the same thing despite knowing that able-bodied males are capable of moving in this manner.

The following instances, in which scar-tissue is triggered by embodied performances, illustrate how previous ways of doing/performing continue to impact on and disrupt my current ways of doing/performing: I tend to feel awkward and uncomfortable when dancing in another male's arms, especially in mainstream public contexts (through my enculturation, the notion of males dancing together was perceived as deviant); the act of sitting with legs neatly crossed feels awkward and unnerving, especially in mainstream public contexts, for reasons pertaining to years of self-policing myself not to sit in this manner and to my understanding of how men should not sit.

Scar-tissue can be inhibiting. The discomforts that the accumulative resurfacing of scar-tissue arouses may inhibit how individuals allow themselves to accept or appreciate the embodiment of gender of others, as well as inhibiting ways in which they embody, or desire to embody, themselves. Scar-tissue is a symptom. Social pressures that lead one to perceive or perform in certain ways are the cause. Tackling the cause and exposing perceptions and taste as socially constructed impositions that affect how we view and perform embodied activity is an avenue that needs to be pursued in order to perceive and perform gender with less restriction. This will be discussed and investigated in subsequent chapters.

I end the discussion of scar-tissue and taste with a snapshot of a recent scar-tissue episode, the personal discomfort of which remains vivid in my mind: I was visiting some friends one day. Their young son, aged nine, asked if he could perform for us. Out came a CD player, and the boy sang along to Kylie Minogue's *Can't Get You Out of My Head*. As he did so, he moved his body in a slinky and feminine manner, not dissimilarly to Kylie herself. I was taken aback and was very uncomfortable watching this performance, unlike the boy's parents, who appeared to find it cute.

My discomfort upon watching the young boy's performance is tied up with and confused by scar-tissue. I believe it illustrates how my habitual ways of seeing/perceiving continue to impact on and interfere with my current ways of perceiving. This episode reflects the pervasive nature of old and fossilized remnants of taste that had become my habitual way of seeing.

In my opinion, the boy had 'negotiated' where and when and before whom he felt he could perform this. He may not have done so at school or before others. For me, however, the young boy's actions contrasted sharply with the multitude of normative images of male bodies in pose, repose, and action that I have been exposed to through my life, both in formal performance arenas and in the everyday. The boy's performance was aligned with performances that in my experience and enculturation are performed by females. Despite a change in my mindset that would have argued for a male's right to embody in any way, and despite being in the company of the boy's parents, who were relaxed about their son's performance, I still experienced major discomfort at the boy's feminine embodiment. This reiterates my previous point that the strength of scar-tissue in the form of gut reactions to what we may see (or perform) is not simple to erase or ignore. Despite my ability to reason about the boy's right to move and choreograph his body in any way it could physically move, something of my ingrained ways of reading (my scar-tissue) resurfaced, signaling to me that this embodied performance was

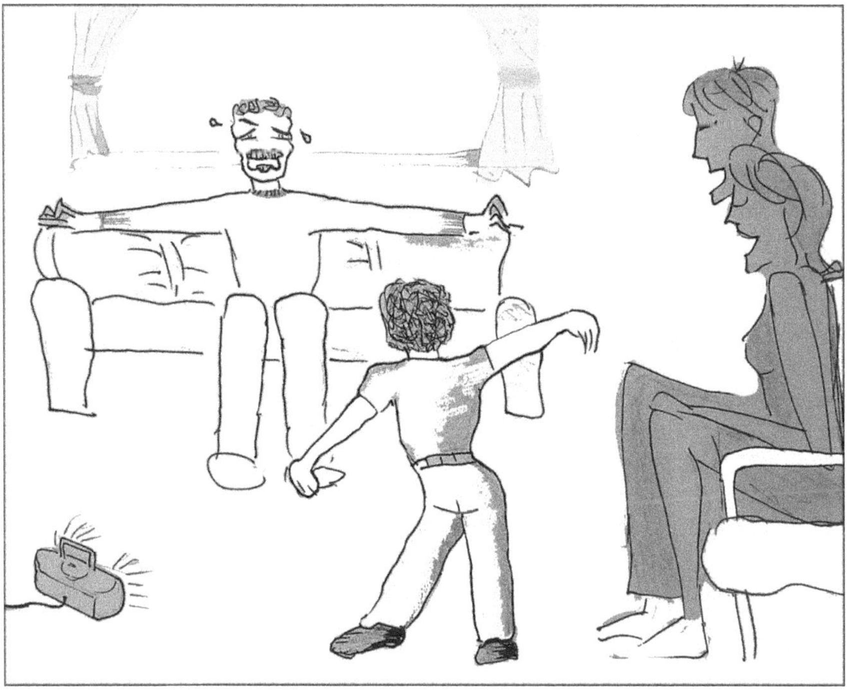

Figure 7.3 Look at me. Artwork by Jack Migdalek.

not suitable for a male. I imagine I would also have felt uncomfortable seeing a small girl perform the same vampy, suggestive motions, but for reasons connected to age and maturity and not biological sex.

As a gay man who has spent a lifetime self-policing his embodiment, I am aware of how feminine embodiment in a male can be the brunt of humor, pity, scorn, and discrimination. It saddens me to think that a young boy's embodiment may lead to him being singled out in these ways. My feelings are those of compassion and empathy concerning the social consequences that a young boy will be subject to if he embodies in this manner. Given all that has been argued concerning social conditioning and the social construction of gender in previous chapters, it is doubtful that my finding such embodiment distasteful is a 'natural' response that is discrete from my socialization and enculturation.

TAKING UP DANCE AND THEATRE

In the previous chapter I investigated how my enculturation positioned my male body against transgression of masculine forms of embodiment and against the idea of embodying in a feminine manner. I now explain and explore how and why I took up theatre and dance, occupations that in the Western world are commonly perceived to be effeminate (Burt 1995, Foster 2001, Cohan 2002, Gard 2003a, Buchbinder 2004, Stoneley 2007, Fisher & Shay 2009, Hanna 2010). Taking up these activities came about through my own agency, as did finding ways to make these chosen activities/occupations accepted and acceptable.

My parents had a respect and appreciation for the arts and regularly took my sister and me along to cultural events, including theatre, which I loved. My parents were keen to have us appreciate and experience performance arts and fine arts. However, they did not conceive or desire that either of us might consider the arts as a livelihood or full-time practice. I knew from an early age that I wanted to be involved in theatre. My initial involvement came through participating in performance activities in school and in a youth movement that my parents sent me to. The options of attending drama or dance classes were not offered to me by my parents. At the age of about fourteen I asked my parents if I could join Saturday morning drama classes, which they allowed me to do. My doing drama as a hobby did not bother my parents. However, I was aware that they would not have wanted me to pursue it beyond that. They did not regard the theatre as a stable profession, especially for a male, who according to their aspirations for me—and their cultural assumptions of gender roles—would need to support a family. They never implied that they saw the profession as an effeminate pastime, just as a pastime that was unstable and not secure. I got messages that the profession was an effeminate pastime for males from other sources such as peers and the mass media.

Looking back, I realize that I contrived ways that I might enter the world of theatre so as not to evoke the disapproval of my parents. First, I decided that I wanted to be a set designer and aspired to do so through becoming an architect, a profession that I knew my parents would find respectable. I did not want to study physics (a pre-requisite for architecture) and soon found another avenue. I decided to become an English teacher as I discovered a teaching college in my city that offered a double major of English with drama. Becoming a teacher was also a profession that would meet with my parents' approval.

Drama students at my college were to take contemporary dance during the first year of study. My male body was lean and flexible, and the dance staff at my college gave me plenty of encouragement and support. I loved what I was learning and undertook dance as a third major. Gradually I ventured beyond the contemporary dance classes offered at the college and took ballet and jazz classes too. In all of these dance styles my body was trained and choreographed to move in ways that were not feminine. I became proficient and realized that this could be an entrée into professional music theatre. By this stage my parents were placated that at least I would have English teaching to fall back on. I was also able to boost the social and physical capital of my dance training by trading on my fitness and taking part-time work in a gym as an aerobics instructor. This embodiment was an obvious demonstration of muscularity and physical power that served to make the dance training I was undertaking more worthy of respect and less suspect.

My enculturation did not promote males entering the world of theatre. Transgressing my enculturation and entering that world was at my instigation and involved agency and self-regulation. Ironically, while I may have transgressed my enculturation and entered the world of mainstream theatre as an agent of my own actions, it was a world that had its own strict preferences in regard to male embodiment that I would never have thought to transgress at the time.

THE DANCER/ACTOR AND/OR CHOREOGRAPHER/DIRECTOR AS AGENT

I believe that the process of induction into performance arts practices can blind the would-be performance arts practitioner to inherent gendered aspects of their performance arts heritage. This induction is in turn likely to exert an influence on work that the performance arts practitioner might create. To illustrate, the following sub-sections briefly chart my own experience as a dancer/actor and choreographer/director in formal performance arts arenas. Despite my agency in these roles over my own body and the bodies of others, I was ignorant of the machinations of my directorial or choreographic habitus. As already raised in the previous chapter, the way in which I cast, directed, and choreographed my own male body, as well as the bodies of male and female actors/dancers, was significantly shaped by the casting, direction, and choreography that I, through a lifetime of exposure to and experience of mainstream examples, perceived and took for granted as appropriate to male and female bodies. Inherent gendered ways in which I cast, directed, and choreographed male and female bodies felt appropriate, natural, and also tasteful to me and came to be my 'directorial-choreographic habitus'.

I was well aware that males performing in a feminine manner elicited laughter or sniggers from mainstream audiences, just as in many cases females embodying in a masculine manner did too. Drawing on my growing kinesthetic experience, knowledge, and aesthetic sensibility of dance and drama, I did not direct or choreograph males to move in a feminine manner unless it was to project as comic, ludicrous, or strange. It never occurred to me why female bodies that I choreographed and directed to move in a feminine manner did not project in these ways.

Directing and Choreographing Dancers

An early experience of choreographing bodies took place in the 1980s, when I and a female friend choreographed our own male and female bodies to perform weekly at a popular Melbourne discotheque (Migdalek 2014). How we choreographed our bodies was informed not only by the ways in which our own male and female dancer bodies had been trained and choreographed by others but also by what we perceived that our employers and audiences wanted and expected of us. Our personal agency as choreographers worked in tandem with social controls and mechanisms. We operated according to our 'male/female dancer habitus': female embodying in a feminine manner, male embodying in a masculine manner. As testimony to habitus being non-conscious (Bourdieu 1990) it never occurred to us to move our bodies any differently.

Together with two other dancers, I choreographed and performed in a national and state funded dance education company that toured to Australian public and private schools during the 1980s (Migdalek 2014). Our company included two male dancers and one female dancer. I recall how we deliberately choreographed and directed our male bodies so as not to move in a soft or feminine manner. We wanted to be received favorably and also wanted our audiences to respect the notion of males dancing. Aware that males performing in a feminine manner were received negatively or as objects of suspicion or ridicule by mainstream audiences (Burt 1995, Foster 2001, Gard 2003b, 2006), we aimed, like many male dancers before us, to alleviate anxieties around how audiences might read our masculinity and sexuality as male performance artists (Burt 1995, Gard 2001, 2006, Buchbinder 2004). Therefore, much of the choreography we created for the two males in the company was hyperathletic and hypermasculine, involving expansive steps that took power, space, and a high degree of athleticism. Any physical contact between the male dancers in our choreography was athletic and robust. I recognize that we also imbued our action with extra vigor and aggression in the substantial number of schools visited where we sensed and feared that students may have come to the performance with hostility to the notion of males dancing.

On the whole, our choreography was effective in that our performances were positively accepted. Retrospectively, I realize that we were playing into notions of male dance being accessible and acceptable only when perceived as a highly athletic feat on a par with sports (Burt 1995, Foster 2001, Gard 2001, Gorely et al. 2003, Risner 2007). Tactics such as these were evident in the political agenda of the 1950s and 1980s television specials *Dancing: A Man's Game,* choreographed by and featuring Gene Kelly, and *Dance Is a Man's Sport Too,* choreographed by Twyla Tharp (both produced by Omnibus), which aimed to parallel the pursuits of sport and dance and dispel stigmas of effeminacy that clung to the latter (Keefe 2009). The male dancer posited as an athlete or sportsperson denies the male dancer as artist who might also move delicately or perform with great sensitivity (Gard 2006). In trying to get by as male dancers, we worked directly toward combating students' gendernormative preconceptions of dance. However, in doing so, we denied the artistry, validity, and aesthetic qualities of male bodies that might also move in a soft, gentle, delicate, or feminine manner.

Our highly self-conscious effort to legitimize dance as a suitable pursuit for a male was not without cost. My male body—as well as the male bodies on whom I came to choreograph—became further distanced from the notion of male bodies performing motion that was delicate and graceful.

Moving in such ways was regarded as effeminate and associated with homosexuality. It was an exhausting charter to keep proving to others that

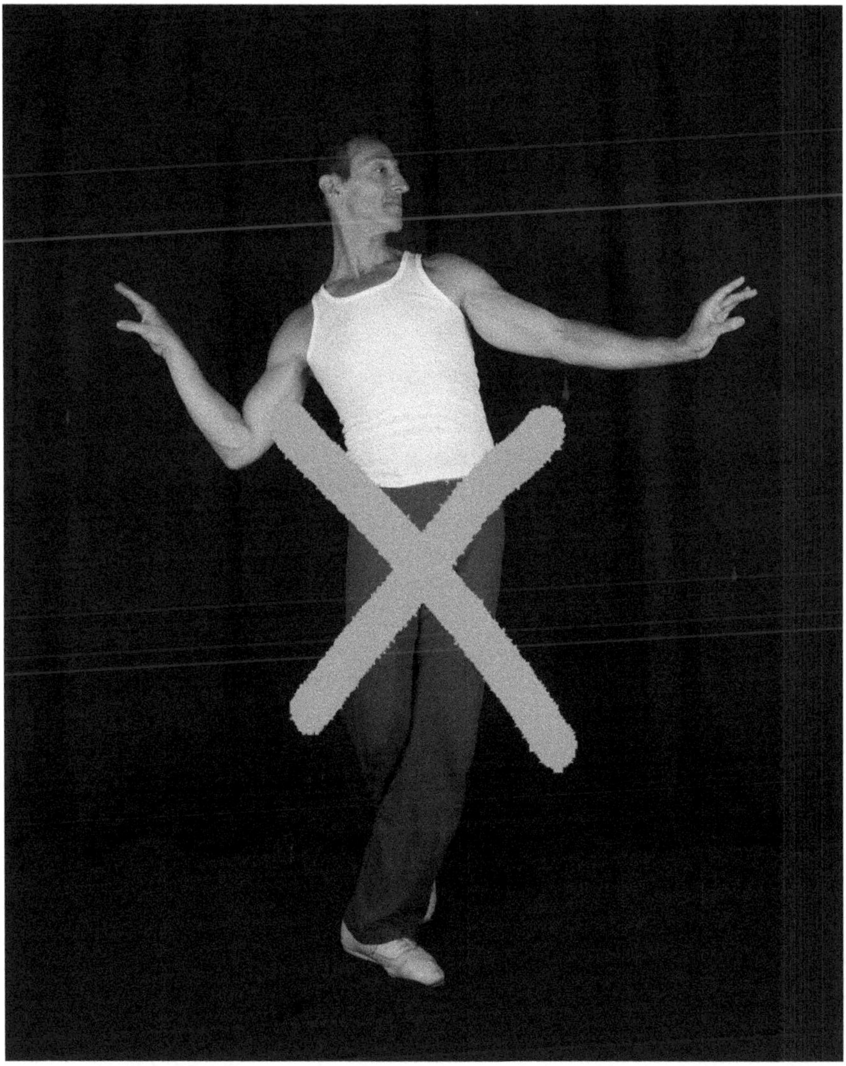

Figure 7.4 Feminine demeanor. Photograph by Rob Chiarolli (www.photosthattell.com).

dance, through its very athleticism, could be seen as an appropriately masculine pursuit for males, while all the time negating and neglecting the possibilities of ever moving in ways that might be deemed feminine.

In addition to choreographing for the stage, I taught jazz classes for adults at dance studios, fitness establishments, and community centers. As is often the case, most of the students who attended were female. I would prepare routines in advance of classes, and I recall how I automatically adjusted these whenever males joined my class. Where choreography may have been slinky and feminine, I adjusted it to be performed with straighter lines, a wider stance, more force, and less fluid hip and shoulder motion. I did so because I presumed that moving in the feminine manner of the choreography as I had intended to teach it would be uncomfortable and unbecoming for male students to execute (Migdalek 2014). To my culturally constructed and habitual ways of perceiving, a male dancing in a feminine manner was unattractive and un-aesthetic. Strangely, whereas performing in a feminine manner on stage before a viewing audience caused me discomfort and anxiety (as articulated in the previous chapter), playing into existing gendered norms and choreographing/teaching this style of movement to females in the context of a dance studio did not.

Directing and Choreographing Actors

The romantic male lead in Rogers and Hammerstein's musical *Oklahoma,* Curly, is a farm-dweller who in the course of two acts woos, wins, and fights for his love, Laurie. It can be argued that the character of Curly has both feminine and masculine personality traits: he is firm and resolute but also sentimental and romantic. As the curtain rises on *Oklahoma* (first produced on the stage in 1943, for the screen in 1955, and for DVD in 2003), Curly enters the stage (a meadow) and sings the ballad *Oh What a Beautiful Morning*. The sentiment of the song, proclaiming that "all the sounds of the earth are like music", is that of a daydreamer: reflective, romantic, optimistic. As a director, it is likely that I would have directed the character of Curly, at some stage while singing this song, to straddle his foot on a haystack or tree stump while leaning his forearm on his elevated thigh. Directing the character of this heterosexual romantic hero in this arguably masculine way would have seemed normal and would have come to me 'naturally', even though it should be appropriate for Curly to embody in both or either feminine or masculine manners. Why not direct the character delivering these thoughtful and sensitive lyrics to stand with one foot placed in front of the other and tilting his head toward the sky with hands over his heart?

Given my exposure to norms of embodiment for heterosexual male leading characters in conventional musicals and dramas, it is unlikely to occur to me to direct the body of the romantic male lead in ways other than masculine. Were I to direct the character to embody in a feminine manner, he may not come across to audiences as a strong, resilient character that would

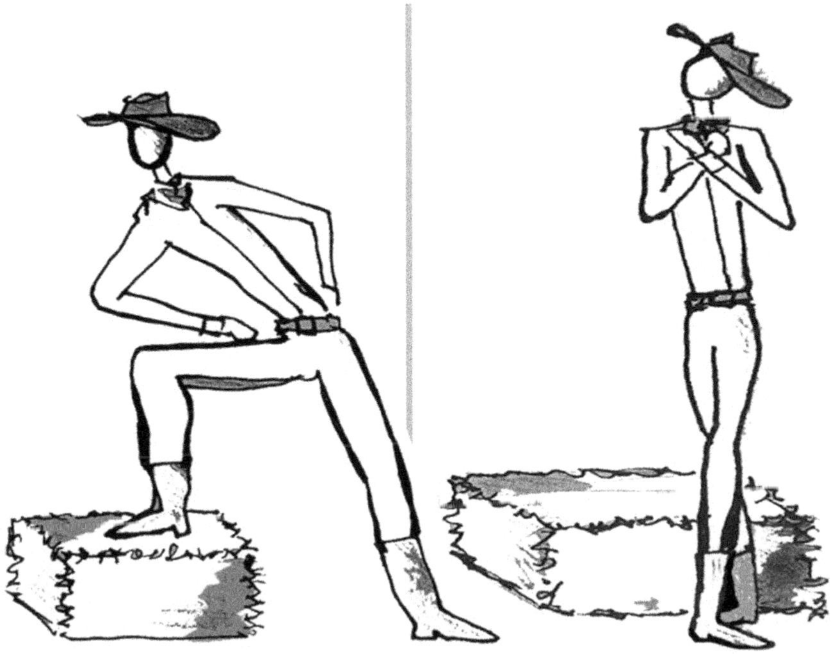

Figure 7.5 Cowboy character. Artwork by Jack Migdalek.

stand up for himself. More to the point, he may not come across to audiences as heterosexual.

I found employment choreographing and directing plays and musicals for professional, community, and youth theatre groups. In choreographing production numbers in musicals and other theatre performances, my choreography would invariably be different for male and female bodies. I choreographed in line with socially established ways in which males may acceptably dance (Buchbinder 2004, Gard 2006), norms wherein male bodies support and lead female bodies and move powerfully with straddled legs and splayed hands. Although I may sometimes have choreographed female dancers to move strongly and powerfully, I never choreographed male dancers to move delicately or femininely. This was not a mindful practice but a habitual one. Breaking from it risks the chance of producing work that will not have mainstream appeal. As such, it would impede my further employment as director or choreographer for mainstream audiences.

In directing plays and musicals, I cast and directed the roles of male and female characters very much in line with already established stereotypical gender conforming patterns. Generally, the deportment of lead romantic male roles would be strong and masculine; the deportment of lead romantic female roles would be graceful and feminine. On the other hand, I realized

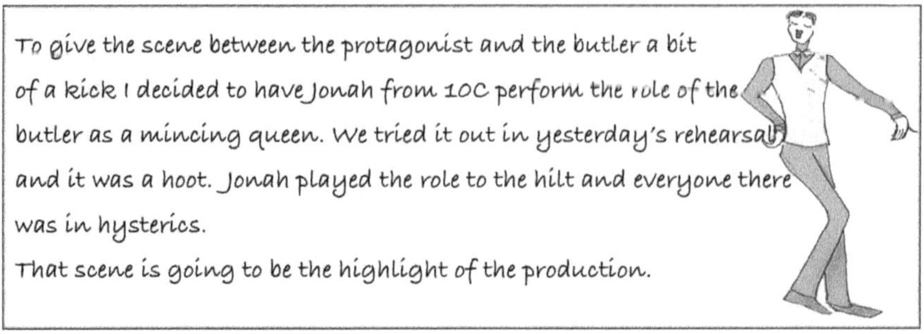

Figure 7.6 Director's journal entry (fictional). Artwork by Jack Migdalek.

that directing comic or oddball male and female supporting roles to embody against gendered norms of embodiment evoked audience laughter, which as a commercial director was often what I desired. Lightweight supporting male roles could be played to comic effect by having actors playing those roles embody in a feminine manner; lightweight supporting female roles could be played to comic effect by having actors playing those roles embody in a masculine manner. In casting and directing roles in this way, master-signifiers, such as that which is understood to be romantic, straight, or normal, become more fixed because of how they contrast with that which is understood to be comical, oddball, or queer (see Zizek 1999, R. Butler 2005)

Individuals sitting among audiences who laugh and guffaw at characters whose embodiment goes against conventional norms of gender can glean that those who embody in these ways, both on stage and in the everyday, are to be regarded as objects of amusement.

REINFORCING OPPRESSIVE GENDER NORMS OF EMBODIMENT

It is at this point in my life that I question the force and ideology with which my habitual ways of perceiving have set what I find to be tasteful and tasteless, aesthetic and un-aesthetic (Migdalek 2014). My habitual ways of perceiving have guided and shaped what became my 'directorial and choreographic habitus'. It was experiences such as consciously adjusting my choreography whenever male students came to my dance classes that highlight for me how embedded my gendered notions were of 'suitable' movement for male as opposed to female bodies. Choreographing and teaching females and males to move in distinctively different ways serves to perpetuate and reinforce the notion of females moving in a feminine manner and males moving in a masculine manner as normal. The recurring theme that arises here is that where males and females moving in these ways come across, in the mainstream, as aesthetic, popular, or normal, they serve to mark transgressions of these norms as marked and/or remarkable performances that come to project as tasteless, un-aesthetic, comic, tragic, ugly, or other.

Retrospectively, I realize that my choreography and direction of male bodies (as illustrated by my hypothetical direction of the character of Curly in *Oklahoma*) adhered to and reinforced notions of male embodiment and characterization being heterosexual or 'normal' only when perceived as masculine. An abundance of representations such as these serve to delimit the range of options by which the male dancer or actor, who might move delicately or femininely, can operate or define himself.

It is ironic and frustrating to me that my directorial habitus operated in such gender conforming ways given that my own embodied inclination and tendencies as a youngster tended to be gender non-conforming. Gender conforming ways by which I came to operate are testimony to the force of my social conditioning. The ways in which I came to direct and choreograph male and female bodies simply reinforced oppressive gender norms that had themselves been oppressive to me. I believe that other directors and choreographers—even liberal minded ones who might hate to think of themselves as gendered—also do so unwittingly. Even though directors, choreographers, and casting directors may be agentic, embedded habitual ways in which they *do* and *view* male and female bodies are so ingrained that they are likely to be unaware of how these affect the ways in which they perceive, cast, direct, and choreograph the bodies on whom they work. These agents' casting, direction, and choreography of bodies in mainstream performance arenas such as cinema, theatre, and television are likely to have an effect on the minds and bodies of those who see their works. Where these agents predominantly cast, direct, and choreograph male characters who embody in a feminine manner as marginal, oddball, comic, or deviant, such representations are likely to affect how audiences perceive males who embody in a feminine manner in the everyday. These representations are also likely to affect how males in the everyday may monitor and self-police their own embodiment to ensure that they are not perceived similarly.

My directorial and choreographic habitus grew out of what I had come to see as 'normal' embodiment for male and female bodies. I believe that I would not have continued to get employment directing and choreographing for mainstream audiences had I transgressed the gendered norms that seemed so natural to me, apart from where I did so for comic effect. In order to work in the mainstream and to earn a living from their art, performance arts practitioners are in a bind. If one wants one's work to be successful and appreciated by mainstream audiences, then it is a bind that is difficult to operate against. Although I still admire much about mainstream theatre, I am no longer financially dependent on an income from working in that area. This makes it possible for me to create, direct, and choreograph performance art in ways that I had not previously had the opportunity or dared. Indeed, in the theatrical work I have produced since 2003, I have been much warier of the presence and workings of my gendered enculturation and habitus, as well as the relationship between personal control, theatrical conventions, and social influences on the material that I produce.

In this chapter I have considered strategies by which individuals inclined to transgress mainstream gendernormative modes of embodiment may get by. I have also focused on the effects and impacts of the habitual ways that we come to operate in various cultural contexts and settings. A recurring theme that has arisen is the social, emotional, and physical vulnerability of those whose performance inclination is not aligned with socially prescribed gender norms of embodiment, and the need to safeguard these persons from marginalization or alienation. There is a need for social change wherein diverse or multiple expressions of masculinity and femininity are permissible (Connell 1995, Martino & Pallotta-Chiarolli 2001, Monro 2005, Paechter 2006). The following chapter is concerned with how such social change in regard to the embodiment of masculinity and femininity might come about and how, for the individual, pressure to comply, the fear of standing out, and/or the force of 'scar-tissue' may be diminished.

REFERENCES

Anzaldua, G. (1987). *Borderlands, La Frontera: The New Mestiza.* San Francisco: Spinsters/Aunt Lute.

Anzaldua, G. (1990). *Making Face, Making Soul: Creative and Critical Perspectives by Women of Color.* San Francisco: Aunt Lute.

Bourdieu, P. (1990). *The Logic of Practice.* Oxford: Polity Press.

Buchbinder, D. (2004). *The Sign of the Dancing Men: Negotiations of Masculinity in Film Musicals.* (Conference Presentation). Masculinities: Gender, Art and Popular Culture Symposium, The University of Melbourne. [Retrieved 4/4/06 from www.art-museum.unimelb.edu.au/events_transcripts]

Burt, R. (1995). *The Male Dancer: Bodies, Spectacle, Sexualities.* London: Routledge.

Butler, J. (1990). *Gender Trouble, Feminism and the Subversion of Identity.* New York: Routledge.

Butler, J. (1993). *Bodies That Matter.* New York: Routledge.

Butler, R. (2005). *Slovoj Zizek: Live Theory.* London: Continuum.

Cohan, S. (2002). 'Feminizing' the Song-and-Dance Man: Fred Astaire and the Spectacle of Masculinity in the Hollywood Musical. In Cohan, S. (Ed.). *Hollywood Musicals: The Film Reader.* New York: Routledge.

Connell, R.W. (1995). *Masculinities.* Sydney: Allen and Unwin.

Fisher, J., & Shay, A. (2009). *When Men Dance: Choreographing Masculinity across Borders.* New York: Oxford University Press.

Foster, S.L. (2001). Closets Full of Dances: Modern Dance's Performance of Masculinity and Sexuality. In Desmond, J.C. (Ed.). *Dancing Desires: Choreographing Sexualities On and Off the Stage.* Madison: University of Wisconsin Press.

Foucault, M. (1977). *Discipline and Punish: The Birth of the Prison.* London: Peregrine.

Gard, M. (2001). Dancing around the 'Problem' of Boys and Dance. *Discourse: Studies in the Cultural Politics of Education.* Vol 22, No 2, pp. 212–225.

Gard, M. (2003a). Being Someone Else: Using Dance in Anti-oppressive Teaching. *Educational Review.* Vol 55, No 2, pp. 211–223.

Gard, M. (2003b). Moving and Belonging: Dance, Sport and Sexuality. *Sex Education*. Vol 3, No 2, pp. 105–118.
Gard, M. (2006). *Men Who Dance: Aesthetics, Athletics, & the Art of Masculinity.* New York: Peter Lang.
Gee, J.P. (2008). *Social Linguistics and Literacies: Ideology in Discourses*. London: Routledge.
Gere, D. (2001). Effeminate Gestures: Choreographer Joe Goode and the Heroism of Effeminacy. In Desmond, J.C. (Ed.). *Dancing Desires: Choreographing Sexualities On and Off the Stage*. Madison: University of Wisconsin Press.
Goffman, E. (1959). *The Presentation of Self in Everyday Life*. New York: Anchor.
Gorely, T., Holroyd, R., & Kirk, D. (2003). Muscularity, the Habitus and the Social Construction of Gender: Towards a Gender-Related Physical Education. *British Journal of Sociology of Education*. Vol 24, No 4, pp. 429–448.
Hanna, J.L. (2010). Dance and Sexuality: Many Moves. *Journal of Sex Research*. Vol 47, Nos 2–3, pp. 212–241.
Keefe, M. (2009). Is Dance a Man's Sport Too? In Fisher, J., & Shay, A. (Eds.). *When Men Dance: Choreographing Masculinity across Borders*. New York: Oxford University Press.
Kirby, S., & Hay, I. (1997). (Hetero)Sexing Space: Gay Men and 'Straight' Space in Adelaide, South Australia. *The Professional Geographer.* Vol 49, No 3, pp. 295–305.
Kroeger, B. (2003). *Passing: When People Can't Be Who They Are*. New York: Public Affairs.
Mac an Ghaill, M., & Haywood, C. (2007). *Gender, Culture and Society: Contemporary Femininities and Masculinities*. London: Macmillan.
Martino, W., & Pallotta-Chiarolli, M. (2001). Gender Performativity and Normalizing Practices. In Haynes, F., & McKenna, T. (Eds.). *Unseen Genders: Beyond the Binaries*. New York: Peter Lang.
Martino, W., & Pallotta-Chiarolli, M. (2005). *Being Normal Is the Only Way to Be*. Sydney: University of New South Wales Press.
McKenna, T. (2001). Enactments of Difference. In Haynes, F., & McKenna, T. (Eds.). *Unseen Genders: Beyond the Binaries*. New York: Peter Lang.
Migdalek, J. (2002). Performing English: The Classroom as Rehearsal Space. *Prospect: An Australian Journal of TESOL*. Vol 17, No 2, pp. 53–61.
Migdalek, J. (2014). Mincing, Striding, Stomping, Gliding: Messing with Gender Choreographic Taboos. In Pallotta-Chiarolli, M., and Pease, B. (Eds.). *The Politics of Recognition and Social Justice: Transforming Subjectivities and New Forms of Resistance*. New York: Routledge.
Monro, S. (2005). *Gender Politics*. London: Pluto.
Paechter, C. (2006). Reconceptualizing the Gendered Body: Learning and Constructing Masculinities and Femininities in School. *Gender and Education*. Vol 18, No 2, pp. 121–135.
Pallotta-Chiarolli, M. (2004). Weaving Textual Tapestries. In Scarparo, S., & Wilson, R. (Eds.). *Across Genres, Generations and Borders*. Newark, NJ: Delaware Press.
Pallotta-Chiarolli, M. (2010). *Border Sexualities, Border Families in Schools*. Lanham: Rowman and Littlefield.
Plummer, D. (1999). *One of the Boys: Masculinity, Homophobia and Modern Manhood*. New York: Harrington Park Press.
Risner, D. (2007). Rehearsing Masculinity: Challenging the 'Boy Code' in Dance Education. *Research in Dance Education*. Vol 8, No 2, pp. 139–153.
Savigliano, M. (1995). *Tango and the Political Economy of Passion*. Boulder, CO: Westview.
Schirato, T., & Yell, S. (1996). *Communication and Cultural Literacy.* St Leonards, NSW: Allen and Unwin.

Shilling, C. (2003). *The Body and Social Theory.* London: Sage.
Stoneley, P. (2007). *A Queer History of the Ballet.* London: Routledge.
Taga, F. (2005). East Asian Masculinities. In Kimmel, M.S., Hearn, J., & Connell, R.W. (Eds.). *Handbook of Studies on Men and Masculinities.* London: Sage.
Threadgold, T. (1994). Performing Genre: Violence, the Making of Protected Subjects, and the Discourses of Critical Literacy and Radical Pedagogy. *Changing English.* Vol 1, No 1, pp. 2–31.
Turner, B. (1984). *The Body and Society.* Oxford, UK: Basil Blackwell.
Turner, B. (1992). *Regulating Bodies: Essays in Medical Sociology.* London: Routledge.
Wex, M. (1979). *Let's Take Back Our Space: Female and Male Body Language as a Result of Patriarchal Structures.* Munich: Frauenliteratur Verlag.
Zizek, S. (1999). *The Sublime Object of Ideology.* London: Verso.

8 Challenging Norms

Connell (2000) claims that masculinities and femininities are actively constructed, not simply received. If this is so, then change in how notions of masculine and feminine are constructed should be possible. However, while individuals may have agency to alter how they perform within an existing regimen, it is another thing again to change the regimen itself (Foster 1998). As proposed in Chapter 2, social change does not happen automatically, nor does it occur simply as a result of purely intellectual motivation (Shilling 2003). Despite the forceful nature of enculturation and educational practices in positioning individuals toward the embodiment of gender, "corporeal creativity and change is possible" (Shilling 2004, p. xxi). In this chapter, I ponder how individuals might challenge norms of embodiment in their everyday lives. And on a larger platform, I ponder the potential of mainstream performance arts in challenging these same norms.

MINDFUL EMBODIMENT

There are multiple ways in which an individual is able to perform any action. However, frequently the ways in which individuals *do* perform is limited as a result of habitual patterns of embodiment (see Callery 2001, Feldenkrais Method 2008). Recognizing such limitations may be a means to being open to alternative embodiment, both on one's own body and the bodies of others. In much the same way that the Feldenkrais technique, referred to in Chapter 2, combats movement patterns and muscular habits that may be physically damaging, I believe that habitual patterns of embodiment that are gendered are damaging. This is because they limit and restrict the ways in which we allow ourselves to move, as well as the ways in which we regard those who embody differently from our expectations of how they should embody. For example, the male who holds back from embodying in a delicate, graceful manner is denied a whole spectrum of embodied and kinesthetic experience. He may also find it impossible to appreciate such embodiment performed by the bodies of other males.

It is only relatively recently that I have become mindful of ways in which my own embodiment is grounded in habitual patterns of embodiment that are gendered. I recognize that ways in which I have come to embody are compliant with, limited by, and reflective of dominant patriarchal ideologies embedded-as-nature in the cultures from which I hail. In time and through re-embodiment, the machinations of gendered ideologies pertinent to embodied behavior may be disrupted (Butler 1990, Monro 2005). Anzaldua (1987) lauds the courage of individuals who challenge dominant forms of masculinity. Individuals willing to engage in such practice may be closer to understanding and overcoming the taboos concerning the embodiment of gender than those who unthinkingly accept, and operate according to, dominant norms as norms of nature and not culture.

Akin to the Feldenkrais Method (2008), which promotes enabling one to know and do things in other ways, I have become mindful in regard to gendered performance that there are alternative ways in which I can embody and alternative ways in which I can appreciate the embodiment of others. I have been consciously endeavoring to bring myself to practice these alternatives in the everyday. For example, I now sometimes stand contrapposto (with hip cocked, weight resting on one leg, the other leg bent); through years of self-regulation it had been my habitus not to stand in this way. I now sometimes cross my knees neatly when I sit; through years of self-regulation it was not my habitus to sit in this way. I now sometimes embrace platonic male friends without back-slapping and sometimes embrace female friends with back-slapping; my usual habitus had been to punctuate embraces with males with back-slaps, and to embrace females with no such punctuation. I now sometimes walk allowing my hips to move from side to side; my usual habitus had been to keep my hips level. Although these practices feel unfamiliar and are sometimes uncomfortable, I am coming to appreciate, and at times enjoy, the foreign, fresh, strange, and sometimes liberating feeling of performing against my habitus. The experience of practicing alternative ways of sitting, standing, walking, and embracing is a means of recognizing other ways one might embody, ways that are not constricted to socially imposed manifestations of gender ideology. As regards alternative ways in which I can appreciate the embodiment of others, sometimes when I see individuals whose embodiment goes against dominant gendered norms—such as males whose embodiment is particularly effeminate or females whose embodiment is particularly masculine—I consciously combat my former preconceptions of the aesthetic and the surfacing of 'scar-tissue', and attempt to take in and appreciate such alternative embodiment afresh.

OPPOSING EMBODIED GENDER INEQUITY IN THE EVERYDAY

Even when we become aware of a habitual way of performing a practice, and even when we might desire to affect or alter that practice, effecting change is not necessarily easily or comfortably achieved (Bourdieu 1990, Shilling 2003). From a very young age, we develop habitual ways of doing as well as viewing bodies. These are so entrenched that they are in effect invisible to us. Were individuals to become aware of and perhaps wish to change habitual ways of performing something, how easily might a change of habitus be achieved?

CHALLENGING THE HABITUAL: BUTTONING HABITUS

Exercise: If like me, you have always worn shirts that button up on one side as opposed to the other, put on a shirt that buttons up the opposite way. How does it feel to button the shirt up differently? What degrees of difficulty does doing so present? Why might this be? How might the practice of buttoning up on the opposite side to the usual become habitual or feel natural?

Predominantly shirts (a cultural construction) have buttons on the right for males and on the left for females (a gender construction). Buttoning up a shirt is a practice we are not likely to think about nor pay attention to. It is an action that we, in the Western cultural world, are likely to have performed countless times in our lives. When we put on a shirt, it is likely that our hands automatically go to the side that we are used to buttoning from. It is a practice (like many practices) that for many will feel 'natural', whether we happen to be left or right handed, even though it is a cultural and gendered construct.

CHALLENGING THE HABITUAL: LINKING ARMS HABITUS

Together with a female friend who identifies and presents as female, I conducted the following exercise. We assumed the traditional arm in arm pose: the female's arm resting on and supported by the male's proffered arm. We looked at ourselves in a mirror. We tried walking in this way along a public street. We then reversed the link of our arms (my female friend's arm proffered, my arm supported) and repeated the activity. We asked ourselves how it felt performing the choreography according to and opposing the traditional roles of our own biological sex. We found that where my male body assumed the male traditional role and my friend the traditional female role, we both felt fairly comfortable performing the choreography. Despite feeling that the practice itself was rather archaic and outmoded, the practice did not feel otherwise odd to perform. On the other hand, where my body assumed the female traditional role, and my female partner the traditional male role, the action felt decidedly uncomfortable to both participants. This sense was both conceptual and corporeal. Given that we were as physically capable of performing both permutations of the choreography, our discomfort can be understood to be the result of social conditioning. Apart from instances where the supporter is elderly, frail, ill, or infirm, we in Western society are not likely to come across versions of this choreography with a male resting his arm on the proffered arm of a female partner.

For those who are products of cultures that repeatedly reinforce the sex-specific traditional configuration of a female's arm resting on a male's arm, the act of physically performing according to that choreography is likely not to be uncomfortable. Inversely, the conventional configuration is so naturalized that to perform against it *is* likely to be uncomfortable, despite the physical capability to do so.

The example of arm placement raises questions concerning the power of heteronormative and gendernormative choreography and what comes to seem and feel natural. Although a person's head may tell them that there is no logical reason why arm placement should not be reversed from the conventional choreography, changing roles is not easily adopted, even where one regards oneself as an agent of one's own actions. Such is the power of heteronormative choreography that deviations of the usual choreography tend to stand out and are marked as 'other'. Unless deconstructed by performing the practice in ways that oppose the usual sex-specific choreography, be it performed by same-sex or opposite-sex pairs, the gendered and inequitable make up of such traditional practices is likely to escape notice.

CHALLENGING THE HABITUAL: EVEN-HANDED PLATONIC KISSES

The following episode illustrates my struggle with trying to greet male and female friends to whom I am equally close in the same way.

> I was to meet four friends at a cinema in a central suburb. When I arrived, my friends Sue, Ben, Gail, and Ted were already there, clustered in a circle outside the foyer. I know Sue and Ben very well and Gail and Ted (a married couple) not all that intimately. As I joined their circle, I kissed Sue and Ben. Next to them was Gail, who I also kissed, and next to Gail was her husband Ted. '*Well*', I thought in that split second, '*I know and like Ted just as well as I know and like Gail*', and so, with a mass of thoughts swimming in my head that were itching to challenge how unequally we relate to people according to their biological sex, I went to kiss Ted. What followed still irks me as a highly awkward moment. Ted and I found ourselves hovering between what was going to become a kiss or a *biff-slap*-on-the-shoulder embrace. I imagine that the moment was as uncomfortable for Ted as it was for me. The really pitiful thing is that, in order to be even-handed, the next time I met Gail and Ted, I controlled and regulated my body and kissed neither of them.

While I might see the logic of a platonic kiss of greeting between two males as no different from a platonic kiss of greeting between two females or a male and a female, the 'scar-tissue' of my previous understanding of and positioning toward the male to male kiss surfaced. As a result, the embodiment of that kiss was not easily taken on or executed. The episode illustrates how one's conditioning toward embodied performance becomes so habitual that it is not easily or comfortably changed, even in the case of a practice that one might desire to perform. That the moment described was so awkward for me (and for Ted also, I believe) illustrates that changing embodied norms in one's everyday life involves far more than intellectual justification. If people are more ordinarily exposed to a range of embodied performances that transgress gender norms, then images and notions of 'other' embodiment of gender may lose their otherness and come to be less marked and less remarkable.

CHALLENGING THE HABITUAL: WHAT WE FIND REPUGNANT

If taste is culture turned into nature (Turner 1992), then changing or revising ways that I *naturally* perceive, appreciate, and perform gender is not an easy proposition, especially where my positioning toward a practice is aversive. Where a lifetime of established models—via culture/s that formed my taste and my embodiment as nature—have positioned me to regard feminine embodied practice on a male as repugnant or distasteful, then questioning or changing what I feel to be my own natural responses toward certain styles of male embodiment will not even be likely to come to mind. Even in cases where I do come to question why I find certain practices to be unaesthetic, altering my habitual responses will be a difficult proposition.

The reasons that an individual finds particular embodiment on a male or female to be repugnant and distasteful may connect to the 'Sesame Street mindset' (introduced in Chapter 6), where that which is 'other' comes to be regarded or pigeon-holed as odd, ludicrous, subordinate, suspect, or deviant. It may well be harder to shift the 'Sesame Street mindset' that manifests in aversion than it is to shift the 'Sesame Street mindset' that manifests in amusement. Either way, I take Connell's (1995) suggestion that in order to broaden what is considered to be acceptable gender behavior, individuals need to come to empathize with and take on the viewpoint of the other. Achieving this might lead individuals to understand the potential consequences of what it is to be scorned at or trivialized.

Putting images of *other* embodied gender practices out there as that which is not ab-normal or ludicrous may be a threatening undertaking for individuals in the everyday. The individual who transgresses norms, deliberately or not, carries the risk of negative consequences such as aversion, ridicule, and alienation. What follows are considerations of the performance arts as a potential medium through which steps toward understanding or empathizing with the viewpoints of others, and steps toward social change in outlooks on the embodiment of gender, may be achieved. I will look at performance arts first in terms of formal theatrical performances as created by performance arts practitioners, and then as the province of performance arts educators within sites such as schools.

OPPOSING EMBODIED GENDER INEQUITY IN PERFORMANCE ARTS

Representations of male and female forms as they predominantly exist in mainstream performance artworks are likely to continue to inscribe, perpetuate, and reinforce gender oppressive notions: that masculinity is a male quality and femininity a female quality. Some change in mainstream performance artworks is necessary in order to effect change in the social mindset concerning what comes to be considered as appropriate and aesthetic embodiment for males and females. The following pages speculate on the various ways such change may be achieved.

Dealing with the Politically Incorrect

Performance artworks that represent male and female bodies in gender oppressive ways could be banned! Doing so would ensure that the public is not directly exposed to ideological sentiments that go against the political agenda of a governing body that promotes gender equity. At various stages of Chinese history, specific operas and ballets were banned because they were seen to be in opposition to the political rule of the time (Mackerras 1975). Although it may be desirable for people to lose their gender bias regarding embodiment as derived and reinforced through forms such as classics of Western dance and drama, it is debatable whether controlling, censoring, or banning expressions of art is an appropriate or moral means by which to do so.

Conventional performance arts classics, with males embodying in a masculine manner and females embodying in a feminine manner, are worthy of being re-presented in their traditional form. However, some kind of contextualization and critical deconstruction is warranted, wherein audiences, and especially young audiences, are made aware of the archaic gendered ideologies that underlie the embodiment presented in such works. Exposure to performance arts pieces that represent male and female bodies in gender oppressive ways could be accompanied by presentations, demonstrations, and/or exhibitions designed to expose the embedded and invisible gender oppressive ideology that underlies the direction, choreography, and costuming as constructed on male and female bodies within the pieces. Propaganda such as this could be used in an attempt to change people's mindset.

In 1937 a touring exhibition titled *Entartete Kunst* (Degenerate Art) was mounted by the Nazis in Germany and Austria. The exhibition displayed artworks in styles of Cubism, Dadaism, Surrealism, Expressionism, Impressionism, and Fauvism and deemed them, through hand written captions and slogans displayed beside the works, as depraved, subversive, degenerate, and contaminated by Jewish influences (Petropoulos 1996). Although I would like to change the way that people perceive the embodiment of males and females as directed and choreographed in mainstream performance artworks (both classic and contemporary), I believe that this should be done with an openness to debate or analysis, and not via blatant, manipulative labeling, slating, and denigrating as in the aforementioned *Degenerate Art* propaganda or the captioned graphics that follow.

Using the example of dance, it can be argued that classics of the ballet (such as those referred to in Chapter 5) are worthy of being re-presented in their traditional form. However, audiences, especially young audiences, should be made conscious of the deep-rooted gendered ideologies underlying the plots, choreography, and design that mark and control the male and female bodies on show. Audiences should understand and make connections between fossilized and iconic sex-specific representations of ideals of embodied masculinity and femininity and contemporary notions that continue, in many aspects, to be sustained. The overwhelmingly consistent and repeated representations of valorized masculine male bodies and valorized feminine female bodies unduly pressure males and females to perceive, value, and embody maleness and femaleness with reverence to such

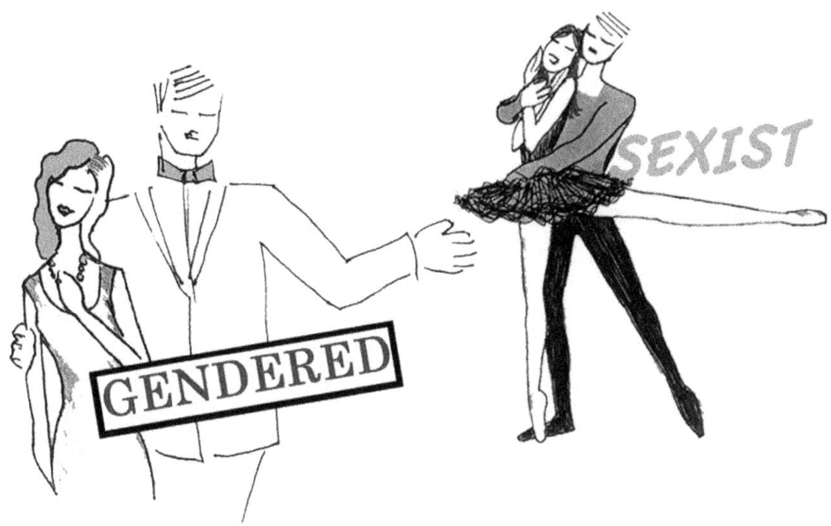

Figure 8.1 Labeling. Artwork by Jack Migdalek.

distinctive gendered ways. Without contextualization, traditional, limited, and idealized representations of males and females will be reinforced as that which is normal and natural, marginalizing or subordinating that which differs or is in opposition. Positioning audiences at a critical distance from dance works may lead audiences to analyze, understand, and challenge gendered ideologies inherent in Western societies (Burt 1995, Gard 2004). This line of thinking can apply to inequitable embodiment of gender as it occurs not just for dance but for drama too.

Challenging Deep-Seated Ideology

It is possible for performance arts work—even mainstream performance arts work—to challenge deep-seated ideology and cause audiences to think about their worlds from other perspectives. However, the effects of deep-seated patriarchal, sexist, and heteronormal ideology and attitudes toward human embodiment frequently escape scrutiny.

The song lyrics of Richard Rogers and Oscar Hammerstein's *You've Got to Be Carefully Taught* from the musical *South Pacific* (first produced on the stage in 1949, for the screen in 1958, and for television in 2001) serve as a hard-hitting critique against discrimination and prejudice pertaining to the interracial relationships within the storyline (*Broadway: The American Musical* 2005). The lyrics tell us that discrimination is taught to us from when we are young ("Before you are six or seven or eight"); that indoctrination to discriminate is handed down to us ("You've got to be taught . . . [t]o hate all the people your relatives hate"); that that which is different is noteworthy as being odd or misfit ("people whose eyes are oddly made . . . people whose skin is a diff'rent shade").

While the verbal text and storyline of *South Pacific* may be critical of and highlight discrimination against that which is considered 'other' in regard to race, the embodied visual text within productions of the musical is oblivious to its own discriminatory machinations against that which is 'other' in regard to the embodiment of gender. For example, in the *Thanksgiving Follies* production numbers, the characters of Luther, a male moving in a feminine manner, and Nellie, a female moving in a masculine manner, are presented as objects of comedy—and ridicule in Luther's case—in comparison to the other females and males, who are moving in feminine and masculine ways respectively within the same production numbers.

The drive behind the groundbreaking *South Pacific* was to put forward and challenge the notion that discrimination according to race is taught and is not something that is inherent (*South Pacific* Twentieth Century Fox DVD commentary 2008). However, the idea that the choreography and direction of male and female bodies in *South Pacific* overlooks the notion that females embodying in feminine manner and males embodying in masculine manner may also be taught—as opposed to being natural states—is entirely ignored.

This raises the issue of temporal context, where some discriminations are recognized and others are not.

Alternative Choreography

It can be argued that in contemporary times, norms of gender and sexuality are being challenged, but, in my opinion, this is not happening in ways that disrupt norms of gender choreography and embodiment. There are more and more contemporary dramas and musicals being produced that put forward positive images of homosexuals. It has become more socially acceptable and not particularly remarkable for heterosexual males to display feminine qualities, such as sensitivity, sentimentality, or gentleness, in their personality and character, as evidenced in the qualities of male protagonists in motion pictures such as *Edward Scissorhands* (Twentieth Century Fox 1990), *Sleepless in Seattle* (Tristar Pictures 1993), *American Beauty* (Dreamworks 1999), and *The Green Mile* (Castle Rock Entertainment 2000). However, male characters who display feminine qualities in their physical disposition and embodiment, in contrast to master-signifiers of males who display masculine qualities in their physical disposition and embodiment, continue to be marked and remarkable—turning heads, raising eyebrows, provoking comment. As identified in Chapter 5, consistent and pervasive gendered casting, directing, and choreographing of male and female bodies leave transgressive embodied representations labeled as 'other'. There is still little deviation from stereotypical norms of representation when it comes to the embodiment of characters as being homosexual or heterosexual. There is a marked absence of representations of heterosexual male characters who embody in a feminine manner who are not deemed to be figures of suspicion, pathos, or amusement.

My contention is that males and females should be free to move in feminine and/or masculine manners without being labeled in terms of personality or sexuality. In order to realize social freedom as regards embodiment of gender, archaic ideologies that limit notions of what is appropriate embodiment for male and female bodies need to be exposed and deconstructed. Formal performance arts arenas where embodied representations of males and females are deliberately displayed as objects of gaze may be one area in which, through alternative choreographies of the body, the machinations of ideologies of embodied behavior may be disrupted. It needs to be noted that simply transgressing norms of direction and choreography will not necessarily serve to challenge existing norms. Indeed, parodic transgression is not only capable of empowering but also capable of reinscribing heterosexist norms (Butler 1990, Burt 1995). For example, where a comedian might embody the characterization of a 'straight' male in an effeminate manner, this is likely to only reinforce notions of how absurd and ludicrous the straight, mincing male is.

In order for a staged reconstruction of male or female embodiment to affect or change the social mindset, it needs to disrupt the categories of the body, sex, gender, and sexuality beyond the binary frame (Butler 1990). Simply reversing what is is not necessarily effective deconstruction (Davies 1993). There is a difference between parody or transgressive representation that challenges an audience to think, and parody or transgressive representation that trivializes that which is being displayed and simply reinscribes and validates restrictive heterosexist norms (see Bollen et al. 2006, 2008). In order for alternative choreography of gender in a mainstream public performance arena to be thought provoking or confronting, it is necessary to drive a message to audiences that exposes and deconstructs the ideological binds of a dominant mindset that has over a long period prescribed and regulated how *normal* males and females embody. Acts of transgressing gender norms need to be presented as food for thought and not as easy laughs. While defying norms of representation and casting roles such as Edna Turnblad in *Hairspray* (New Line Cinema 2007) and Lady Bracknell in *The Importance of Being Earnest* (Melbourne Theatre Company 2011) as drag roles—played by John Travolta and Geoffrey Rush respectively—may be admirable in theory, the roles are sadly still merely caricatures of larger than life characters of amusement. They do not validate alternative ways in which those who present as males might embody.

As referred to in Chapter 5, the masculine embodiment of the two gay protagonists in Ang Lee's *Brokeback Mountain* (Alberta Film Entertainment 2005) provoked and challenged mainstream audiences' preconceived notions concerning the embodiment of gay males. It can be argued that the performances caused mainstream audience members to question connections made between embodiment and sexual orientation—a positive step toward change in the social mindset. On the other hand, although there have been movies in which male heterosexual protagonists have feminine emotional characteristics, we have yet to see movies in which male heterosexual protagonists embody in a feminine manner. I hope for a time when embodied representations of male and female characters in performance artworks that go against gendered and sexist norms of embodiment are no longer regarded, or marketed, as remarkable (as those of the protagonists in *Brokeback Mountain* were). Achieving this will be indicative of a shift toward a more equitable social mindset toward the embodiment of alternative masculinities/femininities.

I applaud and admire theatrical works such as *Cloud Nine* (written by Caryl Churchill 1979), *29 Effeminate Gestures* (choreographed by Joe Goode 1987), and *Relic* (choreographed by Adrian Burnett 2005) that, in my opinion, challenge audiences to think about and question gendered norms of embodiment. These works have not achieved notable popularity with mainstream audiences. Can it be that work that is deconstructive must necessarily sit outside of mainstream taste? Not so. Works such as the enormously popular *Gentleman's Agreement* (Twentieth Century Fox 1947),

South Pacific (Broadway 1949, Twentieth Century Fox 1958, Buena Vista 2001), *West Side Story* (Broadway 1957, United Artists 1961), *Philadelphia* (Tristar 1993), *Hairspray* (Broadway 2002, New Line Cinema 1988, 2007), and *Transamerica* (IFC Films 2005), which have been lauded for serving to critique issues such as racism, prejudice, gender, sexism, body size, and/or homophobia, indicate that mainstream works are also capable of exposing and deconstructing existing norms. Creating performance pieces that might challenge *embodied* norms of gender, while at the same time being accessible to and appreciated by mainstream audiences, is something I believe performance arts practitioners should strive for.

Until such a time as opposing models of embodied gender performance become unmarked and acceptable, traditional representations of heterosexual males and homosexual females as masculine, and heterosexual females and homosexual males as feminine, will continue to project as that which is normal and natural. It is problematic when this kind of signification positions that which transgresses those norms as ab-normal, subordinate, and not natural, a theme that continues to surface in this book. It is also problematic when ideals of the 'natural' are embedded in often-revered arts disciplines. I take these concerns with me into the fieldwork described in Chapter 10.

Neutral Bodies and Gender Bias

Even though bodies are visible, there are blindspots to inequitable and discriminatory ways of doing and viewing bodies according to biological sex. The workings of gendered ideologies in dominant norms of embodiment are so embedded through our enculturation that they are rendered virtually invisible. These ideologies also operate within established and revered disciplines of dance (classical ballet) and drama (Lecoq technique).

In classical ballet training all over the world, male and female dancers may do identical technique classes, yet they are then given specific tuition appropriate to the choreographic demands of the classics of the art form, and these differ for male and female dancers (Australian Ballet 1993). For example, it is rare for *pointe, pas de bourre couru, pose pirhouettes en tournant, petit develope,* or *fouette ronde de jambe en tournant,* steps involving intricate and contained footwork, to be taught to male dancers. It is rare for continuous *grande pirhoette a la seconde* or *batterie entrechat huit,* bravura steps propelled by extreme muscular power, to be taught to female dancers. Whereas females may not be taught the latter steps because of the amount of muscle power required in the legs, the same does not apply to why males are not taught the former steps, which appear to be more feminine and delicate.

Likewise, in drama training, gender bias exists in regard to the notion of the neutral body. The neutral body is primary to the Lecoq technique, as introduced in Chapter 2. Lecoq's rationale for the neutral body is that the actor should be able to construct a character from a position of innocence or neutrality. For this reason, the Lecoq technique strives to rid the actor of deeply ingrained and conditioned habits and attitudes reflective of the individual's personal or cultural history (Callery 2001, Sears & Hollos 2002). Lecoq defines these habits and attitudes as 'traces' of what actors have lived and experienced in their day to day lives and upbringing (Lecoq 2002). In order for actors to be able to work from a neutral state, Lecoq trains actors in

> stripping away learned behavior patterns which do not belong to them, eliminating everything which might hinder them from rediscovering life at its most authentic. We have to divest the students of some of what they have learned . . . in order to . . . create for them a blank page.
> (Lecoq 2002, p. 27)

I respect this acknowledgment of the invisible presence and restrictive potency of habitual patterns of behavior and temperament, which Lecoq wants actors to be able to shed in the drama workspace. However, the Lecoq technique stops short of realizing this acknowledgment in practice.

In order to achieve this neutral state, Lecoq training commences with mime work in which actors wear what he calls 'neutral mask' (Lecoq 2002). These leather masks that Lecoq co-designed with sculptor Amleto Sartori are different for males and females. The following reasons are given for this: "Since the male and female bodies have different centers of gravity, the masks that will be carried by them must also differ" (Sears & Hollos 2002, p. 142); "our skeletal and facial architecture is determined by our biological gender" (Callery 2001, p. 34). These explanations strike me as absurd: First, if male and female centers of gravity differ from one another, then it is the spine and not the face itself that determines the axis, angle, and pitch of facial features. Second, the skulls of biological males and females differ only in the attachment of muscle to skeleton, bone, and tissue surfaces, as well as the mastoid process that occur behind the ears, and not on the surface of the face as such (Ecker 1868). As for facial architecture, not all female faces are what could be considered feminine, just as not all male faces are what could be considered masculine. If "a neutral mask puts the actor in a state of perfect balance and economy of movement . . . [equipping] . . . the actor to express a character's inbalance or conflictual states" (Lecoq 2002, p. 38), then why is it that Lecoq bypasses notions of gender and biological sex as non-conflictual by insisting on different masks for male and female actors? If actors are to approach their craft from a neutral state devoid of learned behaviors, then surely the stripping away of learned male and female behaviors should be just as much a part of finding that neutral state.

It is hypocritical to strive to recognize and achieve states of innocence or neutrality yet overlook gendered behavioral differences as though they are differences of nature and not culture. Given that the shapes and sizes of the surfaces of male and female faces are not fundamentally different, the imposition of different masks for the faces of males and females respectively implies that the Lecoq method regards gender behavior as steeped in biology and nature and not as behavior that is learned.

According to the Lecoq technique (2002), learning to acknowledge the presence and potency of habitual and invisible patterns of behavior and temperament is a key toward rediscovering a position of innocence or neutrality that is free of preconception or bias. This line of thinking is not just relevant to actors in performance arts arenas but also to individuals in the everyday. If effecting positive change in both mindset and behavior is to be a viable possibility, then it must involve a questioning of and sensitivity as to why embodied patterns of behavior might be perceived and performed differently according to the biological sex of the performer.

Much of this discussion hinges on that which comes to be 'taken for granted' as theorized by Alfred Schutz (1972). We are effectively blind to the workings of that which is 'normative' until such time that the make up of the normative becomes blatantly obvious—as pointed out to us by Schutz' (1944) 'stranger', who questions what we might previously have viewed as being unquestionable. As a result, from such time on, it may be impossible to see things as they were. This kind of deconstructive work could be an endeavor of performance arts practitioners through avenues of performances and education. For this type of work to eventuate, performance arts practitioners/educators first need to be open themselves to the notion that there may be inequitable aspects of their own practices and disciplines that they may unwittingly take for granted.

For positive social change to occur in this regard, performance arts practitioners need to take an inventory of their own unwitting gendered casting, directing, and choreographing of male and female bodies. They need to question what they take for granted as natural for male and female representation, and to be mindful that the male and female representations they create can have a negative impact on the social and emotional well-being of those whose embodied inclinations transgress the norms of embodiment prescribed according to biological sex. Where norms of gender representation position that which is 'other' as marginal and ab-normal, they may cause embarrassment, self-consciousness, and even self-hate for males and females whose embodied inclination is transgressive or 'other' than the norm.

PERFORMANCE ARTS EDUCATORS AS AGENTS OF CHANGE

I now bring my focus to performance arts educators (dance and drama teachers particularly) and how they might practically address questions concerning what is involved in effecting change in regard to the perception and performance of embodiment of gender that differs according to the biological sex of the performer. As put forward in Chapter 2, I endorse applying means of critical literacy (frequently used to expose inherent ideologies in spoken and written language) to visual, embodied text, wherein focus is placed on the signification of embodiment prior to and distinct from plot or storyline. I also referred to Gard's (2003) as well as Gorely, Holroyd, and Kirk's (2003) hopes for schools' dance and physical education sites to problematize gender and sexuality and encourage students' recognition and use of their full and real bodily capacities. I contend that schools' drama sites too, as well as design and music sites, can serve as vital settings for addressing and exploring the embodiment of gender. Indeed, these art forms all connect with embodiment and the projection of femininity and masculinity, which, in mainstream arenas, customarily differs according to biological sex. Performance arts activities may be a positive means of finding and exploring a broader range of embodied states of self.

As a drama educator, I conduct activities where students are invited to focus on and explore the semiotics of bodies in pose, repose, or action prior to or independent of the storyline, plot, or spoken text (Migdalek 2014). To illustrate, I have students execute everyday sequences, such as closing a door, sitting on a chair, and drinking a beverage. They then identify together the type of character or demeanor that different performances of the sequence suggest. We then explore whether, how, and why an identical performance of the same sequence projects differently if performed by a person who projects as a different biological sex. I then invite students to create and explore dramatic ways of destabilizing and challenging the normalized, stereotyped representations of gender that are so pervasive in popular culture. In cases where this work evokes laughter from students, I endeavor to draw their attention to what made them laugh, and the differences between embodied parody that challenges an audience to think and parody that trivializes that which is being displayed. As mentioned, embodied parody is not only capable of empowering but also capable of reinscribing heterosexist norms (Butler 1990, 1993, Burt 1995). It is possible to also apply these principles to the staging and direction of school productions, wherein issues of transgressing gender norms might be presented as food for thought and not as easy laughs.

Imagine that I am directing a school production of a conventional musical. As mentioned previously, it is likely that I would choreograph and direct heterosexual male and female characters to embody in typically masculine and feminine manners. I claim that directors of school productions should be mindful of the messages that the direction and choreography in their/our school production may be sending out regarding gender norms of behavior to students under their/our direction, as well as audiences who see the production (Migdalek 2009, 2014). Favorite conventional school productions such as *Grease, Oklahoma, Pirates of Penzance,* and *South Pacific* may involve depictions of males and females situated in gendered times and locales, but unless contextualized in some way, these depictions serve to reinforce and valorize gendered and inequitable norms of embodiment that differ for males and females. Even in the high school production rehearsal room, males and females are likely to be commended/censured for gender conforming/non-conforming modes of embodiment, be it via the authority of the drama teacher/director or from the unauthorized but nevertheless potent authority of students themselves.

I have seen and continue to witness school productions in which certain characterizations have been directed to transgress gender 'norms' of embodiment for easy laughs from the audience, such as the male character who minces daintily or the female character who strides with straddled legs. Really, the situation is not so laughable when one considers the impact these 'amusing' embodied performances may have on the self-perception and well-being of the male or female within the production, or in the audience, who may not be inclined to perform according to dominant norms of sex-specific gender behavior. As previously pointed out, those individuals who are made to feel that they do not fit the heteronormative bill will either resist and be marginalized, resulting in social alienation and perhaps harassment, or self-police and play to 'pass' (Kroeger 2003) and embody masculinity or femininity as socially prescribed for their biological sex. Whereas 'passing' may assist individuals to avoid conflict, danger, prejudice, discrimination, or rejection, this kind of self-editing may also cause depression, hostility, anxiety, and low self-esteem (Kroeger 2003).

Performance arts educators need to search for and question gendered elements in their own practices and the impact that these may have on school and other populations with and for whom they work. Although respect for diversity is commonly promoted and prescribed in staff and student codes of conduct (for example, Department of Education and Early Childhood Development Victoria 2014), it is possible that inherent gendered elements in the work of performance arts practitioners and educators may serve to reinforce established inequitable attitudes that hinge on biological sex. It is crucial that the training and professional development of educators draw attention to such a likelihood. The drama/dance classroom and school productions should be seen and utilized as sites in which students might explore, experiment with, challenge, disrupt, and transform modes of embodiment that may be restrictive and differential according to biological sex. I bring these concerns to performance arts practitioners/educators in the fieldwork discussed in Chapter 10.

GENDER ICONS—PERFORMING AGAINST MY EMBODIED HABITUS

Performance artworks and performance arts education may challenge norms of gender embodiment. However, it is not just the content and effect of performances that challenge norms that warrant attention, but also that which is involved for performers—especially live performers—as objects of the gaze in the actual performing of pieces.

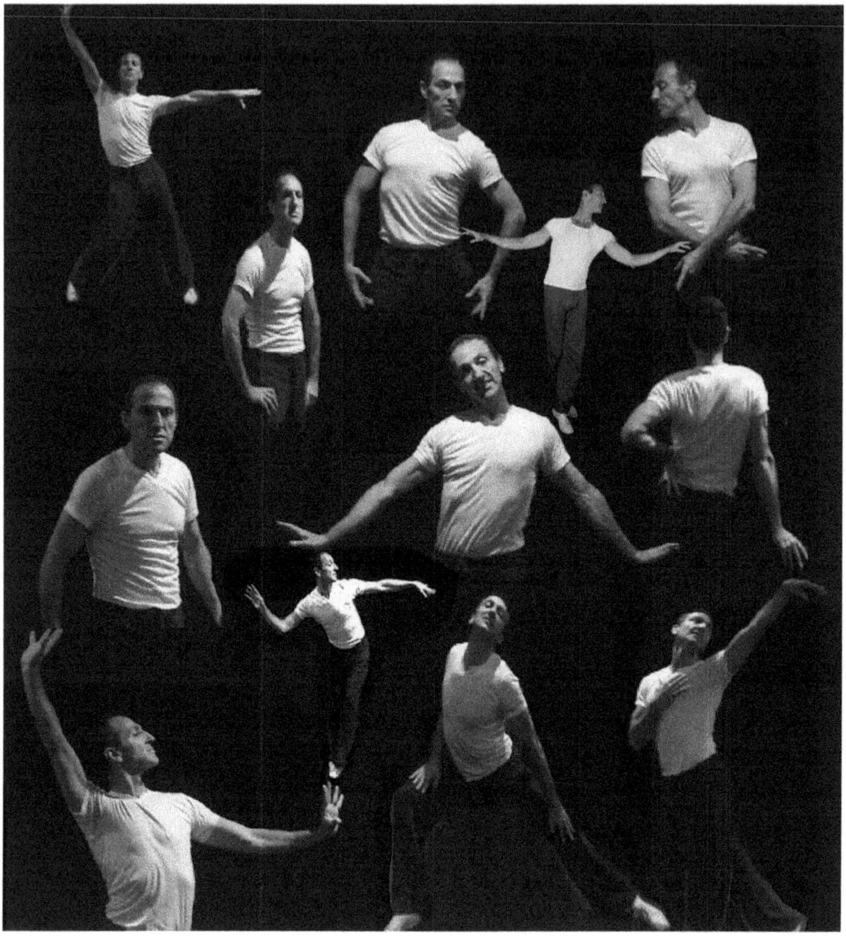

Figure 8.2 *Gender Icons*. Photograph by Rob Chiarolli (www.photosthattell.com).

I now want to shift attention to forces that might inhibit or discourage live performers or performance artists/educators (like myself) who want to present work that challenges embodied norms of gender from placing themselves in a position of having to endure or deal with the reactions of live audiences that might be mocking or aversive. Here I refer to my performances of *Gender Icons,* a solo that I created and performed on my own body, as a prominent component of my fieldwork. *Gender Icons* was created as an embodied articulation of my concerns. I created the piece as an exploration of elements of my own lived experiences and sense of consciousness of embodiment and gender. The piece was choreographed to an eleven-minute sound collage that I put together, a combination of thirty linked music excerpts, each of which projected or signified to me as distinctively feminine or masculine. In working on the piece I was mindfully exploring and acknowledging repertoires of embodiment that in my own lived experiences and consciousness had become natural for me, as well as those that were corporeally uncomfortable to me. *Gender Icons* was an exploration of uncharted areas of consciousness, confusion, frustration, anger, dilemma, and desire.

Preparing sections of *Gender Icons* in which my body danced in feminine ways involved deliberately embodying against what had become my 'male dance habitus'. Although I was confident that I was physically and technically capable of performing the sequences of movement that I had choreographed, moving my body in the feminine manner required by particular sections of my choreography felt unfamiliar and uncomfortable to me. It was not my habit to move in such ways, unless choreographing for females, and I found it difficult to let myself go in ways I could when performing action that was not feminine.

I decided to incorporate *Gender Icons* into my fieldwork because it would trigger personal reflections on issues of embodiment and gender in others. As Leavy (2009) contends, performance work can evoke emotional responses, raise consciousness, educate, and empower. A performance may pull audience members not only into the experiences of the performer/researcher but also into their own experiences (Snowber 2002, Ellis 2004, Leavy 2009). Stacy Holman Jones (2005) refers to the potential of (autobiographical) performances not only to make participants and audiences glimpse who and what they are and desire but also to be avenues through which they might come into contact with different identities, positions, and desires. As a choreographer, my interest was to challenge audience perceptions of what is fitting embodiment for male and female bodies. At the same time, as a performer, I was anxious that I would feel embarrassed or be confronted when moving in a feminine manner in front of others. This was contingent on my sense of the audience reaction to me—the male performing the piece—during the moments of performance itself.

My initial performances of *Gender Icons* were held and contextualized as academic events for peers and academics in lecture theatres, university classrooms, and a metropolitan bookshop. In pre- or post-performance discussions with adult participant groups, I spoke of everyday and formal situations and contexts in which I felt uncomfortable moving in a feminine manner (such as those referred to in Chapter 6) and was therefore asked how I had felt performing the feminine sections in *Gender Icons*. I answered that performing those sections of the piece was not too disconcerting because my audience comprised academics in an academic site for whom the piece had been contextualized prior to viewing. My sense of confidence was contingent on the audience knowing something of the context of the piece prior to viewing it. Even when audience members laughed at the content, I felt that their responses were grounded in the knowledge that the piece had a purpose. Audience members acknowledged that the piece would evoke very different responses from spectators in non-academic contexts. The view was that I would be laughed or sniggered at.

As my investigation progressed, it seemed appropriate to incorporate *Gender Icons* into fieldwork that I had planned to conduct with high school student groups. As a choreographer, my hopes were that the piece might touch or trigger something in the minds of teenage audiences that would challenge inequitable gendered ways in which they perceived masculine and feminine embodiment differently according to the biological sex of the performer. However, as a performer I was anxious about performing *Gender Icons* for those students because of how uncomfortable I thought I would feel dancing before an audience who might not be attuned to the intended tone of the piece. As I said, and recorded, in discussion with adult fieldwork participants regarding how I might feel performing *Gender Icons* for high school audiences, "The sniggers and giggles would really probably tear me up".

I was aware through my enculturation and extensive first hand experience as a performance artist who had performed before school audiences at all levels, in both private and public institutions, that a male moving in a feminine manner elicited sniggers and laughter from audiences. To be dancing, and to continue to dance, through an awareness of such reactions before an audience of high school age students was something I was reluctant to put myself through. Fellow male performance arts practitioners to whom I had spoken of my anxieties verified that they too would feel similarly about performing a piece such as *Gender Icons* for high school students. Being constantly on guard and anticipating reactions that might be mocking, aversive, or offensive is hardly an appealing situation in which to place oneself, particularly when the performance requires deep immersion into a persona or emotion.

As it happened, despite my anxieties, most student groups before whom I performed were sufficiently respectful of me as a performer to not be disruptive in ways I had feared. Perhaps my earnestness on introducing myself and the fact that the sessions occurred in sites of learning set a tone that communicated that the piece was not intended to be comic. Even so, I was aware of several students sniggering during my performances, and, as expected, these moments were difficult for me to work against.

My fears and anxieties regarding how high school students *might* respond to me embodying in a feminine manner in a staged performance surfaced and continue to resurface on every occasion that I perform before high school students. I acknowledge that perhaps not contextualizing the piece prior to performing it would allow for audiences' unguarded reactions to the performance and subsequently make post-performance reflection a more provocative learning experience for audiences. However, at the same time, in addition to my own anxieties as a performer, I am unwilling to take the risk that the piece might be misinterpreted and received in a way that might reinforce already existing discriminatory and potentially aversive attitudes. I do not want to present the piece at the risk of reinforcing for high school student audience members what they already find weird, bizarre, different, gay, or 'other' about males embodying in a feminine manner.

It seems to me that my anxieties over performing the feminine sections of *Gender Icons* may be parallel to those that inhibit me in a large number of everyday contexts from embodying in ways that are transgressive of gender norms. In both cases, transgressive performances that challenge gender norms of embodiment run the risk of being the brunt of others' scorn or ridicule. Deliberately transgressing gendered norms of embodied practices may be difficult, if not uncomfortable, for an individual to do personally in the everyday. Despite my anxieties, I believe that transgressing gender norms in formal performance arts arenas is potentially a safer and more effective means toward destabilizing the social mindset toward the embodiment of gender. For these reasons I reiterate my proposal that performance arts as a medium have the ability to challenge and deconstruct existing dominant gendered norms regarding the representation and perception of male and female forms. A staged performance, being steeped in 'play' and being more detached from the viewer than a performance that occurs in the everyday, may protect the performer from bearing the personal brunt of scorn or ridicule, and may also make it possible for viewers to see the performance with more objectivity. There is the chance that through involvement in performances and performance arts workshop situations that transgress gender norms, notions of 'other' may lose their potency and come to be less marked and remarkable. These views were taken with me in the implementation of the fieldwork that is the basis of the next chapters.

REFERENCES

Anzaldua, G. (1987). *Borderlands, La Frontera: The New Mestiza*. San Francisco: Spinsters/Aunt Lute.

Australian Ballet. (1993). *A Window on the World of Classical Ballet*. Sydney: ABC Video Arts, Roadshow Entertainment.

Bollen, J., Kiernander, A., & Parr, B. (2006). *What's a Man Gotta Do? Masculinities in Performance*. Armidale: University of New England.

Bollen, J., Kiernander, A., & Parr, B. (2008). *Men at Play. Masculinities in Australian Theatre since the 1950s*. Amsterdam: Rodopi.

Bourdieu, P. (1990). *The Logic of Practice*. Oxford: Polity Press.

Broadway: The American Musical. (2005). DVD, directed by Michael Kantor. Sydney: Australian Broadcasting Corporation.

Burt, R. (1995). *The Male Dancer: Bodies, Spectacle, Sexualities*. London: Routledge.

Butler, J. (1990). *Gender Trouble: Feminism and the Subversion of Identity*. New York: Routledge.

Butler, J. (1993). *Bodies That Matter*. New York: Routledge.

Callery, D. (2001). *Through the Body: A Practical Guide to Physical Theatre*. London: Nick Hern Books.

Connell, R.W. (1995). *Masculinities*. Sydney: Allen and Unwin.

Connell, R.W. (2000). *The Men and the Boys*. St Leonards, NSW: Allen and Unwin.

Davies, B. (1993). *Shards of Glass*. St Leonards: Allen and Unwin.

Department of Education and Early Childhood Development Victoria. (2014). *Unity through Diversity.* [Retrieved 07/30/14 from http://www.education.vic.gov.au/Documents/about/programs/cultures/unitydiversity.pdf]

Ecker, A. (1868). On a Characteristic Peculiarity in the Form of the Female Skull, and Its Significance for Comparative Anthropology. *Anthropological Review.* Vol 6, No 23, pp. 350–356.

Ellis, C. (2004). *The Ethnographic I.* Walnut Creek, CA: Altamira Press.

Feldenkrais Method. (2008). *The Feldenkrais Method.* [Retrieved 02/11/08 from http://www.feldenkraismethod.ca]

Foster, S.L. (1998). Choreographies of Gender. *Signs: Journal of Women in Culture & Society.* Vol 24, No 1, pp. 1–33.

Gard, M. (2003). Being Someone Else: Using Dance in Anti-oppressive Teaching. *Educational Review.* Vol 55, No 2, pp. 211–223.

Gard, M. (2004). Movement, Art and Culture: Problem-Solving and Critical Inquiry in Dance. In Wright, J., Macdonald, D., & Burrows, L. (Eds.). *Critical Inquiry and Problem-Solving in Physical Education.* London: Routledge.

Gorely, T., Holroyd, R., & Kirk, D. (2003). Muscularity, the Habitus and the Social Construction of Gender: Towards a Gender-Related Physical Education. *British Journal of Sociology of Education.* Vol 24, No 4, pp. 429–448.

Holman Jones, S. (2005). Autoethnography: Making the Personal Political. In Denzin N.K., & Lincoln, Y.S. (Eds.). *The Sage Handbook of Qualitative Research* (third edition). Thousand Oaks: Sage.

Kroeger, B. (2003). *Passing: When People Can't Be Who They Are.* New York: Public Affairs.

Leavy, P. (2009). *Method Meets Art: Arts-Based Research Practice.* New York: Guilford Press.

Lecoq, J. (2002). *The Moving Body: Teaching Creative Theatre.* New York: Routledge.

Mackerras, C. (1975). *The Chinese Theatre in Modern Times.* London: Thames and Hudson.

Migdalek, J. (2009). Masculine Moves: The Measure of a Man. *N J Drama Australia Journal.* Vol 32, No 1, pp. 45–54.

Migdalek, J. (2014). Challenging Gendered Practices through Drama. In Meyer, E.J., & Carlson, C. (Eds.). *Gender and Sexualities in Education.* New York: Peter Lang.

Monro, S. (2005). *Gender Politics.* London: Pluto.

Petropoulos, J. (1996). *Arts as Politics in the Third Reich.* Chapel Hill: University of North Carolina Press.

Schutz, A. (1944). The Stranger: An Essay in Social Psychology. *American Journal of Sociology.* Vol 49, No 6, pp. 499–507.

Schutz, A. (1972). *The Phenomenology of the Social World.* London: Heinemann.

Sears, A., & Hollos, W.H. (2002). Actor Training in the Neutral Mask. In Zarrilli, P.B. (Ed.). *Acting (Re)Considered: A Theoretical and Practical Guide.* London: Routledge.

Shilling, C. (2003). *The Body and Social Theory.* London: Sage.

Shilling, C. (2004). Educating Bodies: Schooling and the Constitution of Society. In Wright, J., Davies, B., Shilling, C., & Evans, J. (Eds.). *Body, Knowledge and Control: Studies in the Sociology of Physical Education.* London: Routledge.

Snowber, C. (2002). Bodydance: Enfleshing Soulful Inquiry through Improvisation. In Bagley, C., & Cancienne, M.B. (Eds.). *Dancing the Data.* New York: Peter Lang.

South Pacific. (2008). DVD, directed by Joshua Logan. Moore Park: Twentieth Century Fox.

Turner, B. (1992). *Regulating Bodies: Essays in Medical Sociology.* London: Routledge.

9 Embodied Performance of Gender in the Worlds of High School Students

I wanted to gauge whether and how issues of gender and embodiment that resonate with me personally were of relevance to others, particularly contemporary youth. To this end, I conducted fieldwork with high school students, educators (performance arts and other disciplines), graduating youth-work and healthcare trainees, and members of the general public, in which I put a mirror of my experiences and outlook before others. I did so in a combination of forums, including professional development sessions, workshops, and performance-presentations. Data that I draw on in reporting on my fieldwork (conducted between 2007 and 2010) are taken from observational and reflective field notes, narrative accounts, audio recorded group discussions, and participant response sheets. The medium of anonymous response sheets made it possible for participants to voice ideas that may otherwise have been silenced and/or not come to my attention (see Lincoln 1995, Fontana & Frey 2005). Indeed, a number of participants, especially school students, put forward sentiments that had not been voiced or were contradictory to those that were offered publicly. I include direct quotations from participants to illustrate common as well as disparate perspectives that circulated during the fieldwork sessions. These have been pared down from a larger collection of quotes to represent a distillation of the attitudes expressed. In quoting participants, ". . ." indicates that I have made a break in what was a longer quotation; "—" indicates that the speaker did not finish or has paused mid-utterance; and text in *italic* indicates word emphasis.

Ethnographic fieldwork that I conducted with some four hundred high school students occurred in one government public high school, two non-government private schools, and two international summer schools, all in Melbourne, Australia. Each of these co-educational groups included students born in Australia and those born in regions of North America, Europe, Asia, Africa, and/or the Middle East. Fieldwork sessions comprised a combination of a performance of *Gender Icons,* group discussion, a movement workshop activity, and the filling in of anonymous response sheets. On the whole, a similar range of responses to issues of gender and embodiment were expressed across each of the various groupings of students. I will point out a particular participant group or state the biological sex, age, or nationality of any individual student only where I feel these points of difference are noteworthy.

I address students' views on the following themes that arose in open group discussions and students' anonymous written response sheets: socially acceptable male/female embodiment, culture and globalization, embodiment as social construction or nature, differing aesthetics for male/female embodiment, binary versus continuum, consciousness of how embodiment is perceived by others, connections between embodiment and sexual orientation, connections between saying and doing, social and emotional consequences for the individual inclined to transgress embodied gender norms, and possibilities of change in the social mindset toward the embodiment of gender. In addition to views expressed by students, my analysis also draws on my reporting and reading of how they engaged in a practical workshop activity.

SOCIALLY ACCEPTABLE MALE/FEMALE EMBODIMENT

Students' comments on performances of gender focused on differences between embodied behavior that is deemed socially acceptable for males and embodied behavior that is deemed socially acceptable for females, as well as the power and pressure that society exerts on the individual:

> Gender stereotypes are influenced by the society or culture we live in.
>
> Males can only behave in a certain way, . . . Once a male moves in a certain way their sexuality and I suppose competence and dominance is somewhat questioned.
>
> If you walk along and you see a man with his legs crossed, like sitting (demonstrates effeminate crossed leg pose), you're bound to have a giggle . . . It's just the way it's—I don't know—the way it's always been. You just kind of learn from how it used to be.

The last quote indicates a passive yet mindful acceptance of the existing and inherited status quo. A similar sense of acquiescence to social mores is expressed by a male who was prompted to ponder why it is he does not embody in a feminine manner: "I imagine that I do at a sub-conscious level move my body in a way deemed masculine. This . . . upon reflection seems somewhat irrational, but these are things that have developed over time, out of habit". It makes sense that where particular ways of embodying become habitual, the individual is not likely to be conscious of *gendered* aspects of such embodiment. What these students are used to is what seems natural and normal to them.

For some, the juxtaposition of conservative and transgressive gender embodiment staged in the performance of *Gender Icons* disrupted their perspectives regarding the embodiment of gender, causing them to perceive/question embodiment in ways that they had perhaps not considered before:

> The performance was intriguing and made me realize things I see everyday but never think about.
>
> [The performance] was a great way of opening people's eyes and making them see and think of the world with a new view. It was an enlightenment to watch and I can't see the world the same again.
>
> For me, it really highlighted the fact that there are so many rules in society that people abide by just because they're male or female, even if we actually don't notice them. But now . . . I think I'm probably going to start recognising how much people look down upon a girl doing things that they shouldn't because that's usually what a guy does, or a guy doing what a girl usually does.

For those students whose perspectives were disrupted, it is as if what the master-signifier (Zizek 1999) has caused to stand out as negative or abnormal has shifted, foregrounding that master-significations are not stable or beyond change. That the embodied theatrical performance provoked audience members' consideration of issues in ways that they may not necessarily have considered before is testimony to the power of the theatre as a medium that can lead people to see themselves in new ways (see Saxton & Miller 2009, Sinclair et al. 2009). Questions arise concerning distinctions in attitudes toward transgressions of gender embodiment as portrayed on a stage and those that occur, or are 'staged', in the everyday. The idea that something portrayed on a stage is contrived might allow the performer more license and freedom to transgress norms of behavior—albeit temporarily. On the other hand, performances that occur, or are 'staged', in the everyday may be regarded as 'unstaged', and as such place more pressure on the performer to ensure that what they perform is socially acceptable. Audiences too may be inclined to be more open to accepting transgressive embodiments of gender that occur, or are 'staged', on a stage than those that occur, or are 'staged', in the everyday, such as by a person sitting beside them on a bus.

CULTURE AND GLOBALIZATION

Issues were raised as to whether and why there are differences in cultural perspectives toward acceptable male or female embodiment. Some students held to the line that views regarding acceptable embodiment for males and females were world-views or part of the natural order: "The whole world agrees on the 'acceptable' way for males and females to act"; "I feel that male should be masculine and female should be feminine because this is just the way it is".

Regarding the performance of *Gender Icons,* one Chinese Singaporean student in an international summer school observed:

> It's interesting how the audience from different countries and ethnic groups responded in similar ways to the movements . . . Today's diverse

> audience did respond in the same way and laughed at the same moment. I think we're very much moving toward a global culture.

Whether the commonalities in reaction were the result of a natural response, or, as the student suggests, because "we have been so used to western perspective", is worthy of contemplation. As a non-Western subject, the student is questioning Western domination over world-views and globalized perspectives.

Other students expressed the view that differences in perspectives on what embodiment was appropriate/inappropriate for males and females varied according to culture. Several non-Western students commented from cultural points of view that they were not comfortable with behavioral role reversals between males and females. Such comments were impervious to Asian and other cultures' pre-Christian and pre-colonial openness to gender and sexual diversity (see Taga 2005). One student in an international summer school made direct links between his own perceptions as a Peruvian subject and the cultures that had colonized his country:

> Being a Peruvian, I think that my perception of gender and society in general has been influenced by the Western culture, as my country was conquered by the Spanish empire. So our culture carries the perception of European people since the conquest.

This comment connects to the discussion of postcolonialism in Chapter 2 and commentary on the influence of dominant Commonwealth cultures put forward in Chapter 5.

It is too simplistic to talk about outlooks as being shared across any particular culture. Two international summer school students of the same age, biological sex, nationality, and high school expressed opposing personal views on cultural attitudes in their home-country, New Zealand, toward the embodiment of gender. One of the students referred to her society as being accepting of transgressive gender behavior. Her counterpart sensed discriminatory attitudes that a male in her culture would suffer for the same behavior. Where one student recognizes prejudice in her culture, the other does not. Clearly there can be variations in individual perspectives despite some aspects of culture that are shared. These may stem from differences in family/home life, socio-economic factors, and their own life experiences of prejudice and discrimination.

EMBODIMENT AS SOCIAL CONSTRUCTION OR NATURE

Students demonstrated a variety of viewpoints concerning whether male and female differential embodiment was a social/cultural manifestation, a matter of biology, or a combination thereof. Some students saw differences in male and female embodiment as being biologically determined: "A male lacking a particular hormone may lead him to serious hormonal imbalance such as feminization"; "I guess it is also the way genes are in humans. For example, during puberty, males become more muscular and thus almost naturally they will behave more rough"; "I find it perfectly fine with guys being more feminine . . . Guys who does this mostly have something different with their hormones as compared to normal guys thus resulting in their action". Despite the accepting tone of the last quote, it counterpoints hormonal imbalance and feminine action against 'normal' biology and the action of 'normal' guys, thus pathologizing such differences as ab-normal.

Other students indicated an awareness of an interconnection between individuals' perceptions and their upbringing: "It's the older generation that has caused the stereotypes. We're just continuing it on"; "It's just been drilled into us". Students also indicated an awareness of interconnections between how they perceive things and their saturation from media representations and ascriptions: "Media impacts on how we see certain movements".

During my discussion with the public high school participant group, I instigated the following dialogue in reference to gendered embodiment and nature:

ME: Is femininity more suitable to females? Is masculinity more suitable to males? Is that a natural thing or a cultural thing do you think?

STUDENT: It's more natural than cultural . . . because when you go and live that life, the way you get raised and the way people around you, it's just how you get influenced, it's how you inform yourself.

ME: But being raised is a cultural thing, isn't it?

STUDENT: Yeah . . . it's a bit of both.

In this interaction, lines are blurred between culture and nature, with cultural and social influences being understood to be by-products of nature. The student's inability to distinguish between nature and culture is concerning. The feeling of resignation to the way things are leaves no scope for resistance. Other students held hardline views in which readings of embodied gender performance were hardly negotiable: "If a woman moves in a masculine way they must be a lesbian or frigid. While when a male moves in a female way he must be gay or lacking".

DIFFERING AESTHETICS FOR MALE AND FEMALE EMBODIMENT

Across my fieldwork with high school students it was evident that most students had clear thoughts concerning the type of embodiment that was suitable/unsuitable and aesthetic/un-aesthetic for male or female bodies, whether it be from the perspective of scrutineer and/or subject of scrutiny: "I might stop myself from sitting with my legs open because it doesn't look good for girls to sit like this"; "Women are attracted to men with biceps and masculine ways". Modes of embodiment that these comments espouse—be they in response to external ascriptions and/or self-ascribed—align with forms of embodiment as valorized for male and female bodies in mainstream media (referred to in Chapter 5).

Most students did not question why they found a particular male or female embodiment to be personally aesthetic. However, the following comment put the onus on society and culture:

> It's all down to . . . the people around us who influence our thoughts. From an early age the difference between gender has been established for us and we'll always think with that ideal we were brought up with.

BINARY VERSUS CONTINUUM

Students across all participating student groups positioned masculine and feminine as binary opposites seen to suit male bodies or female bodies respectively: "Males have their own way to move their body and so do females . . . that allows people to differentiate you as male or female". Comments were made regarding how children are raised to understand notions of male and female as binary opposites: "Around Year 1 and Year 2, teachers and parents start to put these stereotypical images of the boy and girl as being two completely separate things". Consistent with the notion that children need boundaries of difference to be clear-cut (Paechter 2007), one student commented that seeing gender in binary terms is simply less complicated than dealing with multiple categories: "It's easier to just work with two different values . . . Anything in between gets divided into either this group or that group".

For some, notions of male and female and masculine and feminine as binary opposites, as discussed in regard to binary classification and hierarchical dualisms in Chapter 2 (Davies 1989, Butler 1990, 2004, Monro 2005, Mac an Ghaill & Haywood 2007, Pallotta-Chiarolli 2010), was desirable:

> We like the contrast . . . We like to stay with males being strong and females being elegant and dainty, because we're comfortable with being different in the fact that he's a male and I'm a female because of the way that we are, our genetic make up.

In stating "we like", this student's comments are blind to understanding that her personalized aesthetic preferences may be interconnected to deep-rooted ideologies that have become embedded as second nature or habitus

(Bourdieu 1990). While the student voiced a preference for a clear demarcation between male and female, she added, "At the same time I don't think there should be anything wrong with breaking that mould". Despite this sentiment, the student's preference for males to be strong and females to be dainty leaves the individual who *does* break the valorized mold as being marked, if not un-aesthetic.

There were other students who voiced objections to being forced to adhere to binary models of gender, claiming that "stereotypes are forcing people to conform and stay in the barriers of female and male which isn't really right". The following arguments were made for a differing mindset concerning the divide between masculine and feminine: "You don't really have to have this line that differentiates whether this person is acting like a male or like a female . . . Somewhere along the line we really need to stop differentiating so much"; "I can be both masculine and effeminate and that's ok!"; "It doesn't have to be always 'this is masculine, this is feminine'. There are things that blur between the lines, and it *should* be like that". These voices are advocating a kind of gender continuum (see Monro 2005, Pallotta-Chiarolli 2010) where an individual might operate and shift between cultural and gender extremes/polarities ranging through masculine and feminine and not have to feel the need to behave one way or the other. Despite these sentiments, there is still a slippage into a binary mindset when one student, on advocating being "able to act any way that you feel", limited the range of acceptable *'act'*-ion by qualifying her statement with the binarily constructed addendum "whether it be male or feminine".

One student noted that although she recognized that it was possible for an individual's embodiment to shift across a gender continuum, doing so "might be hard for some people". Questioning why this is so may illuminate the degree to which social/cultural constraints regarding masculinity and male as a binary opposite to feminine and female cause such difficulties.

CONSCIOUSNESS OF HOW EMBODIMENT IS PERCEIVED BY OTHERS

In a group discussion that occurred during my public high school field visit, the view was put forward that individuals should not care about how others regard them. One male student firmly advised, "You've got to not care what people think". I followed this by asking, "How many people don't really care what people think?" In response, around 50% of the group put their hands up, indicating to me that these students would themselves be tolerant and accepting of alternative behaviors. It may be that those who raised their hands did so as the result of panopticonic anxieties, so as not to appear to be unaccepting, politically incorrect, old-fashioned, or uncool. Nevertheless, the strength with which this view was put forward could be encouraging to those in the group who may feel conscious of how their behavior is perceived by others. However, I found that what appeared to be a very accepting school culture was at odds with privately expressed anxieties articulated in response sheets to the question of if/when one might stop oneself from moving in masculine/feminine manner. These indicate significant panopticonic fears and concerns hinging on how one's embodiment is perceived by others: "I might stop myself from moving in masculine ways whenever there's friends or others present because I don't want them to laugh at me"; "I am really a person that cares about what people think"; "People will think I'm gay and they will laugh".

Despite the strongly expressed view that individuals should not care about how others regard them as put forward during the public high school group discussion, comments in anonymous response sheets make it clear that a number of students in the group did not take comfort in such rhetoric. My observations of the limits to which this student group was able to practically engage in and commit to the ensuing workshop activity also indicate a gap between what students may espouse and what they practice. What people *think* or *know* on a cognitive level is not necessarily akin to what they *do* impulsively or habitually (see Paechter 2007). How students handled the practical workshop activity will be commented on shortly.

Several students in other high school participant sites were also bold in advising individuals not to care about what others may think of how they embody. In promotion of an individualistic stance, students' proclamations were loaded with media-driven commercially popular jargon and self-help rhetoric such as *"go for it"*, *"be what you want"*, and *"build a bridge and get over it"*, which in themselves may be cool to declare. Although these pieces of advice may be well intended, sentiments expressed via anonymous response sheets by a far greater number of students (across all student fieldwork sites) indicate that consciousness of how others would perceive their embodiment should they embody in gender transgressive ways figures as a major obstacle to being comfortable embodying in ways that may go against the norm. Acute self-consciousness pertaining to embodied performance can be understood through concerns over decency and not making the wrong impression:

> As I am a female I would certainly move my body in a decent feminine way and not in a masculine way at any point of time. If you're a girl you act like a girl. It applies the same for a boy.
>
> A lot of the time, I will be conscious to not look butch, so I will emphasize my feminine movements. I do this so that people don't get the wrong impression of me.
>
> I will feel embarrassed if I do some effeminate ways even if nobody is looking at me.

The fact that the student who wrote the last comment envisages feeling embarrassed even when not being observed is testimony to the force of panopticonic self-monitoring.

The responses of students across all fieldwork sites indicated a concern about being labeled: "Society can automatically put you into categories based on how you present yourself". It was made clear that being labeled for embodying in gender transgressive ways has undesired consequences, such as being frowned on, made to feel culturally insensitive or misfit, marginalized, physically policed or discriminated against: "We need to act according to the 'norm' or else people will not accept us"; "My dad would give me a right beating". It is clear from these anonymously made comments that connections were being made by students between transgressive embodiment of gender and ensuing discrimination. This was in contrast to one student's comment to me that "society is not nearly as oppressive as you portrayed it to be". In regard to homophobia—which will be dealt with in a subsequent section—her claim that "jokes about gay people are light hearted and shouldn't be taken to heart as discrimination" displays an insensitivity to what those who are trivialized may feel but not say, as well as the lengths to which some may go in order to avoid standing out as different. Where students spoke of modifying or self-policing their embodiment, it was in order to feel safe and avoid negative reactions from those around them: "If I felt threatened by people around me, or pressured to act a certain way I would change the way my body moves".

Although advice that individuals should not care about how others may regard their embodiment was strongly expressed by several students, data that emanated from anonymous response sheets indicate that a great many high school students are indeed very conscious of and concerned about how their embodiment is perceived by others. One wonders whether the same students who had brazenly purported that individuals should not care about how others regard them were the same ones who in the anonymous response sheets had expressed anxieties over how others regard them. Indeed, those in communities such as schools may operate according to "mutual panopticism" (Paechter 2007, p. 20) and publicly conform to collectively constructed concepts of masculinity or femininity, despite their private views. Could it be that publicly espousing that individuals should not care, while at the same time self-policing how they allow themselves to perform gender, serves to protect members of communities, such as schools, from marginalization?

Altogether, sentiments expressed in anonymous response sheets that differed from sentiments shared in discussion indicate students' reluctance to reveal aspects of themselves before others. For example, a male student who wrote of *almost falling into tears* during the performance of *Gender Icons* made no mention of this in the post-performance discussion. If social change toward embodied gender equity is to occur, then it is necessary to foster environments in which it is possible to transfer what is privately felt and believed into a public realm where individuals might openly advocate, declare, and act on their private feelings without fear or anxiety. There must surely be ramifications for the well-being of those whose position and behaviors in public realms are in conflict with their private feelings and inclinations.

EMBODIMENT AND SEXUAL ORIENTATION

"I don't want people to think I'm gay". Anxieties about being perceived to be gay were frequently expressed as reasons to self-police one's physical deportment. This correlates with the findings of a national report on the well-being of same-sex attracted youth in Australia, which spoke of young people making changes in their embodiment as a means of avoiding homophobic abuse (Hillier et al. 2005). Consistent connections were made by fieldwork participants between feminine embodiment on a male and homosexuality, which for these students did not carry much weight as cultural or physical capital:

> I would always stop myself from moving in a feminine way with the exception of when I am joking or impersonating someone. This is possibly because I am 16 years old and all a 16 year old really wants is to be accepted, to know that he's okay. Not be ridiculed or called 'gay'.
>
> Any masculine movement may mean others challenging my sexuality or even integrity as a female and hence lose the attraction others may have for me.
>
> I would dance like a female only when dared to or while imitating someone. However while doing so I wouldn't feel conscious/awkward cause I know and so does everyone else that I am straight.

It appears that the student who made the last comment is secure in transgressing only as a result of being secure in his heterocapital.

Many of the students whose comments connected femininity on a male with homosexuality understood homosexuality as undesirable and negative:

> I think if a person shows feminine habits and behavior (such as the lecturer) he is bound to be gay. I do not accept homosexuality . . . I am a male. It will look awkward if I start behaving like a female. I rather die than act like a female (or be gay).

One student who complimented me on my presentation even felt the need to qualify his admiration by making it clear that he was not homosexual: "By the way, I love your talk and performance Jack, and I'm not gay 'ha ha'". My reading of his need to append his compliment with a *'ha ha'* declaration that he was straight implies to me that for him, being gay, though possibly acceptable, is something he would not want to be. Perhaps he felt the need to add this declaration in order to allay a fear that his *loving* my performance might lead me to assume that he was gay and attracted to me.

Some students admitted to self-policing their embodiment because of pressures and prospects of being thought of and/or pathologized as gay: "I used to have a habit of swaying my butt whenever I walk. My parents thought I was 'gay'. They actually sent me for a full body check up . . . That's when I stopped. I couldn't take that kind of pressure"; "I tend to avoid acting in an effeminate manner when I am around other males for fear of being thought of as gay". These sentiments should not be surprising given that levels of homophobic abuse, particularly in school sites, have been on the rise (Hillier et al. 2010).

A number of students admitted to self-policing their embodiment to varying degrees, even in cases where they felt that they were capable of resisting pressures to conform. The student who said, "I am comfortable doing things b/c I don't care what people think, but sometimes I restrain myself b/c people will judge me", oscillates between what is felt and what is actually practiced.

Responding to the strongly expressed view that people should not care what others think of how they move (as articulated in the group discussion), a dance teacher at the public high school questioned why the boys in her dance class were discriminatory in the types of dance steps they were willing to do, adding that this had forced her to choreograph 'boy alternatives' for them. She asked, "Can some of the boys in my dance class talk about some of the steps that you don't want to do?" The boys then described and parodied certain styles of motion ("those hippy movements") as those that they don't do. When asked why, the only answer offered was "I don't know, it doesn't really feel that masculine". The students were unable to articulate why feeling un-masculine felt uncomfortable for them. They lacked the skills to critically analyze the machinations at work that led to these discomforts.

The prospect for these males of dancing in ways that might not feel masculine implies that for a male to feel anything other than masculine is undesirable. Surely having a hang up about feeling feminine when moving in certain ways is connected to concerns about how one's embodiment projects to others. Why else would feeling feminine when moving in certain ways matter? It concerns me that what comes to *feel* comfortable for these males to do—or dance—is so pervasively promoted and prescribed that it becomes ingrained, effectively obliterating the potential to experience alternative options. Although they may think themselves open to embodying in ways that might be transgressive of gender norms ("I wouldn't stop myself because I don't care what people think"), this seems not to be the case in practice.

The dance teacher made the comment that pop star Ricky Martin used his hips a lot when dancing and looked great doing so. Although several girls offered comments of "He's hot", one male offered, "Isn't he gay or something?" reinforcing connections between such motion on a male and homosexuality. Here, the straight-presenting male uses the trope of 'gay' to demean, subordinate, and denigrate the way another male moves, degrading what the girls had positioned as Ricky Martin's physical capital into social or cultural poverty instead. Questions were raised as to whether all gay men wiggled their hips. A different male answered that this was not so "cos when you're gay one's got to be a bloke, one's got to be a chick". Here the student imposes heteronormative and heteropatriarchal constructions of gender roles in a heterosexual relationship onto a same-sex relationship. The comment acknowledged that not all gay men embody in a feminine manner (in this case the 'bloke' in a relationship). However, it also illustrates the fixed mindset that the male who *does* move in that way must be homosexual. There is a discrepancy here between intellectual reasoning and socially/culturally cultivated perspectives. Essentially, the dogma that these males held true was that straight men do not move in a feminine manner.

A handful of students expressed that they made no connections between manner of embodiment and sexual orientation: "I see no problem in acting effeminately and do not draw a parallel between this and homosexuality". Despite sentiments such as these, views expressed across students' response sheets and also in discussion overwhelmingly associated transgressive gender embodiment, particularly effeminacy on a male, with homosexuality: "Apart from homosexuals, you don't see males/female acting the opposite way". What I find problematic are the assumed connections made between gender behavior and sexual orientation. Despite some concern for the well-being of those who may embody in gender transgressive ways, assumptions that such persons are gay illustrates fixed preconceptions concerning the embodiment of the homosexual. Many comments made by student participants presuppose that the feminine moving male is queer, which is very much in line with DePalma and Atkinson's concerns about the conflation of sex, gender, and sexuality, which ignores "that these are in reality separate aspects of human identity and experience" (2008, p. 127). Students' assumptions of how queer males embody can also be related to Zizek's (1999) master-signifier theory in that they are determined in counterpoint to notions of how straight males embody.

SAYING VERSUS DOING

What was most telling about sentiments expressed by those student participants who argued that individuals should embody in any way they want to was how they, along with a majority of other students, handled a practical workshop task that I conducted with them. This was preceded by my performance of *Gender Icons* and a discussion around students' responses to the piece and issues that they thought it raised. For the workshop activity that followed, I read out to the students a quote from the second series of the popular, high rating Australian version of the US television program *So You Think You Can Dance* (Network 10), which was still airing at the time. The comment was made by one of the judges (Jason Coleman) to a female hip-hop dancer (Pania Taku):

> What you showed me is very aggressive and very masculine actually. It's very masculine. At the end of today you are a dancer that I will remember and that's a credit to you. I enjoyed you.

I asked students to imagine the inverse being said to a male dancer, whereby a male might be complimented for moving in a feminine manner. Then I organized students to work in mixed groups with four to eight students in each group. With the female students working as choreographers and the males as dancers/subjects, the brief was to create and choreograph a dance sequence for a male body that was feminine in manner that would be admired and get the following positive comment from a judge on a mainstream television program such as *So You Think You Can Dance: "What you showed me is very soft and very feminine actually. It's very feminine. At the end of today you are a dancer that I will remember and that's a credit to you. I enjoyed you".*

Students were given time to work on the task and then were asked to perform their choreographed sequences before the whole class. In running the workshop activity, I was interested in observing how students would conceive of, approach, and physically perform embodiment for males that was transgressive of norms of male embodiment. In each of the school fieldwork sites where I conducted the workshop, female students created and taught their male counterparts short dance sequences that for the most part involved swaying of hips, wafting arms, and limp wrists. In the public high school and in one of the private high schools there was a lot of laughter in the room during the workshop session, and the atmosphere was, on the whole, playful. However, in both sites it was apparent that moving in feminine ways was uncomfortable, embarrassing, or amusing for the males concerned. For example, boys laughed or groaned as their female choreographers showed them steps to perform; boys held back physically from accurately reproducing steps that they were taught; boys stood with hands in pockets until prodded by their female choreographers to *do* the steps they were being taught; boys added parodic embellishments such as pouting lips and/or vocalized flourishes that mocked the choreography they were executing. This included the males in the public high school who had indicated that they did not care about how others regarded them. In the same school, one group of three males refused outright to do the activity. They told me that they were too uncomfortable to move in feminine ways. I did not insist on their participation and allowed them to observe the activity, leaving their female choreographers to work on the task on their own. I was surprised that the boys in question did not cajole or ridicule other males in the class for moving in feminine ways as I feared they might. Perhaps this was a result of being let off the hook from having to do so themselves.

I found that girls too, in the public high school and one of the private schools, did not handle the workshop task in the previously endorsed spirit that individuals should be able to embody freely. Their peals of laughter denoted what felt to me as boorish pleasure at challenging their male choreographic subjects to tackle steps that they put together for them to execute, enforcing notions that males moving in a feminine manner were incongruous and ludicrous.

After some preparation time, groups presented their sequences for one another. In each case audiences were supportive of the males performing 'on stage', and in the two schools mentioned there was a sense of fun as audiences whooped for the males dancing before them. Despite earlier expressed and supported sentiments that "You've got to not care what people think" and "I don't care what people think", it was clear to me from my observations of the workshop activity that doing so in practice was a different thing altogether. It was as if 'mutual panopticism' (Paechter 2007) in the form of the disciplinary gaze between peers ensured conformity to lived embodiment of gender.

It was clear to me that in all but one school there was a contradiction between what the students could articulate rationally or cerebrally about embodied gender equity and how they could actually engage with embodied performance that did not match prescribed norms of gender behavior. Performances were very self-conscious and unanimously carried out in fun and parody. Male and female audience members whooping for their male classmates moving in a feminine manner before them made clear that, despite earlier expressed sentiments, the male moving in a feminine manner continues to be positioned and regarded as an object of amusement. There was no sense that any of the dance sequences that were created were actually aesthetic as executed by a male body, despite this having been the challenge of the task. I was dismayed that collectively two of the high school student groups with whom I conducted the workshop were unable to earnestly commit to the physical problem-solving task they were given, especially given that the context was a staged or 'unreal' performance for the stage. Although the students in question claimed to have enjoyed the session—"Really enjoyed"; "Awesome Dude!"; "Excellent"—I believe that only a handful of them came away from it with a practical critical perspective or understanding of transgressive embodiment of gender.

Harking back to Gard's (2004) theories on critical reflection of embodiment, I tried to use the experience of the practical workshop as a vehicle to encourage reflection on why it may have felt good or bad to move in certain ways; why people do not more readily break out of corporeal expectations that hinge on biological sex; how ways in which we move may be influenced by a consciousness of how our performances are perceived by others. I mentioned that I thought that for male students, the workshop task might not have been as easy to execute as they may have thought it would be. One male student claimed that the execution of the task hinged on what he referred to as the "care factor", the extent to which a performer cares about what others think. The male in question contended that he had a *"zero"* care factor, even though from my perspective on the way he held back in the performance of the choreography he had been given, he very clearly did care about how he projected to others.

My impression was that the extent to which males in this particular group were willing to enter into embodied expression that was transgressive of socially prescribed norms was marred by a lack of respect and support for one another to take a risk, even within the context of an exploratory workshop. The threat of being mocked or ridiculed by peers appeared to prevent these particular students from engaging with the set task in a way that was earnest and without inhibition. I believe that this was due to deep-seated attitudes toward and perspectives on transgressive embodied performances of gender, which wield an influence over the school culture. While productive on a rational level for many, it saddens me to think that the outcomes of this particular workshop may have reinforced the restrictive and inequitable gendered codes of embodiment by which they operate, and the threat of social ridicule, alienation, or harassment that might result from transgressing these norms. The boys' discomforts at moving in a feminine manner in a staged or 'unreal' performance for the stage would have been even more acute if they had been performing in 'real' contexts of the everyday.

Comparing students' spoken and written responses to their practical execution of the workshop activity reveals that there can be a dissonance between reasoning/rationalizing/knowing and acting out/behaving/doing. Established habitual ways of *viewing* and *doing* gender, and scar-tissue of what particular styles of action may have previously meant, can weigh on our ability to effect change in a practical sense, even when we are able to argue for/articulate embodied gender equity. Whereas students expressed sentiments that appeared to be accepting of and able to physically adopt a loosening of embodied gender-based constraints regarding *adornment* for male and female bodies (such as those in fashion and grooming), there was little sign that—for males especially—they were open to or able to adapt respectfully, at this stage, to a broadening of *embodied performance* possibilities of gender. This may have been the first time these students were challenged in this way, and it would be interesting to investigate how they would handle subsequent opportunities that contested notions of gender embodiment.

A large number of students spoke in theory of having no issues with transgressive embodiment of gender. However, it was clear that for many students, even in the arguably 'safe' bounds of a structured workshop activity within the cultural confines of school, to directly deal with or actually embody in ways that were transgressive of gendered norms was a complicated and problematic practice. With this in mind, I argue that it is vital to foster an atmosphere in which students feel confident that school sites are safe places in which they might explore or play with gender possibilities without risk of being ridiculed, being squealed at, or losing face. How those in two of the three school groups handled the workshop session I conducted with them may have been specific to tensions relating to an exploratory workshop on transgressive embodiment of gender, not necessarily to problem-solving activities dealing with other issues.

Following the conclusion of my fieldwork sessions with students, many of them complimented and thanked me for my performance of *Gender Icons*. My sense was that they thought me brave and courageous as a male to have performed before them in a feminine manner as I did:

> It was a good performance and a good show of confidence and a very good attitude towards people who would judge your body because you don't care.
>
> The performance to me represented the performer's confidence. The performer initially came across as someone who had a slightly feminine side. However, his confidence in himself seems to make it seem alright—even though it is anyway.
>
> I think that it took a real man to do what was showed at the performance today. Many people would not dare to portray that kind of performance in today's society. Kudos to you.

As complimentary as the last comment is, the male student who made it displays clear discriminatory ideas on qualities, such as daring, that make a 'real' man. The implication here is that other men with other qualities are not real men and as such subordinate. These comments verify that for these students, transgressing norms of gender embodiment takes courage and the overcoming of fear and, if done with confidence, earns respect. At the same time, the comments maintain a distance between what I, the performer, a man, was daring enough to do in transgression of gendered norms of embodiment and any notion that they themselves might follow suit.

I find it interesting that students did not think that I cared about how I projected. I wonder with what esteem students would have regarded or admired me had I shared my apprehensions about performing feminine sections of *Gender Icons* before them. I wonder if in exposing my fears, or what some might regard as weaknesses, I would still have been regarded as a 'real man'. I cannot explain why it was that I did not express these fears, but I wonder if having the nerve to do so would have made me even *more* of a man in their eyes. Somehow I do not think so.

It was noteworthy for me that one of the participating private high school groups (an outer suburban private high school) handled the workshop very differently from the other high school groups. When both rehearsing and performing the feminine choreography that they were given, all of the boys in the group took the task seriously and focused on executing the choreography that they were given by the girls as well as they were able. They appeared to perform the moves given to them by their female choreographers without inhibition or self-consciousness of how others might respond. They performed with neither laughter nor any sense of parody, as opposed to the males in the other high school groups. I was impressed with what I witnessed. On discussion with the school teacher and the vice-principal, I learned that this particular school earnestly advocates respect, both of self and of others, an outlook that seemed to operate in practical and not just theoretical terms within this school culture.

In post-workshop discussion, students in the group in question were vehement that all persons should be able to move in any way that they wish. Although students in the group advocated the acceptability of a broad range of embodiment for all persons, it surprised me, in group discussion, that nobody took exception to one student's declaration that in general males who move in a feminine manner are homosexual. Here too connections were made between an individual's performance of gender and their sexual orientation.

SOCIAL AND EMOTIONAL WELL-BEING

Where students expressed concern for the social and emotional well-being of those who transgress norms of gender embodiment, comments centered on discriminatory repercussions that would follow as a consequence of such transgression: "They will alienate me and isolate me because I am different than how a true male or female should be, so I will refrain from behaving differently". In all participant groups, discussion concerning repercussions for males who embodied in a feminine manner moved seamlessly to discussion of repercussions for homosexual males, again connecting with sex/gender theories put forward in Chapter 2.

Comments that students made regarding the embodiment of gender and social and emotional well-being centered on the repercussions for the individual who actually embodies in gender transgressive ways. What students' considerations appear to overlook are the social and emotional repercussions that occur for the individual who, while 'passing' as gendernormative, goes through life self-policing an inclination to embody in gender transgressive ways. Also overlooked are social and emotional repercussions for the individual who may embody, or be inclined to embody, in gender transgressive ways and who may not be gay.

The fieldwork sessions referred to in this chapter led some students in all participant groups to reflect on their own outlooks on life with shifted perceptions: "I had a preconceived notion or perception of what each gender is supposed to behave like. I had never questioned this or even thought about it because it was just something I always believed without thinking or questioning it". This comment is indicative of the force of that which is taken for granted (Schutz 1944, 1972) and fixed schemes of perception as habitus (Bourdieu 1990).

In making direct reference to fieldwork sessions and the performance of *Gender Icons,* the following comments reinforce the notion that performance arts (performances and workshops) can be used as vehicles toward achieving attitudinal change (see Sinclair et al. 2009): "[the session] made me a little more sensitive toward males who are feminine"; "The performance was intriguing and made me realize things I see everyday but never think about"; "[the session] has helped me realize that I am what I am and I should do what I want to do. Thanks".

CHANGE

A variety of views were expressed by students on whether and how social change in mindsets toward embodiment of gender might come about. Several students expressed attitudes that change was seen as fundamentally undesirable: "It's kind of like a cat say pretending to be a dog. You think that's extremely strange. It's not how it should be, because everything has to be as it should be, because we can't deal with difference and change".

There were those who demonstrated resignation to the established order or status quo and advised submission to the hegemonic line, as a system that they did not deem to be in need of change: "This is how our society is and although it may not be terrific it is still how things are and it works well". Other students were more optimistic and committed to the need for change to occur:

> People just need to start accepting the fact that we shouldn't make these stereotypes. It's okay to do something feminine, like to move in a feminine way, to move your hips even if you're a male . . . People just have to accept the fact that it's not wrong. They have to move on from these old views.

A student who claimed, "It doesn't matter if you're straight or gay", also claimed that "it doesn't matter if you walk or talk in an unnormal way". The student's use of the term 'unnormal' to describe a way of walking does not indicate an affirmation of differences. If anything, it betrays an attitude that sustains a gulf between *we* who are all the same and those who might behave differently.

One student saw a difference in the gender equity needs of males and females, stating, "Gender equity needs a new focus. Previously it has been about a women's movement and elevating females to the level of men, but there have been few efforts on the other end to say to males that it's okay to be feminine". Another student noted that whereas change in regard to acceptance of those who may be 'different' may be occurring, perceptions of behavior, appearance, and embodiment of that which is homosexual remain fixed and in need of attention: "I think society is starting to accept gays and stuff, but I think it will take much more time to change the perception of what we think is gay".

Some students thought that change in the social mindset toward the embodiment of gender would occur in time, although not through deliberate lobbying or effort. The language they use speaks of changes in the world/society, yet with no indication of their personal attachment to it: "I feel gradually the society would accept guys having girlie postures and vice-versa" (female student). This comment, while seemingly open to change occurring, is problematic. The student's descriptor of certain postures being 'girlie' indicates how fixed her perceptions are, making clear links between particular embodied forms of gender and female biology. Use of linguistic descriptors, such as 'girlie' and 'manly' as indicative of feminine and masculine, coined by individuals within each participant group, illustrate how fixed perceived interconnections between gender and biological sex can be.

A number of students espoused active intervention in areas such as education as ways in which social change in mindsets toward transgressive gender embodiment might come about. At the same time, it was acknowledged that influencing change comes at a personal cost to those brave enough to effect it, through reference to taking risks, getting hurt, and paying a price for such bravery: "If you never make a change it's never going to happen . . . if nobody gets hurt it probably can never evolve".

The tone of discussion among the private high school students who had handled the workshop without inhibition or self-consciousness about how others might respond was generally indignant regarding discriminatory attitudes in the broader community. One student in the group spoke of effecting social change through pro-active intervention in the form of "social revolution". Despite reservations about change coming quickly, several students in this group endorsed deliberate acts of resistance and advocated for young people to "start pushing the boundary of what they can and can't do": "Instead of asking 'Why can't we?' I should consider 'Why shouldn't we?'" None of these students commented on the consequences or forces that might deter an individual from taking such action.

There were students who were not hopeful of social change coming about any time soon, even in situations where individuals *appear* to be more open to changes in norms of gender embodiment. Although there were students across each of the participating student groups who expressed a readiness to accept changes regarding transgressive embodiment of gender in a broad social sense, students' comments illustrate that such changes are perceived differently when it comes to personal and familial contexts. There was a sense of wanting to protect intimates from embodying in gender transgressive ways: "Let's say like you have a child, you wouldn't want him to act like feminine right? . . . You encourage other people and you don't discriminate against other people, but you don't want your own children to act this way". This comment indicates a significant delineation that discriminates between what these students feel should be condoned within society and what they would find problematic to accommodate within their own families.

FIELDWORK WITH HIGH SCHOOL STUDENTS: ISSUES AND OUTCOMES

My fieldwork revealed that despite sentiments that transgressive embodiment on a male may not be problematic in theory for most students, in practice it was. Students in most participating high school groups spoke of having no issues with transgressive embodiment of gender. However, apart from the workshop output of the students in one of the private schools, it was clear that even in the arguably 'safe' bounds of a structured workshop activity within the cultural confines of the school, to actually embody in ways that were transgressive of gendered norms—for the males particularly—was problematic and uncomfortable. There is a dissonance between reasoning/rationalizing/knowing and acting out/behaving/doing (see Paechter 2007).

Quotes from high school aged youth that have been used in this chapter connect certain styles of gender embodiment with cultural poverty, physical poverty, and homosexuality. The personal fears, and feelings of discomfort and disquiet, expressed and implied within these quotes lead me to believe that the fears and anxieties pertinent to the embodiment of gender that touched me in my youth are still relevant to high school aged youth of today.

Harking back to students' reactions to my performance of *Gender Icons,* several students commented on how differently transgressive gender embodiment comes across in formal performance contexts as opposed to contexts of everyday life:

> I was thinking about how the audience seemed to accept it, and viewed it as a comedy of sorts, but I also think that despite this, when we see someone acting this way out of context, AKA on the street we'd probably be discriminating.

The fact that these students can engage with transgressive gender embodiment in a formal performance more willingly than in the everyday indicates to me the potential for performance arts as a vehicle toward effecting change in social attitudes toward embodiment of gender. Staged performances have the potential to challenge and provoke audiences' positioning toward transgressive as opposed to normative embodiment of gender, can lead students to reflect on their own reactions and actions, and can lead students to engage in critical thinking, analysis, and evaluation. The challenge for educators is to motivate students to link what they understand from staged performances with what they see around them in the everyday.

REFERENCES

Bourdieu, P. (1990). *The Logic of Practice*. Oxford: Polity Press.
Butler, J. (1990). *Gender Trouble: Feminism and the Subversion of Identity*. New York: Routledge.
Butler, J. (2004). *Undoing Gender*. New York: Routledge.
Davies, B. (1989). *Frogs and Snails and Feminist Tales: Preschool Children and Gender*. Sydney: Allen and Unwin.
DePalma, R., & Atkinson, E. (2008). *Invisible Boundaries: Addressing Sexualities Equality in Children's Worlds*. Stoke on Trent: Trentham.
Fontana, A., & Frey, J.H. (2005). The Interview: From Neutral Stance to Political Involvement. In Denzin, N.K., & Lincoln, Y.S. (Eds.). *The Sage Handbook of Qualitative Research* (third edition). Thousand Oaks: Sage.
Gard, M. (2004). Movement, Art and Culture: Problem-Solving and Critical Inquiry in Dance. In Wright, J., Macdonald, D., & Burrows, L. (Eds.). *Critical Inquiry and Problem-Solving in Physical Education*. London: Routledge.
Hillier, L., Jones, T., Monagle, M., Overton, N., Gahan, L., Blackman, J., & Mitchell, A. (2010). *Writing Themselves In 3: The Third National Study on the Sexual Health and Wellbeing of Same Sex Attracted and Gender Questioning Young People*. (Monograph series no. 78). Victoria: La Trobe University.
Hillier, L., Turner, A., & Mitchell, A. (2005). *Writing Themselves In Again: 6 Years On. The 2nd National Report on the Sexuality, Health & Well-Being of Same Sex Attracted Young People in Australia*. Victoria: Australian Research Centre in Sex, Health & Society (ARCSHS), La Trobe University.
Lincoln, Y.S. (1995). Emerging Criteria for Quality in Qualitative and Interpretive Research. *Qualitative Inquiry*. Vol 1, No 3, pp. 275–289.
Mac an Ghaill, M., & Haywood, C. (2007). *Gender, Culture and Society. Contemporary Femininities and Masculinities*. London: Macmillan.
Monro, S. (2005). *Gender Politics*. London: Pluto.
Paechter, C. (2007). *Being Boys, Being Girls: Learning Masculinities and Femininities*. Berkshire: Open University Press.
Pallotta-Chiarolli, M. (2010). *Border Sexualities, Border Families in Schools*. Lanham: Rowman and Littlefield.
Saxton, J., & Miller, C. (2009). Opening Pandora's Box: The Ethics of Practice in Multicultural Communities. *N J Drama Australia Journal*. Vol 32, No 1, pp. 35–43.
Schutz, A. (1944). The Stranger: An Essay in Social Psychology. *American Journal of Sociology*. Vol 49, No 6, pp. 499–507.
Schutz, A. (1972). *The Phenomenology of the Social World*. London: Heinemann.
Sinclair, C., Jeanneret, N., & O'Toole, J. (2009). *Education in the Arts: Teaching and Learning in the Contemporary Curriculum*. Victoria: Oxford.
Taga, F. (2005). East Asian Masculinities. In Kimmel, M.S., Hearn, J., & Connell, R.W. (Eds.). *Handbook of Studies on Men and Masculinities*. London: Sage.
Zizek, S. (1999). *The Sublime Object of Ideology*. London: Verso.

10 Embodied Performance of Gender in the Worlds of Adults

The fieldwork sessions I conducted with some 160 adults occurred with educators, graduating healthcare and youth-work trainees, performance arts practitioners/educators, and interested members of the general public. Settings in which these sessions occurred included Australian and international academic conferences, professional development seminars, and university courses, as well as publicly advertised meetings held in community centers and bookshops. Participants harked from Australia, North America, Europe, and Asia. In general, sessions consisted of a talk and/or a performance of *Gender Icons* as a lead in to open-ended discussion on issues relevant to participants' personal and/or professional experiences of gender and embodiment. In addition, practical workshop activities were conducted in sessions for performance arts practitioners/educators. Fieldwork was documented by means of field notes and audio recordings of discussions with participants' permission. Most attendees also filled in post-session anonymous response sheets.

The sessions referred to in this chapter aimed to put a mirror of my experiences and outlook concerning gender and embodiment before others. I had hoped through this fieldwork to expand and enrich my thoughts on whether, and by what means, positive change in the social mindset toward embodiment and embodied performance of gender might come about. I had hoped especially that data from the fieldwork would expand and enrich my thoughts on the potential role of performance arts and performance arts education in effecting such change. Note that I framed the focus of all of these sessions to be on mainstream culture as opposed to unique and uncommon students, communities, or arts education situations.

Fieldwork participants referred to in this chapter responded to sessions I conducted from professional and personal viewpoints. The overlap in viewpoints is acknowledged as inevitable. This chapter addresses participants' views on themes that arose out of group discussions as well as in comments made on response sheets. On the whole I found that a similar range of responses to issues of gender and embodiment were expressed across the various adult participant groups. I will point out the biological sex, nationality, or precise source of responses of any individual participant only where I feel these points of difference are noteworthy.

SOCIALLY ACCEPTABLE MALE/FEMALE EMBODIMENT

From fieldwork group discussions as well as anonymous response sheets, there seemed to be a shared perspective from adult participants across all fieldwork groups that Western mainstream society recognized some forms of motion as feminine and others as masculine. It was understood that in the mainstream, masculine behavior was generally associated with males, and feminine behavior with females, with differing behaviors advocated for and expected from males and females from a very young age:

> So much is set from the time you're 7 . . . If you are girl who sits down you know like that (sits straddle legged) "*Excuse* me" (delivered with an admonishing tone) . . . and similarly for a guy, you know, if he went like that (sits demurely) "You're a bit of a woosie" (delivered with a condescending tone). (trainee youth worker)

The viewing of a performance of *Gender Icons* triggered participants to reflect on their own responses and positioning toward transgressive embodiment of gender; one participant implied the uniqueness of education contexts to other contexts:

> I was quite comfortable viewing it, probably due to the education context it was in, but when I imagined myself performing in a feminine way, I suddenly felt that I would be VERY uncomfortable and embarrassed. (male trainee youth worker via anonymous response sheet)

A number of other participants also articulated feelings of discomfort where aspects of the male embodiment in the performance were at odds with participants' experiences and expectations of how males should move: "I must admit I did find it somewhat uncomfortable at times seeing a male performing effeminate embodiment, not due to prejudice, purely because it is not something I am used to viewing" (trainee youth worker); "It was almost uncomfortable to see a man moving in such a feminine way" (trainee youth worker); "I was actually embarrassed at my own reaction. My reaction was 'But you're a strong man doing these movements'" (educator).

Where the following comments speak of *being caught off guard* and *not knowing where to look*, it is as if exposure to particular styles of action as performed by a man are an affront of sorts that causes observers to feel confined:

> The extremely feminine motions did come across as comedic, while when taken in the extreme . . . left me not knowing where to look.
> (female trainee youth worker)

> It did make me uncomfortable in some parts. Maybe because I never especially considered movement as being gendered, but then when I saw you act the woman parts it put me back a bit and I guess caught me off guard.
>
> (female trainee youth worker)

The latter quote illustrates a mindset that differentiates male from female movement vocabularies. My understanding is that the participant's discomfort was caused because 'woman' parts were performed by a male. That the performance highlighted for some participants their own tendencies to polarize male/masculine from female/feminine indicates the need to draw attention to the notion that an individual's embodied style of performance need not necessarily be 'either-or' when it comes to embodying in gendered ways.

Many participants, upon viewing my performance of *Gender Icons,* articulated their feelings that the piece would not be easily palatable for other audiences. My assumption is that these comments stemmed from my embodiment in the piece:

> If you were to do that in the country . . . you would literally be bashed . . . It's not so much accepted like in the city.
>
> If this was performed in public, exposed to a large variance of people of different ages, cultures and social groups, it would stir up a lot of discomfort and even ridicule.
>
> I was thinking of my partner who is an electrician and thinking how uncomfortable he would be in this performance. His family and work environment are so gender biased that he would find the performance so confronting he would probably just laugh.
>
> (female trainee youth worker)

These quotes are quite definite that the performance would be received by other audiences with laughter and/or derision. Assumptions are being made not only about gender but also about rurality, culture, class, and education. Differences were noted in the ways the performance would be received in contexts pertaining to entertainment, and those of official academic discourse: "If I was with a group of friends and we saw this, I would probably laugh. In a health class however, I don't find it funny" (trainee youth worker). This is consistent with Leavy's (2009) contention that interactions between audiences and performers vary according to context. As several fieldwork participants commented, it is important to acknowledge that those of us who are exposed to a more diverse range of people may have broader perspectives and may be more accepting of difference than others in mainstream Western society.

Consistent with findings from my fieldwork with high school students, a number of adult participants also acknowledged that in contemporary

Western society, females had a broader range of socially acceptable options of embodiment than males: "As a female I feel that I am freer to not act feminine all of the time . . . It is difficult to imagine males feeling happy about embracing more feminine behaviors in this current climate".

EMBODIMENT AS SOCIAL CONSTRUCTION OR NATURE

Fieldwork participants held a range of viewpoints on whether male and female differential embodiment was a social/cultural manifestation, a matter of biology, or a combination thereof. Personal reflections were made on participants' own upbringing and/or the behaviors of children in the participants' lives, concerning whether and in what ways natural behaviors are influenced by nurturing and other social influences: "My sister and I, we grew up as tom boys. We'd be out playing trucks and cars with our brothers . . . Now we've both grown up very girlie girls. Whether that's a matter of society changing us or whether it's just the natural way we've gone . . ." The use of broad definitions of behavior as being 'girlie' does not take into account that such sweeping terminology may itself be a social and linguistic construction.

In relaying the following, the speaker all but exonerates her partner and herself, as parents, from having any cultural influence on their adopted children:

> We adopted 2 Korean children. It was amazing cos we never facilitated or encouraged them to play with certain toys . . . but F (female name) was such a girlie girl . . . whereas M (male name) loves trucks. I don't think we influence them. I think it was just their natural—but then later on I suppose there is that underlying thing.

One participant referred to the sometimes 'awkward' social deportment of blind persons by way of claiming how significant the visual learning of the social body is, and the extent to which our embodied behavior is learned from what we see of other bodies in motion. It would be insightful to study the 'feminine/masculine' embodiment of gestures in those who are blind from birth and whether, and to what extent, these vary according to the biological sex of the individual.

BINARY VERSUS CONTINUUM

Akin to the high school students referred to in Chapter 9, language used by most fieldwork participants positioned male-female and masculine-feminine in binary opposition to one another. This dichotomy of masculine and feminine spills over into a common regard of embodied behavior as either one or the other:

A number of participants who viewed my performance of *Gender Icons* commented with respect to how 'fluidly' my male-performer body transitioned between and across masculine and feminine styles of motion: "The performer was able to move in and out of femininity/masculinity stereotype movements so fluidly". To my mind such transitions are within the capabilities of all able-bodied persons. The fact that viewers found the fluidity of transitions to be noteworthy supports the notion that, in general, our gender performance styles are expected to be situated at a stable point along the spectrum of masculine/feminine and not to traverse and transit along and through a range of gender possibilities. The notion of masculine and feminine being broad points on a continuum that could also include shifting and varying positions was only rarely expressed or promoted.

On the whole, notions of being able to shift between and along a continuum of what could be regarded as masculine and feminine behavior are still not easily perceived/accepted (see Martino & Pallotta-Chiarolli 2001, Alsop et al. 2002, Monro 2005). Even at an Australian national drama conference that I attended in 2009, drama education delegates giggled in a research report on boys and drama education (Sallis 2010) in which a boy was quoted as loving drama because he could play Cinderella one day and the prince the next. Why should playing a range of gender possibilities be amusing?

DIFFERING AESTHETICS FOR MALE AND FEMALE EMBODIMENT

Discussions concerning aesthetics often touched on dance. In theory, many adult participants advocated dance where male and female dancers are choreographed according to their movement capabilities and not their biological sex. However, admissions were made by several participants that indicated a preference to see male dancers moving strongly and athletically, and an aversion to males dancing in a feminine manner. One dance educator spoke with concern of her own fixed sense of aesthetics for male and female forms in regard to a contemporary dance piece: "A lot of the time the women and men were doing the same thing . . . but they had none of the same vibe at all". She went on to speak as a mother about her discomfort with her reactions to the feminine way that one of her sons dances: "So, when he dances and when X (other child's name) dances, I react differently. It's a worry". This kind of reflexive self-consciousness as to why feminine embodiment on a male as opposed to a female might evoke a differential aesthetic response is a positive step toward questioning the root of one's sense of taste. Whereas most participants were clear on *what* they felt was aesthetically pleasing, only several appeared mindful to considering *why*.

ENCULTURATION AND AESTHETIC SENSIBILITIES

To shed light on interconnections between our enculturation and our sense of aesthetic appreciation, I now discuss an improvisation workshop activity that I conducted with different sets of performance arts practitioners/educators (or teacher-artists), whom from this point onward I will refer to as T/As. These male and female T/As had specialist skills in areas of dance, drama, design, and/or music and a commitment to working in their specialist areas with school students. They were predominantly Anglo-Celtic and European in origin and ranged in age from twenty-two to their mid-fifties. For the activity, which I will give the name 'Sound Collage Physical Improvisation', participants were invited to physically improvise in response to an eleven-minute sound collage. I asked participants as choreographers-of-self to draw on and physically explore repertoires of movement that different excerpts of music stirred them to perform. Prior to the activity, participants were randomly paired and asked—in addition to improvising—to observe the work of their partner. Following the improvisation, I had participants share responses to the following points:

- Reflect on shared/common interpretations/readings of music played.
- Reflect on shared/common styles and repertoires of motion.
- What was comfortable/uncomfortable about the improvisation?
- How might school students find this improvisation activity?
- Why might male/female students be more comfortable moving in some ways as opposed to others?

I found overwhelming commonalities in participants' embodied responses to particular music and sound excerpts in physical improvisation activities. For the most part, music that had a strong and powerful beat and was arguably masculine evoked strides, thrusts, and gestures from participants that were also strong and powerful. Music that was delicate, lilting, and arguably feminine evoked footwork and gestures from participants that were delicate and graceful, such as work on tip-toes and wafting of arms. At the same time, several male participants punctuated their feminine balletic moves with parodic grins that bespoke their amusement, embarrassment, or sense of awkwardness with performing in such ways. This was consistent with parodic ways in which male high school students from all but one school participant group performed feminine action in the workshop activity in which they took part.

In discussions that followed improvisations, T/As commented on how easy it was to physically submit to 'cliches' that the music suggested as opposed to finding one's own responses to the music: "The music sort of set up a particular normity of response and it was very hard to find your own authentic response working against the grain of that". Although a handful of T/As argued, "A few of us don't see music in a gender related way", almost all spoke of music evoking stories, states of mind, and feelings that connected with notions of masculinity and femininity:

> We have that aural perception when we are listening to music, that if it has a certain amount of grace or cadences or a general melodic structure or emotional structure, in our hearts I think we feel it's feminine, whereas if it's dominant or pulsating like *We Will Rock You* it then becomes a masculine element.

This line of thought aligns with notions that cultural media, such as music, can have an effect on our positioning toward gender (McClary 1998). In the same way, cultural artifacts that put forward and valorize particular forms of male and female gendered embodiment can affect how we perceive, respond to, and practice the embodiment of gender.

In post-improvisation discussion, many T/As readily acknowledged that how individuals come to read, appreciate, and respond to art forms such as music is influenced by one's enculturation. A person whose upbringing included exposure to kabuki music will have a different understanding and appreciation of that music than a person not used to the sparse rhythm and irregular chords particular to it. I found that very few T/As were as open to the notion that the way they read and appreciate certain forms of male and female embodiment might also be contingent on their enculturation. A person whose upbringing included exposure to certain forms of embodiment will have a different understanding and appreciation of those forms than a person not exposed, or exposed differently, to the same. My sense was that T/As did not question why it was that they found certain forms of male or female embodiment to be personally aesthetic. Nor did they question why, in directing/choreographing male and female forms, they made the aesthetic decisions that they did. My sense was that T/As regarded what they found to be personally aesthetic for male or female embodiment to be organic and instinctive. Even when we think we might be responding to stimuli such as music in an authentic way, it is important to bear in mind that the music we might be responding to (dancing, improvising) is a constructed and orchestrated artifact itself and therefore is likely to have an impact on what we think to be our authentic response/s to it (Gandolfo 2006).

Interconnections between our enculturation and our positioning toward embodiment are not always obvious. For example, the T/A who declared that she did not see music in gendered ways made reference to one particular music excerpt as 'striptease music', a label that stuck throughout her day-long fieldwork session. Here the T/A categorizes a piece of music according to associations with striptease that are necessarily culturally learned and also framed from a perspective of gender. She said of not "ripping into" the striptease music: "As a woman . . . I wouldn't necessarily feel comfortable doing it here . . . with all these people that I don't really know".

The contradiction between talking about music as non-gendered and yet declaring that 'as a woman' she felt uncomfortable physically improvising to particular music implies a blindspot to the impact of enculturation on her sense of what is uncomfortable for her to perform. There appears to be a contradiction between what the T/A *knows* rationally or cerebrally and what she *feels,* which is similar to the contradiction between what student fieldwork participants *said* and what they *did,* as referred to in Chapter 9. I contend that the reasons that the T/A felt it was distasteful—as a woman—to improvise to the piece of music in question were due to culturally embedded connotations of (a) particular genres of melody and instrumentation; (b) what it means for a female form to embody to such music in front of others; and (c) the contexts (such as strip clubs and television programs) in which music and performance such as this occur. Cultural connections such as these can be regarded as a form of 'scar-tissue' that can powerfully and invisibly affect one's sense of 'gender aesthetics' toward certain forms of embodiment as performed by male or female bodies. The reason the T/A may feel it is demeaning, undermining, or shameful for a woman to embody in particular ways is because of the cultural semiotics of such actions. Cultural understandings of gendered styles of embodiment performed by male or female bodies can impact in similar ways on an individual's sense of the aesthetic and, in practical terms, on how and what one might censor/deny oneself from embodying.

ENCULTURATION AND GLOBALIZATION

Commonalities in participants' styles of embodied performances to recorded sound/music in physical improvisation activities indicate either that embodied interpretations of sound are universal and natural responses or that shared types of embodied response are the result of commonalities in culture and enculturation. In post-improvisation discussion, I found that most participants concurred with the latter interpretation: "The music had particular culture and gender significance".

Reflecting on how they were inspired to move to the music, some T/As spoke of the cultural connections they had to various excerpts: "Straight away past experiences of movies or whatever come up. There was a tendency to just drop into repertoire for some people, specific repertoire"; "In terms of ballet music, you either dropped into the repertoire of it or you sent it up". Encounters such as those with ballet and movies are necessarily social and cultural (see Burt 1995, hooks 1996, Crothers 2007) and can therefore be understood to be the result of one's enculturation, as opposed to something organic or universal. Indeed, the point was made by several T/As that persons who had not been culturally exposed to the music stimuli used in the activity in the ways that most of the T/As had would not have necessarily responded in the same way/s: "Culturally all the music was very readily accessible to Western ears, . . . Somebody from the middle of Africa might not have recognized a lot of that music. We did"; "If you were from a different era or a different time you wouldn't have those associations . . . If you come from another country you might feel very adrift because you don't have that repertoire of style or responses".

If the way we come to read and interpret music/sound varies according to our enculturation (Gandolfo 2006), then it can be argued that our physical responses to music, by the ways in which we are stirred to embody to it, must also be contingent on aspects of our upbringing and enculturation. Where our enculturation promotes certain forms of embodiment as fitting or aesthetic for male bodies or female bodies, this may be reflected in how we move our bodies, as well as how we choose *not* to move our bodies. That music can evoke differently according to the cultural background and enculturation of the listener supports the premise that our enculturation has an influence on how we come to view and respond to the world around us. It can be argued therefore that one's enculturation will also have an influence on what can be termed one's sense of 'gender aesthetic toward embodiment', such as our appreciation of forms of masculine/feminine embodiment as performed by male/female bodies. Sensibilities of fitting or aesthetic male and female embodiment need not manifest only in response to music.

Despite arguments that gender aesthetics are contingent on enculturation, I found, at an international drama conference workshop, that physical improvisations performed by non-Australian T/As from a range of cultural backgrounds (T/As from the Philippines, Hong Kong, Holland, the United Kingdom, the United States, New Zealand, and Australia) were overall consistent with those of Australian resident T/As in Australian workshops. Particular styles of sound and embodiment were commonly perceived to be distinctly feminine and female and/or distinctly masculine and male. For example, in reference to a 'Scenario Improvisation' activity in which workshop participants were to create soundscores and improvised physical performances, improvised physical action and sound representing the character of a bulldog were interpreted as being masculine and male, just as improvised action and sound representing a butterfly were interpreted as being feminine and female, regardless of the biological sex of the performer participants. A write up of this activity can be found in the Appendix.

Several T/A participants in the international drama workshop session (held in Hong Kong) commented that shared contemporary understandings of particular sounds and particular styles of embodiment as being male or female respectively may be due to the effects and influence of widespread and globalized representations of gender. This is consistent with the observations of a participant who was an educator of overseas students studying in Australia, who commented that overseas students "come to us already indoctrinated to our gendered ways", meaning Western gendered ways.

This is also consistent with shared interpretations and responses to embodiment as expressed by participating high school students of non-Australian and non-Western origin in Chapter 9.

Participants from Asian countries who took part in the international drama conference session commented on the contrast within their cultures between historic forms of gender representation in their performance arts heritage and more contemporary representations that connect masculinity with that which is male and femininity with that which is female. Their thoughts were that their assimilation to the latter might be due to the influence of mainstream Western media via cultural forms of representation such as cinema and television (see Schirato & Yell 1996). Citing historic forms of theatre where males move delicately and with grace, such as Japanese and Thai dance forms (see Sugiyama & Fujima 1937, Yupho 1956), it seems that shared global understandings of gender, as distinct from local understandings, are a recent and growing phenomenon, and not something dating back beyond the reach of mass media as we know it today. As a result of colonization and globalization, shared and universal semiotics of acceptable and aesthetic gender embodiment, for males especially, have made lines between embodiment that is normal and embodiment that is *other* more rigid. Consequently, pressures to conform are likely to be all the more oppressive. The tone of what was shared in the international drama workshop with T/As from a variety of cultures/countries indicates that the concerns of this book are not exclusively relevant to any particular culture.

EMBODIMENT AND SEXUAL ORIENTATION

Even though it was argued, "If you're a feminine male you don't necessarily have to be gay", for the most part fieldwork participants' comments implied a line of reasoning that made connections between feminine embodiment on a male and homosexuality: "Personally, I associate feminine moves on a male body as 'gay'".

Participants offered stories involving males who they or others labeled or judged as gay due to mannerisms and behaviors considered to be feminine:

> I actually was seeing a guy a couple of years ago who moved extremely effeminate. I broke up with him. He made me extremely uncomfortable. I had never really thought about it so much till now. He didn't police it . . . When he was standing, I remember sitting out at dinner and watching him pay from the table, and I was really uncomfortable. I actually thought maybe he was gay and not coming out with it. He was a really nice guy. I really *judged* him.
>
> (female participant)

> My nephew is 10 now, and the only way he got out of being called gay or camp or all that was because he still played Australian rules football as well as did dance.
>
> Friends of ours have a 10 year old son who is flamboyant . . . He's called a poof all the time.

One individual suggested that prevalent connections made between feminine embodiment and homosexuality served as a behavioral option for gay males who want to be identifiable as gay. Another individual quoted a gay friend's frustrations with not fitting into 'gay' stereotypes: "People don't know that I'm gay, and even gay men don't know that I'm gay, and so how do I deal with that? My body language obviously isn't correct". This is in line with Pronger who speaks of the "popular effeminate image of homosexuality . . . as a point of reference for the sense of identity and behavior of many gay men" (1990, p. 146) and how gay men are able to call attention to their sexuality by behaving effeminately. It was noted that the same connections might be what makes heterosexual males *avoid* embodying in an effeminate manner: "Somebody who identifies themselves as a heterosexual male feels less comfortable perhaps . . . using feminine gestures . . . because they want to portray themselves in a particular way". In response, one heterosexual male, referring to feminine aspects of his physical deportment, exclaimed, "I get it now. I get why so many people think I'm gay . . . What am I supposed to do with my hands now?"

If being categorized as homosexual did not negatively or aversely affect how one is regarded or treated in mainstream society, then the well-being of individuals whose embodiment causes them to be categorized as gay would not be of concern. However, in contemporary mainstream Western society, being categorized as gay leaves such identities stereotyped, pathologized, and 'othered' (Robinson et al. 2002, see also Plummer 1999, Martino & Pallotta-Chiarolli 2005)—as illustrated by the homophobic attitudes of students in the previous chapter—and this can negatively affect the social and personal well-being of those categorized as such (Connell 2000, Drummond 2005, Martino & Pallotta-Chiarolli 2005). For this reason, where and why one's embodiment of gender leads to being categorized as gay needs to be challenged and deconstructed.

PRESSURES TO CONFORM AND THE WELL-BEING OF THOSE INCLINED TO TRANSGRESS EMBODIED GENDER NORMS

In my fieldwork with adult participant groups, I encouraged participants to consider the consequences of inequitable notions of appropriate embodiment of gender on the social and emotional well-being of those not inclined to embody in socially prescribed or socially valorized ways. This led to discussion of pressures on people to behave in certain ways and, after theories of master-signifiers as raised in Chapter 2, the sense that difference (in this case physical difference) draws attention to itself: "It's amazing how in a crowd your vision just . . . as soon as there's something just slightly out . . . it takes one's attention". There was acknowledgment that males and females whose behavior or performance inclination did not fit prescribed norms of masculinity or femininity may be "made to feel inadequate, less worthy, inferior and afraid" within mainstream Western societal contexts.

Stories were shared of relatives or friends who as a result of embodying against gender norms became socially troubled and/or withdrawn. For example:

> My son who's got a lot of feminine gestures, and I adore them, he's got two very non-effeminate brothers and he's now nearly 13, and he's now much more aware of what he looks like . . . And now he's much quieter, and . . . he asks me how—should I wear—does this look gay? So he's changing and . . . no matter what my husband and I do, it's the brothers "Oh you're sitting like a girl", and it's his peers that he's really conscious of now, and he wasn't at all aware of before.

Although it was generally believed that people should feel comfortable to embody in whatever way they may be inclined, many participants recognized that individuals may feel highly self-conscious of how their embodiment and physicality are perceived by others: "What we are facing all the time is other people's judgements". It was noted that even "those who do fit the bill . . . are self-conscious themselves". This outlook is reflective of Foucault's (1977) panopticonic model, where individuals come to self-police in order to be free of potentially adverse scrutiny. This outlook was apparent in the practical workshop activity that I conducted with high school student groups, where even males who appeared to fit comfortably in their school cultures as heterosexual and masculine, found it impossible to allow themselves to embody in a feminine manner unless punctuated as parody. An overwhelming number of student participants commented in anonymous response sheets that they would stop themselves from moving their bodies in ways that went against prescribed norms of gender behavior, which in itself illustrates the desire to appear to conform before others.

One T/A spoke of circumstances where an individual may be in danger should they not conform or adhere to established gender codes of performance:

> It is nigh impossible to be truthful to yourself when you've been coded, and it's nigh impossible not to have all those codings and different experiences and all that kind of thing. But I guess what we're talking about here is the coding of gender and how it may be unnecessarily restrictive

> . . . It might be very well to sort of say "Oh I'm just trying to be truthful", but I might be in danger being truthful. In my particular situation, it became dangerous, I couldn't just express myself and be real.

In this line of thinking, 'coding' is a cultural or social phenomenon that has an influence over how we come to operate. The point being made is that conforming in cases where one's natural inclination does not fit with prescribed social norms is untruthful. The danger to which the T/A refers is that of losing touch with a sense of self as a result. This raises the question of just what being true to oneself may be, and the degree to which that which is regarded as the essential self is a product of how one has been enculturated or conditioned, as opposed to something of nature. Even though one believes that one has agency, it is likely that individuals are unaware of controlling mechanisms of external cultural subjectivities on how we continue to operate (McRobbie 2009). Such mechanisms will also have an effect on how we come to embody and what, in time, becomes our embodied habitus.

Some T/As commented that they see themselves as embodying with full agency. They spoke of acting as they feel with no concern whether they appear masculine or feminine. One female T/A stated, "I operate very masculinely . . . but I don't mind if someone wanted to change a tyre for me. I'd go 'thanks' . . . I don't mind being a masculine woman". This T/A sees herself as not fitting clearly into typical gender behavioral norms, which for her is not problematic. In contrast, other participants saw themselves as subjects whose embodiment was very much regulated by panopticonic controls that came from other individuals, institutions, cultures, and/or societies. Addressing the topic of embodied masculinity and femininity triggered several participants to share personal stories and experiences of feeling pressured to conform to hegemonic gendered norms. One heterosexual female participant who spoke of her consciousness of being perceived as lesbian at a time when she had short hair spoke of *having* to grow her hair as a result. A male participant spoke indignantly of how conscious he is made to feel about being gay on a daily basis as a result of how others classify his embodiment.

One female T/A vehemently interrupted comments being made by other T/As who upheld that individuals should simply embody in ways that feel comfortable. She spoke emotionally of her struggles with being regulated as a female by the values of a male with whom she was involved:

> When I became a teenager . . . I started going out with this man . . . I was used to sitting like this (straddles legs), I had natural body language which he at varying points made remarks about, felt uncomfortable about: my physicality, my poses. And that's why I was kind of jumping up and down, cos you don't realize until you face—It's a particularly good example from my point of view because it's like I all of a sudden

> was faced with a culture I wasn't used to facing. But also it was that time when sexuality became an issue, and I very much got coded by that as an adult . . . and I still try and uncode it.

She spoke indignantly of even now being aware of self policing her embodiment of gender in certain social contexts:

> I cross my legs; I contain myself in certain contexts and social situations; I read the room. I don't have the same body language for every situation. I don't have the same body language here as I do when I'm out on a train or whatever . . . It was the other people that felt uncomfortable that tried to form me to be in a particular way so that they're alright, and that's why I was jumping up and down . . . I needed to say that.

The T/A's *need* to tell this story reflects the power and pertinence that feeling pressured to conform can have.

Adult participants such as the T/A above were able to publicly share personal stories about being made to feel alienated due to pressures to conform to hegemonic norms. This was in contrast to high school participants, who relayed similar personal experiences only anonymously via response sheets and not publicly before others, indicating how threatening such disclosure is at a time of life such as one's high school years.

Adult participants with personal stories of being made to feel alienated due to pressures to conform to hegemonic norms—even when not directly relevant to embodiment or gender—seemed to relate strongly and empathetically to my concerns for the well-being of those not inclined to embody in ways socially prescribed for their biological sex. During or following the sessions that I conducted, these were the individuals who offered comments on how strongly they connected with the issues I was raising. I sensed that these concerns did not resonate in the same way with participants who did not have a direct and personal understanding of what it is to be marginalized. Indeed, those who have been marginalized are likely to be more acutely sensitive to and aware of the workings and repercussions of discrimination (Anzaldua 1987, see also hooks 1994, Pronger 1990, Pratt 1991). They are more likely to empathize with what it may be like to feel oppressed as a result of embodying in transgression of gender norms, than those detached from experiences of being marginalized. A similar division of responses occurred in fieldwork sessions I conducted with T/As when I raised the idea that through their work, performance arts practitioners and educators could or should challenge existing norms of gendered embodiment. T/As who had themselves experienced forms of discrimination or marginalization—be it connected to experiences of gender, race, age, or body shape/size—were the most openly supportive of the idea of actively trying to expose, interrogate, and deconstruct existing gender oppressive norms of embodiment within and through their art forms. If, as hooks (2001) argues, making progress toward positive social change needs the active involvement of those who are not oppressed or marginalized, then it is vital to ensure that those who are not oppressed come to an understanding of what it is to feel alienated and 'other' (see Pease 2010).

GENDERED PRACTICES AND BLINDSPOTS

> It's so important for us to keep reminding ourselves to be aware. We might think we are conscious but I don't know. We all need to keep reminding ourselves.
>
> (educator participant)

In fieldwork sessions with adults I suggested that we may be unwittingly sustaining existing gender inequities through our habitual practices. One female T/A participant drew attention to the view that concerns of inequitable gendered embodiment that were the focus of her fieldwork session were being played out in the embodied signaling occurring within fieldwork session discussions:

> I really felt an acute inner urge to nod and smile and offer encouragement and lean towards—and I thought it's so physically embedded. And I noticed the other women doing it too: that when anyone was speaking, male or women, the women are like [nodding positively and leaning into male next to her]. They're so generous with their body language and the men are like [crossed arms, leaning back, stern face] and that's despite all the work we've done, and I'm just offering that as an observation cos I really think that it's through and through us and that's the point of this exercise.

The generosity and affirmation of this kind of "conversational cheerleading" as typically manifested in the faces and bodies of females can be disempowering when unreciprocated, typically by males (Bartky 1990, p. 102). This example also raises the proposition that habitual embodied practices such as 'conversational cheerleading' are so embedded that those performing them are not aware of the cultural messages they may be inscribing/reinscribing for themselves. One T/A who spoke of celebrating the difference in embodiment that occurs between males and females asked whether this was indeed a problem. She acknowledged as 'natural' that "the majority of women *do* respond to the majority of signifiers in society" in similar ways. The problem is not that a majority of women and some males embody in a feminine manner but that mainstream Western society tends to position the performers of such embodiment—particularly if they are male—on a subordinate level to performers who embody in masculine ways. What needs to be considered and exposed is why a society inequitably perceives or positions the person who embodies in generous, affirming, and arguably feminine ways as subordinate, regardless of whether that individual be female, male, or transgender. Through making such positioning visible we might move toward addressing inequities of gender embodiment and gender in general.

My suggestion to T/A participants was that performance arts work that we ordinarily create, as well as the teaching that we ordinarily do, might reinforce gender inequities. Could it be that through their/our training and induction into established art forms, T/As come to operate blindly according to the gendered traditions of these forms? After all, the ongoing employment of most T/As involves the teaching of skills and the creation of work that has traditionally presented, reinforced, sustained, and revered traditional representations of males as masculine and females as feminine. Here I do not refer only to directors and choreographers who direct males to embody in a masculine manner and females in a feminine manner. I also refer to designers and composers who design costumes and music for male and female bodies, which are also decidedly and respectively made to appear masculine and feminine. Aesthetic sensibilities by which we operate can be dictated by deeply embedded ideologies of gender to which we are accustomed and enculturated (as discussed in Chapter 5).

My impression was that a substantial number of participant T/As were confident that in their own cases, their personal practices/perspectives concerning embodiment were not gendered. However, observations I made throughout my fieldwork convince me that although T/As may oppose gender inequity, many still operate in ways that are not necessarily equitable when it comes to the *embodiment* of gender. I refer to these as blindspots and will raise examples in the sections that follow.

AUTHENTIC SELF—ESSENTIAL SELF—NATURAL SELF

In regard to my suggestions that sites of early education may be locales in which embodied gender inequities may be highlighted and challenged, several educators argued the need to respect and sustain the innocence of children and the desire to "provide safe space for students to express their authentic selves" (T/A). The premise here is that sites of early education such as schools are gender neutral.

Despite some recognition of embedded gender inequities and the negative aspects of such inequities within their art forms, there was a reluctance from a number of T/As to interrogate gender readings of such expression through their work with and for students. In an activity in which I asked T/As to explore ways by which young people might be challenged to address where and how it is that they perceive art expression (such as melody, instrumentation, choreography, and costume) to be masculine and by default male, or feminine and by default female, one music T/A worried that this would be "creating more problems than solving them":

> I felt like I was opening this can of worms that might be breaking down an innocence of just being able to listen to a piece of music and going 'that makes me feel . . .'

The T/A questioned, "Why do I want to destroy that innocence?" by perhaps illuminating the machinations of melody or instrumentation that in the adult world come to be commonly associated with male or female attributes. The T/A was defensive that childhood was a pure and natural state as opposed to a state regulated very early on by adult worlds (see Renold 2005, Taylor & Richardson 2005, Paechter 2007, DePalma & Atkinson 2008).

Rhetoric concerning the innocence of childhood as a natural state fails to recognize hidden but prevalent agendas of heteronormativity and gender-normativity (Taylor & Richardson 2005, Curran et al. 2009) and the heterosexual matrix (Butler 1990), to which children are exposed even before attending school. The use of the term 'authentic' to describe the innocent state of primary school youth signifies as a blindspot to cultural forces that affect the way we view and do bodies from very early in life and socialization. I contend that in mainstream Western culture we are taught, very early on, to match certain sounds, images, and actions with particular meanings and feelings, positioning even the youngest of children into discourses that are reflective of particular ideological points of view. For example, I would argue that notions of skipping being suitable for girls, or more specifically not for boys, are set in motion from infancy and not later in life. As argued in Chapter 6, enculturation within mainstream Western societal contexts teaches children very early on that some forms of embodiment are more suited to one biological sex than the other. This dichotomous mindset is verified in the use of descriptors of embodiment such as 'girlie' and 'manly' that arose constantly in the language of both adult and high school participants. Struggles over what the 'authentic' self could be indicate how troublesome the notion is: "Is the authentic self the embedded self or is it something other than that?" The question here is whether the embedded self is something fixed and resultant of nature or something that comes into being (see McRobbie 2009).

The T/A who spoke of 'natural', distinctive, and similar ways in which the majority of women respond reasoned that representing women in the performance arts according to these norms was justified. Where notions of natural and normal are bandied around in regard to gender, we need to consider how this positions that which is 'other' as being unnatural and abnormal by default. Binary thinking such as this has a forceful impact that can itself come to seem natural. We need to consider the impact that notions of *natural* and *normal* embodiment of gender for males and females have on those inclined to embody in ways that do not match the norm.

Consideration should also be given to how notions of 'other' may become further embedded as curious, transgressive, suspicious, ludicrous, and worthy of remark through the prevalent ways in which they are represented and interpreted in forums such as performance arts.

IMPACTS OF ENCULTURATION AND HABITUS

The ways in which our enculturation links to the ways we embody or perceive embodiment, both in the everyday and in formal performance arenas, may not always be obvious to us. To illustrate, I refer to one T/A participant who seemed to be grappling uneasily with issues raised during the day-long fieldwork session in which she participated (Migdalek 2014b). Tanya had been a professional actor and classical ballet dancer. She threw herself into the physical improvisation activity that I conducted at the start of the session. In physically responding to the soft and lilting classical ballet music, it was clear that Tanya drew on a repertoire of motion that was familiar to both her eyes and body as a result of years of exposure and experience as a female student and performer of classical ballet. Although Tanya acknowledged that male and female bodies were positioned differently from one another in the classical ballet, she did not regard this positioning as being gendered, claiming that "art aims to connect people to the deepest parts of themselves" and that "these go *beyond* gender".

In regard to the suggestion that habitual gender norms of embodiment be interrogated, Tanya questioned, "Why the need to unravel?" It seems to me that Tanya did not conceive that her playing into a certain gender performativity, via a lifetime of enculturation into the patriarchal and gender inequitable conventions of the classical ballet, is very much connected to why, from deep within, she is comfortable embodying in a feminine manner. That such embodiment feels natural to her is something I doubt Tanya had ever questioned. I consider that deep-seated and established gender norms experienced and learned via an individual's enculturation render gendered aspects of one's own outlook and behavior invisible. Where a T/A like Tanya might consider particular embodiment as more fitting to a male or female body as an essential or authentic truth, my feeling is that such an outlook is testimony of a blindspot to the force of enculturation as constructive of such sensibilities (see Fuchs 2001).

Although Tanya acknowledged that differences in representations of male and female bodies in the classical ballet may be gendered, she saw these differences as transparent and not relevant to contemporary issues of embodiment. She spoke of the classical ballet as "history" and did not acknowledge connections and influences that representations of classical balletic and other bodies on stage might have with male and female bodies in the here and now of the everyday. She was reluctant to acknowledge that there may be connections between how male and female bodies are represented in arts such as the ballet and how viewers of those bodies come to embody themselves.

> I don't know in this room . . . I can't talk for anybody who has a problem with their own way of being in regards to how they themselves sit, stand, etcetera, etcetera, but they might have a problem with the representational.

Tanya's comments indicate that she could not fathom that embodied representations on stage (the "representational") might have a negative impact on the sense of self of the individual who did not fit that order.

Tanya's lack of empathy with those who may not fit in with established norms and orders of gender embodiment is worthy of further investigation. Tanya is a tall, white, fair-haired, able-bodied, non-masculine-embodying woman who, when she was dancing professionally, had the physical capital that would never have caused her to feel physically disenfranchised or misfit. Due to this privileged positioning (see Pease 2010), it follows that she would not be as aware of or empathetic with what it is like to feel physically impoverished, as would those who struggle with and are tormented by such feelings. Tanya distanced herself from the problems of others by stating that representations of gender seem to be a problem only if an individual has an issue with it: "It's only if you have a problem with it, it becomes a problem. It becomes a problem if you the individual have a problem with it". Implicit in the simplistic line of thinking that sees a problem 'becoming' a problem because the individual lets it become so is the notion that the individual should be just as capable of not allowing a problem to *become* just that. The neo-liberal stance that individuals have such 'agency' and 'choice' is devoid of an understanding of context and systemic constraints and influences (see McRobbie 2009). An educator in another participant group expressed a similar neo-liberal sentiment to Tanya's, arguing that individuals who felt pressured to perform masculinity/femininity in ways that they may not be inclined, would and should be able to work things out for themselves: "That's just a matter of survival though . . . It's part of learning and growing up. You have to process how to adapt . . . like the animal kingdom". In paralleling processes of learning and growing up for humans to matters of survival for animals is the implication that the workings of human social worlds are natural.

These points of view take the position that the problems of those inclined to perform masculinity and femininity against prescribed norms are not the concern of those who do not have such issues. This line of thinking brings to mind Connell's (1995) contention that it is not in the interests of empowered groups, such as white, straight males, to change gender inequities that exist or to defend the rights of 'others' (see also Dyer 1997, Paechter 2007, Pease 2010). Indeed, those who are well positioned within empowered landscapes are not likely to respond well to implications that their own practices are an essential part of networks of oppression and privilege (Fruehling

Springwood & King 2001). There is no vested interest for those whose performances of masculinity/femininity bear elevated physical capital or match dominant norms (such as Tanya's) to seek or effect change.

This line of thinking disengages and exonerates mainstream society from the situations of the marginalized, abandoning all responsibility and connection. What is overlooked here is the possibility that there may be something problematic within the fabric of society that, through sustaining gendered outlooks and attitudes toward other embodiments of masculinity and femininity, causes individuals to feel 'misfit' and experience oppression or marginalization in the first place.

One participant commented defensively that as a female she did not see why she should not act feminine. She assumed that I was suggesting all persons should perform in de-gendered, neutral ways, with each person a "one dimensional android-type human being that doesn't respond to estrogen or testosterone in a way that so many people do". The participant did not consider that embodying in a way that most people do may itself be contingent on social and cultural forces. She did not consider whether 'normal', pervasive gender embodiment, such as her own, may somehow impact negatively on the social and emotional well-being of those whose embodiment is 'other'. My contention is that a society that marks that which is other as subordinate to the norm *does* have a negative impact on those whose embodied inclination differs from the norm. As stated in Chapter 1, I have no objection to females embodying in a feminine manner or males embodying in a masculine manner, and I do not believe that these individuals need to modify how they embody their masculinity or femininity. What needs to be modified is the outlook toward *other* performances of masculinity/femininity and the imposition of a system of hierarchical dualism that accepts, lauds, and privileges certain forms of embodiment over others. That is the way toward overcoming or at least improving the lot of those who do not fit comfortably into societally prescribed norms of gender embodiment.

I return now to Tanya and her apparent lack of concern for the well-being of individuals who embody in gender transgressive ways. When discussion centered on the well-being of individuals who did not walk or sit in gendered ways as prescribed for their biological sex, Tanya dismissed this by exclaiming that people should simply be grateful for being able to walk. Interestingly, eight months after the fieldwork session, I received an apologetic e-mail from Tanya in which she reflected back on the day:

> I just couldn't get my head around worrying about how men are perceived when some people can't even control their capacity to stand. It was just my own issues getting in the way. I do understand the need to be 'you' without too much imposing of stereotypes, I expect dance itself continues to do just that and I am certainly a culprit of continuing tradition. All in all I expect my view is one that is colored and ignorant . . . I am sorry for that.

What strikes and inspires me is that over time, the material that was raised in the day-long fieldwork session stirred something in Tanya's consciousness and made some personal impact or connection, despite having been strongly resisted at the time it was raised. I wonder if, and hope that, activities and performances in fieldwork sessions may have some effect on how other participants (adults and students) came to consider and relate to gendered embodiment following the sessions. As hooks (1994) argues, pedagogy that involves the exposing of biases and old ways of knowing may take months or years to be realized, and in bringing about social shift is likely to cause discomfort, confusion, and pain along the way. Such discomfort may perform a vital role in the process of social shift. In the eight months since the fieldwork, it appears that Tanya has become more sensitive to the situations of those who are marginalized in ways that may not have affected her own life. Individuals may be likely to have more empathy with notions of being 'other' through direct experience of what it is like to be marginalized or different from the norm. On the other hand, one fieldwork participant, a healthcare professional who works with the disabled, noted that the marginalized can themselves be discriminating and unaccepting of that which is 'other' (see Martino & Pallotta-Chiarolli 2003): "Although they yearn for greater acceptance . . . they are very un-accepting themselves of others' differences, i.e. quick to label someone (male) with feminine attributes=gay". This line of thinking aligns with Memmi's (1967) and Freire's (1990) contention that the oppressed can also be oppressors.

TEACHERS ON TEACHING

Fieldwork sessions evoked the sharing of stories from educator participants in which they reflected on professional experiences around embodied performance and gender. Frustrations were aired about students becoming less open to moving in particular ways as they grow older: "In the younger years it's ok for them to do everything, but hit grade four and the boys do this and the girls do that. I just hate it, *hate* it (angrily). They get it so driven out of them".

One primary school teacher declared that the free movement she can ask and expect of both boys and girls in music classes is "impossible" to elicit from boys by the time they get to Year 6. Another educator who teaches creative dance to preschool children bemoaned as "tragic" the gendered physical self-monitoring that occurs as children internalize culturally expected mores through their socialization.

These stories support the contention that even if children come to school or preschool in states of innocence (as suggested by a number of educator participants) this state is short lived. Freire (1990) argues that education processes frequently integrate the young into the logic of present systems. In these cases, the logic being learned by the young is that certain forms of gender expression are not suitable for older females and males respectively. This logic manifests in embodied gendered behavioral patterns. Whereas some T/As expressed their reluctance to disrupt these patterns, I sensed that other T/As felt frustrated and guilty about their inability to challenge or alter inequitable gendered forms of behavior that manifest as normal in their students. For example, a dance teacher spoke of how she can only motivate her male high school students to dance in particular ways, and how conscious she is of ways in which they are *not* willing to embody:

> The boys I've taught will only replicate the kind of dance they've seen in the media. They'll only replicate what they've seen in pop videos or the hip and cool people that they aspire to be. That's all they want to try . . . As soon as I'm doing hip hop or jazz especially, I find myself thinking, the boys aren't going to do these steps . . . Are they going to do this or are they going to just look at me and go "Nup".

The teacher was in a dilemma. On the one hand, she was able to get boys to dance, a province often considered questionable for males. However, in choreographing the boys only in ways she knows that they are willing to perform, she is supporting and becoming complicit in reinforcing existing and restricted norms of what is considered aesthetic, cool, and acceptable embodiment for a male. This aligns with dilemmas over literacy strategies that entice boys to read through promoting the reading of masculinized material (Gilbert 1993, see also Lingard et al. 2009) and, as a result, reinforcing gender stereotypes.

Another performance arts educator, Nanette, shared a dilemma that she faced over how to best handle a situation that exposed her own and her school culture's gendered positioning toward embodiment. Nanette who was organizing musical performances for primary school assemblies was asked by an eleven-year-old boy if he could audition privately for her, which she allowed him to do:

> I drew the curtains in the drama room so nobody could look in at lunchtime, sat down and watched him. And I actually, when I first watched him start to dance, I went "ooh" [uneasy tone]. And I didn't know how to react because it was so feminine.

Nanette's discomfort at the boy's feminine performance was probably because his performance mismatched her own expectations of how boys should/should not embody. Following her initial response, she related that she found the boy's performance to be "amazing" and acknowledged how worthy it would be for him to perform the piece in front of the entire school:

> I just sat there and I thought], well you know what, that just blew me away. And if that's what he wants to show . . . I was really, really keen for him to show that, because anyone with half a brain would have seen the passion in that boy.

In theory, Nanette felt that it was right for the boy to dance in any way he wanted. Nevertheless, she ended up supporting the boy in a decision not to perform the piece for anyone else. Panopticonic consciousness caused Nanette to feel that had the boy performed at a school assembly, reactions to his performance may have led to him being teased and bullied. Here a connection appears to be made between a staged performance on a stage and the life of the boy in the everyday. Protective concern for the well-being of students performing against gender norms on stage or in the drama classroom was also expressed by other T/As: "It might be ok to protect the student. Even though you wish you could let them go out on a limb, you know what's going to happen". In supporting the boy's decision not to perform before the school, Nanette may have justifiably protected the boy from teasing and bullying. However, in doing so, she is reinforcing an already establishing tendency in the boy to self-police his physical expression of gender (he had asked to audition for her privately). I sense that Nanette's major frustration was a feeling that as a teacher she may have failed the boy in not nurturing his talent other than in a clandestine way.

Other drama teachers spoke of male students with feminine mannerisms performing on stage. One rural high school drama teacher spoke of a male student with effeminate mannerisms whom she had encouraged to perform before the school. She related with regret how this resulted in relentless teasing and mimicking of his performance by other students for months following the performance, eventually leading the boy to leave the school. In contrast, another drama teacher spoke of a male student with effeminate mannerisms deliberately playing his femininity for laughs and as a result being lauded for his performance.

In promoting a broadening of acceptable embodied forms of gender, teachers and carers face dilemmas in situations where they feel that there may be repercussions for the student who embodies differently from the norm. How do the repercussions compare between situations in which the student is allowed to embody according to inclination, and those in which the student is encouraged to self-police and *not* embody as inclined? Referring back to my autoethnographic investigation in Chapters 6 and 7, I would argue that while there is the danger of real and tangible repercussions from the former, there is a danger of less obvious repercussions occurring as a result of accumulated experiences of the latter. Together with fieldwork participants, I grappled with questions of how schools might best serve the student inclined to embody differently from the norm, without costs to the student's individual well-being.

When discussion centered on a hypothetical situation raised in *Gender Icons* in which a young male student opts to take on a 'feminine' characterization of a butterfly in a school production, the following options were raised by which a teacher might protect the said male student from the chances of being bullied: arranging/teaching things so that the butterfly role is not made available to the boys in the class; or ensuring that the rest of the class and potential audience have an understanding that a boy playing the role of a butterfly—while perhaps *different*—is not unacceptable or ludicrous. The latter option, if practicable, is more far-reaching in that it might make a positive difference for more than one student. While individual subjects and classrooms may be a good place to start, it is *whole* school cultures that need to positively accommodate and permit a broad spectrum of embodied expressions of gender.

There might have been students in some of the classes that teachers referred to—as well as in some of the fieldwork sessions that I conducted—for whom the broad terms male and female are not adequate. I wish to acknowledge again that while I choose to make do with these categorizations for the purposes and parameters of this book, consideration of individuals who might self-ascribe, or be externally ascribed, as transgender needs to be integral to subsequent research in this field.

Only a handful of teachers spoke of school settings in which they had worked where the students were comfortable doing or trying things differently from the majority of students without fear of being ridiculed or judged. One teacher who said of her students, "They don't edit themselves at all . . . They try things and certainly don't put people down", put this down to the influence of a "huge amount of church going Islanders" in her school population. She thought the respect they afforded one another was linked to their cultural and religious learnings. Whatever the basis, school cultures in which respect of both self and others is earnestly and practically advocated across the whole school—such as the outer suburban private high school referred to in Chapter 9—are to be lauded.

While educators may claim to be intolerant of any forms of gender inequity, I became conscious through my fieldwork sessions of blindspots and inconsistencies in a number of T/As' practices and/or perspectives when it came to *embodiment* of gender. One secondary drama teacher who spoke strongly of not standing for any discriminatory material in her classes, be it sexist, racist, or homophobic, spoke of *having* to teach all the female students playing male roles in her school production how to move in a masculine manner. It is ironic that despite her non-sexist standpoint, the teacher was still subject to the notion that in order to be convincing as men, males need to move in a masculine manner. Another T/A, who proclaimed that males and females should not be restricted in how they embody gender, spoke of her young son who has long hair frequently being mistaken for a girl. She related with irony how people apologize to her when they mistake her son for a girl but added, "I think he comes across—if you pay five minutes actual attention to him—as a boy". Despite her standpoint on gender equity, this statement betrays a deep-seated notion that boys, including her own, *do* behave in particular ways by which their biological sex should be identifiable. Reflecting back on my own practices, I realize that despite my outlook, I too had not been mindful of gendered and inequitable ways in which I positioned the bodies of students and performers under my direction, as I have articulated in Chapter 7.

Education environments impose gendered and sexualized constraints and norms on educators that affect the ways in which they are able and unable to work. These constraints often relate to bodies and embodiment. One male drama educator spoke of panopticonic, institutionalized controls in school environments that restrict him from making physical contact with students (see King 1998, McWilliam & Jones 2005):

> It's a fairly natural kind of thing to do in this kind of work. Suddenly you're having to work within parameters that are fairly unnatural. So being able to think that way and act that way and live that way is the core of how you move and travel through different sorts of societies and groups and institutions.

Beyond the frustration of not being able to make physical contact with students is a sense of realization that the gendered and sexualized ways in which we are conditioned to move and travel through different life situations become habitual ways of *thinking, acting, living,* the machinations of which, through continual repetition, are rendered invisible.

CHANGE IN THE SOCIAL MINDSET

Fieldwork participants were asked to comment on how, and whether, they envisaged a change in the mindset toward the embodiment of gender might come about. There were those who felt that norms of gender embodiment were so embedded that social change in the mindset toward embodiment of gender would be extremely difficult, if not unlikely altogether. A number of individuals expressed the view that social change in the mindset toward embodiment of gender would occur but only very gradually. A variety of views were expressed as to how change in the social mindset toward a broadening of acceptable forms of gender embodiment might come about, with an emphasis and onus on media and education as means of effecting such change. Views were expressed that advocated the destabilization of existing social norms of gendered embodiment through exposure to alternative forms. A participant who worked as a substitute teacher in primary schools spoke of her attempts to make students think about alternative embodiment, such as boys taking part in activities usually regarded as effeminate, by asking incredulously, "Don't you do that at this school?"

The focus for the rest of the chapter is on performance arts and performance arts education as a potential medium for social change.

PERFORMANCE ARTS EDUCATION AND THE DESTABILIZATION OF EMBODIED GENDER INEQUITY

T/A fieldwork participants differentiated work that performance arts practitioners/educators do in education sites such as the drama classroom from work that they produce on stage. The focus of the latter is on acting out for an audience, whereas the focus of the former is on the active participants themselves (Sinclair et al. 2009). Although most T/As who took part in my fieldwork acknowledged that the work they do as arts educators in drama and dance classrooms can affect how their students see and behave in the world around them, there was little acknowledgment that differential ways in which they direct and choreograph the bodies of performers on stage, including in major conventional school productions, might also affect how students see and behave in the everyday (Migdalek 2009). The blindspot here is similar to Tanya's (referred to previously), wherein prevalent ways in which male and female bodies are positioned and represented in classic and conventional formal performance pieces are not understood to have an impact or influence on embedded cultural norms of day to day embodiment for male and female bodies, be it those of audience members or those doing the performance.

Drama educators are advised in *Drama Equity and Diversity Guidelines* to contest and "challenge roles and representations in drama works that reflect restrictive gender codes that exist in popular culture" (Drama Australia 2005, p. 10). Such contestation is not evident when one considers the abundance of conventional and popular major school theatrical productions in which students are directed and choreographed to produce and reproduce gendered norms of embodiment that reinforce—and do not challenge—restrictive and inequitable gender codes and forms of *embodied* representation. An overwhelming number of representations of male and female bodies in school (and other) theatrical productions valorize masculine embodiment on males and feminine embodiment on females. This must surely impact on the sense of aesthetics and the personal physical capital of young audience members as well as cast members. Despite official codes and guidelines that promote respect for diversity in education (such as those espoused by the Department of Education and Early Childhood Development Victoria 2014), how mindful are we, from our power positions as teachers/directors, of what we project onto casts and audiences when we choreograph and direct these public spectacles (see Grady 2000)? I would argue that in directing bodies of cast members in school (and other) productions we frequently and habitually draw on the repertoire of action that *seems* fitting—perhaps through its very familiarity—without deconstructing or contextualizing inherent restrictive and inequitable gender codes within.

In order to highlight these issues, I conducted a workshop activity, which I will refer to as the 'Embodied Characterization' activity, in which participants were to cast, direct, and stage a mimed scenario for a specified male or female character in a particular disposition or state of mind, and then re-present it identically but via a performer of the opposite biological sex (Migdalek 2014a). The scenario was a simple mimed sequence that involved a figure in a café waiting for, and then eating/drinking, an order of coffee and pastry. A write up of this activity can be found in the Appendix.

In the discussion that followed the doing/experiencing/embodying of this activity, participants identified that characters who were masculine or feminine in disposition projected differently according to the biological sex of the performer. Indeed, where actors performed decidedly feminine or masculine blocking that had been set for a body of a performer of the opposite biological sex, these performances frequently evoked laughter from co-participants. I asked participants to consider their own teaching/directing practices in light of the activity. Most participants admitted that in their directorial practice they were likely to direct identical character attributes—such as assertiveness, seduction, humility, sexual orientation—differently according to the biological sex of the performer. Many session participants reflected with surprise that they had not been conscious of these gender inequities in their own directorial practices. What this reiterated for me was how unaware we can be of the inherent gendered habitus within our own directorial practices.

Pushing an Agenda

I had hoped, through my fieldwork with T/As, that T/As would consider the impact that their work, both as performance arts educators and as practitioners, might have on the student/participant, performer, or audience member whose performance inclination did not fit prescribed norms of masculinity/femininity. The degree to which fieldwork participants considered the struggles of such individuals as a domain for educators, particularly performance arts practitioners/educators, to delve into with students/audiences varied significantly.

There was a level of resistance to the notion that we as performance arts practitioners/educators should push an agenda by exposing or deconstructing embedded gender inequities through our work. Some T/As took the view that this was "dangerous territory". Several T/As expressed their discomfort with a workshop task in which they were asked to conceive practical activities for the performance arts classroom that might expose or challenge embodied gender inequities:

> We wanted to be careful . . . that we weren't coming in with an agenda . . . but wanted to be careful of making sure that it was an open discussion and not that we had some moral about types of sexual movement.

This comment belies the existence of dominant societal agendas and implies the group members' political neutrality as educators (see Tierney

1997, Curran et al. 2009). It is likely that these T/As did not conceive that the 'norms' by which they taught and operated could themselves be laden with agendas, precisely because these norms aligned with dominant ways of thinking. T/As' reluctance to expose or tackle a mindset or mentality that discriminates against gendered embodiment with their students fails to acknowledge that the point of drama and other arts education is "not to transmit a particular ideology or to leave unchallenged the things we think we believe, but to see anew, understand ourselves more fully, expand our thinking, and understand how that thinking has been shaped by our social positions" (Drama Australia 2005, p. 37). T/As' talk of focusing students' attention on inequities of gender embodiment as being the 'pushing of an agenda' struck me and frustrated me, because I believe that the same educators would not hesitate to push agendas that would tackle a mindset or mentality that discriminates against racism, sexism, or ageism with their students as forms of discrimination not to be tolerated (see Kehily 2002). Why might inequitable ideologies of gender embodiment be less worthy of being exposed or challenged? It saddens me that promoting embodied gender equity is seen to be 'pushing an agenda', whereas promoting other forms of equity is seen as socially warranted and the right thing to do, and that the system in place is viewed as agenda-less.

This reluctance to challenge existing norms may be explained through reference to Trinh's theories on the tendency to "discard all disturbing subjects so that we don't have to deal with them" (1992, p. 56). I believe that a key issue for T/As who were resistant to delving into how they might challenge embodied inequities of gender may have been a fundamental discomfort concerning their personal submission to the same, or, in other words, their own complicity in sustaining embodied inequities of gender through their personal, professional, and/or everyday practices. It is unsettling to conceive that one's own habitual behavior and practices may be a contributing factor to the continuation of a state of affairs that is inequitable. Furthermore, there may be professional, personal, and peer-group costs to those who issue challenges to existing norms (see hooks 1994, Tierney 1997, Grady 2000). Leaving things as they are is an easier option.

Transgressing Norms

One T/A talked of the need to respect and defend the multitude of ways in which students may present or embody themselves. In reference to her own teaching she spoke of a drama class culture in which *other* views and choices were to be supported:

> For me it's about teaching a certain amount of respect, and how that person is feeling comfortable right now in expressing themselves . . . If they chose typical gestures to their gender, then that's them. I have to respect that. I'm not there to change the world. I'm just there to give them a context and options . . . and support them if they want to be different.

I agree that teachers should be supportive of differing forms of gender expression and other ways of embodying maleness or femaleness. However, it is also important when talking about a student *wanting* to be different (as above) not to overlook what it might take for the individual to *choose* to act on such a desire. One needs to consider what it might take to overcome the pressures of social norms of gender behavior, peer pressure, and anxieties about consequences of deviating from the norm—in students and teachers.

In regard to creating a drama class culture in which alternative ways of embodying are acceptable, the abovementioned T/A added that where a teacher is aware that a student is being "harassed" in a drama activity because of embodying in a manner that is transgressive of gender norms, then the teacher may "need to be an advocate in that case". In such instances the T/A, positioning the teacher as interventionalist, spoke of the need to "stop what you're doing and unpack it". This statement serves as an admission that even in a drama class culture, the individual who performs or expresses themselves differently may be at risk of being singled out and harassed. Social realities in which students find themselves may restrict and inhibit how they are willing to present or embody. The drama class is not necessarily a safe space. Where harassment is a potential reality, one can understand why students might be hesitant to embody differently from commonly accepted gender norms, and by the same token why educators and carers might facilitate activities in such a way that the student whose tendencies are to embody in transgression of gender norms will not be given opportunities or be encouraged to express himself or herself in such ways.

Many T/As expressed the belief that the performance arts classroom was a "safe space for students to express their authentic selves". This harks back to questions of what the authentic or essential self is (as discussed previously) and the likelihood that, in the performance arts class as well, students' *authentic* repertoires of response might simply be artifacts of their enculturation.

Positive reference was made by several T/As to particular instances in performance arts classes where students transgressed norms of embodiment. In recounting episodes in which students cross-dressed or played the opposite biological sex, T/As spoke with satisfaction of how positively such transgressive embodiment was received. For example, one T/A spoke of an airplane scenario in which a male student took on the role of female flight attendant:

> I pointed to this kid and I said "So who are you?" and he said, "I'm the air-hostess" . . . And I said "Okay. Do you want to reconsider that?" And he went "No", so I said "Okay". So we went with it and it was fantastic. It was just great. And he played it to the hilt. All the other kids just laughed and they thought it was great.

Despite the teacher's pleasure at how the boy's characterization was received, it signals a blindspot concerning what the kids' laughter, directed at the boy who "played it to the hilt", signaled about a male in feminine guise, as well as what the students might be signaling to one another. It is likely that what made the performance funny both to the students and to the teacher was the supposed mismatch between the biological sex of the performer and the manner in which he performed.

The emphasis made by T/As in recounting instances such as these was how unproblematic such transgressive embodied performances were. It struck me that although stories of male students embodying in a feminine manner while presenting as female had been unproblematically received, no tales were reported of male students presenting as male but embodying in a feminine manner being received in the same way. Drawing on the responses of high school students in fieldwork sites (as reported and problematized in Chapter 9), it is likely that such representations would be perceived as marked, comic, and/or gay. In contemporary mainstream Western culture this *is* problematic, not only for the social well-being of the object of such classification, but also for those who hold such fixed assumptions.

One T/A spoke of taking a co-educational senior drama class in which students had access to costumes, props, and lengths of fabric. She related how the boys in particular draped and encased their torsos in masses of fabric and how they twirled and pranced around in a feminine manner:

> I was with a group of 12 year old girls and boys, and there was a whole lot of costumes and material and bits and pieces, and I opened up this drama activity where they were able to just get into it and just get out what they wanted and put it on. And I just stood there. I was absolutely amazed . . . Boys in particular could not get enough out. They could not get enough out and they could not put enough on. And some boys went for the swords and the belts and the hats. But there were lots of others that just draped things and got into dresses and put things on. I just couldn't believe it. It was fabulous. It was fantastic! They hadn't had a chance to play.

This episode confirms that the drama/arts space or context can be a liberal place for embodied gender play and exploration. However, the fact that the boys playing and prancing around in dresses and draperies in the drama room and during the drama session was so noteworthy and memorable is a sad reflection of how temporarily such carnivalesque behavior (Bakhtin 1968) is deemed acceptable, and how strongly schoolboys are otherwise denied adorning or moving their bodies in non-masculine ways within non-drama classroom contexts. 'Feminine' practices, such as prancing around with lengths of fabric, are not something that they otherwise have a license to do. Why do established notions of certain practices or behaviors being suitable for female bodies above male ones have such force when it is logical and reasonable to ask why *all* individuals should not have license to deport themselves according to the same range of possibilities?

The fact that the boys referred to in the preceding classroom scenario have license to flounce around in lengths of fabric in drama classes may indeed be transgressive of norms of embodiment. However, on its own, it is not actually deconstructive of embodied norms of gender. To make sites such as the drama classroom more than peculiar and discrete fields in which norms might be fleetingly transgressed, educators need to encourage the questioning of why fields other than the drama classroom (and other rare sites) do not allow for or accommodate transgressions of embodied norms of gender. I contend that occurrences of transgressive gender embodiment in the drama classroom could be utilized as a means by which to focus students' attention on why males would or would not move or dress in a feminine manner in other circumstances, contexts, settings, and times. Students can be challenged to interrogate why transgressive or *other* embodiment of gender is a source of amusement in certain sites. Such questioning could draw attention to other inequitable social forces that impact differently on what is regarded to be appropriate or normal embodiment for male or female bodies. Cultivating the drama classroom as a space where embodied transgression of gender norms is not trivialized or positioned as 'abnormal' or 'other' is admirable. In contemporary mainstream Western culture, achieving this continues to be a rarity. Although the tone in which T/As reported instances where embodied transgression of gender occurred in their classrooms was positive, these instances were related with tones of incredulity, surprise, and amusement ("It was fantastic"; "It was just great"; "I was absolutely amazed"; "I just couldn't believe it"; "It was fabulous"), sustaining the positioning of such transgression as extraordinary and peculiar.

T/A PERFORMANCE OFFERINGS

In my fieldwork, I asked T/A groups to conceive and then present roughed-out examples of performance works suitable for mainstream audiences that they considered might expose, challenge, or deconstruct existing inequities regarding the embodiment of gender. Prior to this task I put forward my concerns that parodic performance in which gender norms are simply reversed, such as the Trocks, did not necessarily achieve these aims. T/As agreed with this point and approached the activity with this in mind. The high energy and intense discussion within T/A groups indicated that T/As were deeply engaged in the task. However, many T/A groups found it difficult to put ideas into practical form. There was a tendency to get stuck in discussion: "Our group . . . talked too much to find the performance to do". When it came time to share ideas, several T/A groups opted to talk about concepts verbally and not actually perform or embody ideas. Of the groups who did devise performance pieces, I found it noteworthy that most of the pieces were heavily steeped in spoken text and storyline. For example, one group proposed a dialogic examination of representations of fairytale characters as gendered archetypes. This struck me as unusual given that the focus was on embodied performance and that at least a third of the participants were dance and/or physical theatre specialists. For me, this implies the challenge, difficulty, and rarity of tackling problems of embodied gender inequity.

One group's presentation that was steeped in embodied communication above speech and verbal expression did stand out for me. The group's performance took the form of a game show in which a contestant was chosen from the audience. The contestant's task was to match five pairs of shoes that sat at the front of the performance space to the bodies of the five actors seated or standing in a line across the stage. Some of the shoes displayed at the front of the performance space were solid, clunky, rugged-looking, and arguably masculine. Others were petite, delicate, ornate, glittery, and arguably feminine. Each of the actor's bodies positioned behind the shoes was posed in ways that could be interpreted as feminine or masculine. Whenever a contestant placed shoes before an actor, the actor's pose gradually shifted to gendered qualities that tended to mismatch the pair of shoes before them. For example, when the glittery shoes were placed before the female seated with legs crossed neatly and hands running luxuriously through her hair, she straddled her legs and burped. This was both comic and telling for the audience.

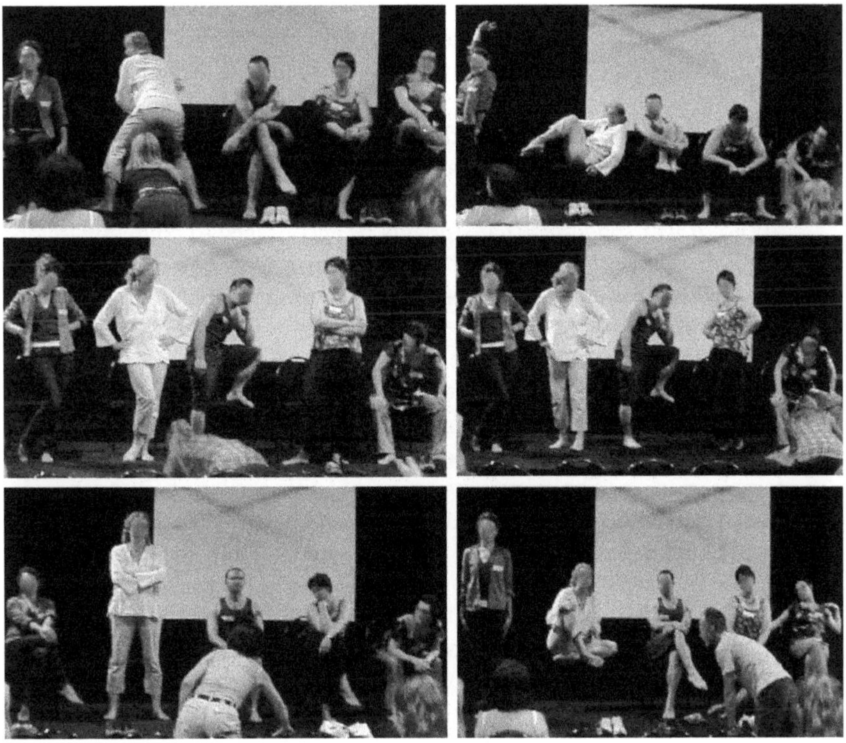

Figure 10.1 Whose shoes? Photograph by Daniel Whyte.

The game show premise of categorizing individuals according to their embodiment suggested how absurd it is to compartmentalize individuals. The mindset of matching a personality with physical articles such as shoes provoked laughter from the audience but also contemplation of how absurd it is to hold expectations of an individual's personality or individual make up according to either the trappings with which they adorn their body or the ways in which they may deport themselves. The changes from feminine to masculine and vice versa made by the actors suggested that gender may be a continuum, a fluid and not fixed phenomenon, and that we are capable of performing the array. The piece, as a work in progress, succeeded in its goal toward exposing and challenging existing inequities regarding the embodiment of gender.

T/A Workshop Offerings

In the same day-long professional development fieldwork session with T/As, I also asked groups to conceive practical activities or workshop programs that could be conducted in education settings that might broaden the ways in which school aged students *view* and perhaps *do* gender. Suggestions made by T/As were focused on bringing students' attention and critical analytic skills to issues of difference. For example: "Expose students to the opposite of the stereotype"; "Assimilate/explore new modalities. Support children in exploring diverse choices"; "Deconstruction of texts, plays, TV shows, commercials".

Practical ideas that were put forward by T/As included the following:

- Drama-dance activity in which students are guided in an exploration of performing everyday actions according to Laban's eight basic effort actions, a system that describes and codifies all ways of moving (Davies 2006). It was suggested that students be encouraged to contemplate/discuss whether particular styles of motion feel and/or look more appropriate for males or females and, if so, why. Having students consider what kinds of males and females are thought to move in particular ways could be used to provoke students to question stereotyping and classification.
- Drama-dance-music-design activity in which students are given the task of creating an advertisement for a 'gender-neutral' product such as a plastic drink bottle, to be pitched specifically to either a male or female market. The suggestion was that this activity be used to provoke students to identify gendered approaches used by the media, the media's binary positioning of male and female, and the promotion of gender 'norms' that vary according to biological sex.
- Dance activity in which students play with and observe the effects of imposing changes to learned routines in specific dance styles via changes in music, changes in whether males or females dance particular steps, and changes in costuming. Doing so and remarking on what felt/looked peculiar, uncomfortable, ludicrous, or 'other' could be used to expose gendered aspects of particular dance forms.

- Design activity in which students explore the history of fashion and design prescribed for male bodies and female bodies at various times. This could be used to highlight the transience of the semiotics of particular designs, textiles, and colors.

FIELDWORK WITH ADULTS: ISSUES AND OUTCOMES

My objectives in the professional development sessions that I conducted with T/As were to (1) draw attention to concerns for the well-being of those whose embodied inclinations did not match those prescribed in mainstream Western culture; (2) elicit reflection on how powerfully our enculturation may position us toward the embodiment of gender; (3) elicit reflection on the interconnections between our enculturation and our own habitual practices as performance arts practitioners/educators in regard to how we direct, encourage, inspire, and teach embodied positioning for male and female subjects; and (4) encourage exploration and a sharing of performance and performance arts workshop activities that might go some way toward challenging and deconstructing gendered and arguably oppressive norms of embodiment.

Reflecting on the outcomes of workshop activities, discussions, and response sheets completed by T/As who participated in my fieldwork, I found that:

1) A number of T/As seemed oblivious to the notion that gendered practices of casting, direction, choreography, design, and composition of bodies and embodiment prevalent in contemporary mainstream Western performance arts might be oppressive to some. T/As who had first hand experiences of being marginalized or alienated tended to be more open to the suggestion.
2) Some T/As did not acknowledge the force of gender enculturation from an early age and did not wish to interfere with what they saw as the innocence and gender neutrality of young students.
3) Despite recognizing gendered aspects of their arts heritage, a number of T/As were resistant to the notion that their own embodied practices might be gendered. I found that even T/As who were open to the idea appeared to be unaware of instances where this occurred.
4) When it came to conceiving performance and performance arts education programs that might go some way to challenging and deconstructing gendered and arguably oppressive norms of embodiment, many T/As found it difficult and challenging to express ideas in practical form. Some T/As were resistant to encouraging young people to question norms of gender embodiment and regarded endeavoring to do so as ‘promoting an agenda’ and overstepping their roles as educators.

In regard to the last point, I would like to think that in our role as arts educators, by presenting students with material that encourages the questioning of embodied norms of gender as inequitable, we "are asking them to reflect on their own reactions and engage in critical thinking, analysis, and evaluation, rather than presenting them with what they should think" (Sinclair et al. 2009, p. 16).

The reasons that I advocate performance arts as a conduit toward effecting social change in mindsets toward the embodiment of gender hinge on the responses of participants to my fieldwork sessions. These sessions were steeped in and encompassed performance arts. They involved participants in responding to a formal performance, *Gender Icons*, and/or actively participating in performance arts based workshop activities. Practical activities in particular revealed to me how powerfully a direct experience can highlight issues of concern as compared to less embodied means such as discussion alone. In the latter, notions are merely articulated. In the former, they are experienced, if not actually embodied. Through practical activities, participants were in a position to see/experience, and not just imagine, what it was that I was trying to have them investigate about their own practices. As with high school student participants' responses to fieldwork sessions, involvement in fieldwork sessions disrupted some adult participants' previous perspectives on embodiment of gender, causing them to perceive/question embodiment in ways that they had perhaps not considered before: "Even though I think I am open minded and not judgemental, the performance made me realize in terms of gender that I really was". The fact that performance arts based fieldwork sessions inspired and triggered shifts in perspectives for some participants is testimony to the potential of performance works and performance arts activities to effect change.

REFERENCES

Alsop, R., Fitzsimons, A., & Lennon, K. (2002). *Theorizing Gender.* Malden, MA: Blackwell.

Anzaldua, G. (1987). *Borderlands, La Frontera: The New Mestiza.* San Francisco: Spinsters/Aunt Lute.

Bakhtin, M. (1968). *Rabelais and His World.* Cambridge: MIT Press.

Bartky, S.L. (1990). *Femininity and Domination: Studies in the Phenomenology of Oppression.* New York: Routledge.

Burt, R. (1995). *The Male Dancer: Bodies, Spectacle, Sexualities.* London: Routledge.

Butler, J. (1990). *Gender Trouble: Feminism and the Subversion of Identity.* New York: Routledge.

Connell, R.W. (1995). *Masculinities.* Sydney: Allen and Unwin.

Connell, R.W. (2000). *The Men and the Boys.* St Leonards, NSW: Allen & Unwin.

Crothers, L. (2007). *Globalization & American Popular Culture.* Lanham: Rowman & Littlefield.

Curran, G., Chiarolli, S., & Pallotta-Chiarolli, M. (2009). 'The C Words': Clitorises, Childhood and Challenging Compulsory Heterosexuality Discourses with Preservice Primary Teachers. *Sex Education.* Vol 9, No 2, pp. 155–168.

Davies, E. (2006). *Beyond Dance: Laban's Legacy of Movement Analysis.* New York: Routledge.

DePalma, R., & Atkinson, E. (2008). *Invisible Boundaries: Addressing Sexualities Equality in Children's Worlds.* Stoke on Trent: Trentham.

Department of Education and Early Childhood Development Victoria. (2014). *Unity through Diversity.* [Retrieved 07/30/14 from http://www.education.vic.gov.au/Documents/about/programs/cultures/unitydiversity.pdf]

Drama Australia. (2005). *Drama Equity and Diversity Guidelines.* [Retrieved 12/12/09 from http://www.dramaaustralia.org.au/assets/files/Equity%20and%20Diversity-.pdf]

Drummond, M.J.N. (2005). Listening to the Voices of Young Gay Men. *Men and Masculinities.* Vol 7, No 3, pp. 270–290.

Dyer, R. (1997). *White.* London: Routledge.

Foucault, M. (1977). *Discipline and Punish. The Birth of the Prison.* London: Peregrine.

Freire, P. (1990). *Pedagogy of the Oppressed.* New York: Continuum.

Fruehling Springwood, C., & King, C.R. (2001). Unsettling Engagements: On the Ends of Rapport in Critical Ethnography. *Qualitative Inquiry.* Vol 7, No 4, pp. 403–417.

Fuchs, S. (2001). *Against Essentialism: A Theory of Culture and Society.* Cambridge: Harvard University Press.

Gandolfo, E. (2006). Making Fictions: A Dialogue. In Martin, E., & Booth, J. (Eds.). *Art-Based Research: A Proper Thesis?* Victoria: Common Ground.

Gilbert, P. (1993). *Gender Stories and the Language Classroom.* Geelong: Deakin University.

Grady, S. (2000). *Drama and Diversity: A Pluralistic Perspective for Educational Drama.* Portsmouth: Heinemann.

hooks, b. (1994). *Teaching to Transgress.* New York: Routledge.

hooks, b. (1996). *Reel to Real.* London: Routledge.

hooks, b. (2001). Men: Comrades in Struggle. In Kimmel, M.S., & Messner, M.A. (Eds.). *Men's Lives.* Boston: Allyn and Bacon.

Kehily, J. (2002). *Sexuality, Gender and Schooling: Shifting Agendas in Social Learning.* London: Routledge.

King, J.R. (1998). *Uncommon Caring: Learning from Men Who Teach Young Children.* New York: Teachers College Press.

Leavy, P. (2009). *Method Meets Art: Arts-Based Research Practice.* New York: Guilford Press.

Lingard, B., Martino, W., & Mills, M. (2009). *Boys and Schooling: Beyond Structural Reform.* Basingstoke: Palgrave Macmillan.

Martino, W., & Pallotta-Chiarolli, M. (2001). Gender Performativity and Normalizing Practices. In Haynes, F., & McKenna, T. (Eds.). *Unseen Genders: Beyond the Binaries.* New York: Peter Lang.

Martino, W., & Pallotta-Chiarolli, M. (2003). *So What's a Boy? Addressing Issues of Masculinity and Schooling.* Maidenhead: Open University Press.

Martino, W., & Pallotta-Chiarolli, M. (2005). *Being Normal Is the Only Way to Be.* Sydney: University of New South Wales Press.

McClary, S. (1998). *Feminine Endings: Music, Gender, and Sexuality.* Minneapolis: University of Minnesota Press.

McRobbie, A. (2009). *The Aftermath of Feminism.* Thousand Oaks: Sage.

McWilliam, E., & Jones, A. (2005). An Unprotected Species? On Teachers as Risky Subjects. *British Educational Research Journal.* Vol 31, No 1, pp. 109–120.

Memmi, A. (1967). *The Colonizer and the Colonized.* Boston: Beacon.

Migdalek, J. (2009). Masculine Moves: The Measure of a Man. *N J Drama Australia Journal.* Vol 32, No 1, pp. 45–54.

Migdalek, J. (2014a). Challenging Gendered Practices through Drama. In Meyer, E.J., & Carlson, C. (Eds.). *Gender and Sexualities in Education*. New York: Peter Lang.

Migdalek, J. (2014b). Mincing, Striding, Stomping, Gliding: Messing with Gender Choreographic Taboos. In Pallotta-Chiarolli, M., & Pease, B. (Eds.). *The Politics of Recognition and Social Justice: Transforming Subjectivities and New Forms of Resistance*. New York: Routledge.

Monro, S. (2005). *Gender Politics*. London: Pluto.

Paechter, C. (2007). *Being Boys, Being Girls: Learning Masculinities and Femininities*. Berkshire: Open University Press.

Pease, B. (2010). *Undoing Privilege: Unlearned Advantage in a Divided World*. London: Zed Books.

Plummer, D. (1999). *One of the Boys: Masculinity, Homophobia and Modern Manhood*. New York: Harrington Park Press.

Pratt, M. (1991). *Rebellion: Essays 1980–1991*. New York: Firebrand.

Pronger, B. (1990). Gay Jocks: A Phenomenology of Gay Men in Athletics. In Messner, M.A., & Sabo, D.F. (Eds.). *Sport, Men, and the Gender Order: Critical Feminist Perspectives*. Champaign, IL: Human Kinetics Books.

Renold, E. (2005). *Girls, Boys and Junior Sexualities*. London: Routledge Falmer.

Robinson, H., Irwin, J., & Ferfolja, T. (2002). *From Here to Diversity: The Social Impact of Lesbian and Gay Issues in Education in Australia and New Zealand*. New York: Harrington Park Press.

Sallis, R. (2010). The Drama Boys. (Conference Paper). Australian Association for Research in Education, Melbourne. [Retrieved 28/4/14 from http://www.aare.edu.au/data/publications/2010/1844Sallis.pdf]

Schirato, T., & Yell, S. (1996). *Communication and Cultural Literacy*. St Leonards, NSW: Allen and Unwin.

Sinclair, C., Jeanneret, N., & O'Toole, J. (2009). *Education in the Arts: Teaching and Learning in the Contemporary Curriculum*. Victoria: Oxford University Press.

Sugiyama, M., & Fujima, K. (1937). *An Outline History of the Japanese Dance*. Tokyo: Kokusai Bunka Shinkokai.

Taylor, A., & Richardson, C. (2005). Queering Home Corner. *Contemporary Issues in Early Childhood*. Vol 6, No 2, pp. 163–173.

Tierney, W.G. (1997). *Academic Outlaws: Queer Theory and Cultural Studies in the Academy*. Thousand Oaks: Sage.

Trinh, T. (1992). *Framer Framed*. New York: Routledge.

Yupho, D. (1956). *The Preliminary Course of Training in Thai Theatrical Art*. Bangkok: National Culture Institute.

11 Conclusion

Limited social notions of what is fitting or aesthetic embodiment for bodies that project as male or female serve to suppress and denigrate 'other' possibilities of embodied gender expression. Despite positive changing cultural attitudes toward notions of multiple masculinities and femininities, and an expanding suite of understandings of what heteronormative, and also homonormative, is, the workings and consequences of differential embodied expression and stylization of gender remain hidden from obvious view.

In this book I have critiqued not only the inflexible ways in which individuals view and do the embodiment of gender but also a reluctance on the part of educators to reassess the ways in which they teach, train, choreograph, and direct those with whom they work within fields such as dance and drama. Perspectives of queer theory that advocate the questioning and disruption of normative modes of understanding have informed suggestions I have made toward social change, and particularly deconstructive work from within performance arts and education fields.

In Chapters 4 to 8, I investigated ways in which—as a subject of particular cultures—I was positioned toward the embodiment of gender, and

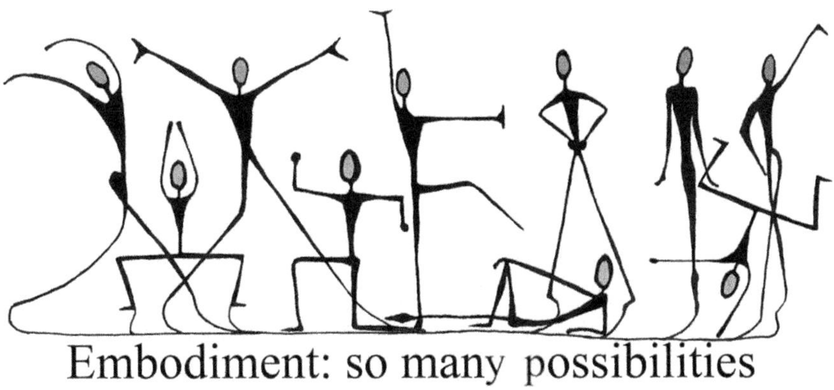

Figure 11.1 Options. Artwork by Jack Migdalek.

how this positioning affected the ways in which I came to operate in the world, both as a person in the everyday and as a performance arts practitioner/educator. Recollections of externally imposed delimitations placed on my embodiment, and my own panopticonic self-regulation, highlighted the delicacy of the relationship between social and personal control of my embodiment of gender.

Through autobiographical and fictocritical vignettes I described my sense of alienation, my introversion, and the 'scar-tissue' that resulted from feelings of embodied dislocation from, and resistance to, parts of myself that I experienced and understood as being feminine and taboo. These feelings were affected by prevalent connections, made in wider society between male embodied femininity and homosexuality, each of which were considered as suspect. With reference to Bourdieu (1990), I demonstrated that, in time, my desire and compulsion to project in certain socially valorized ways—and not to project as 'gay'—manifested in habitual ways of embodying gender, which further developed into dancing, acting, teaching, choreographing, and directing habitus that were fundamentally gender inequitable. This investigation highlighted the impact on and consequences for social and emotional well-being that mainstream dominant culturally promoted norms of what is seemly gender embodiment for male and female bodies have on those whose embodied inclinations do not fit—or do not fit comfortably—with such norms. The limited set of options given and taken up as representative of heteronormative and homonormative embodiment for males and females can adversely affect the self-image and self-esteem of those who do not feel comfortable taking up the embodied subject positions prescribed for them by societies/cultures/institutions to which they aspire or belong. The precarious and oppressive situations of such persons will persist unless there is some change in the social mindset of mainstream society.

In order to ascertain if these issues were pertinent to contemporary youth, I carried out empirical ethnographic fieldwork with high school students through a combination of performance, discussion, a practical workshop, and avenues for anonymous response. I also undertook fieldwork with educators, performance arts practitioners, and other adult participants in the form of presentations, seminars, professional development sessions, and/or workshops, with the aim of exploring and devising arts based educational activities (with an emphasis on visual critical literacy) through which to engage youth, both conceptually and practically, in challenging and deconstructing gendered and inequitable discourses of embodiment.

The performance arts, as powerful media of communication, influence, and education, tend, in mainstream incarnations, to reinscribe and reinforce existing gendered norms and attitudes toward the embodiment of gender. My intention through fieldwork conducted with T/As was to theorize on the potential role of performance arts practitioners/educators in destabilizing and challenging such mainstream norms through reflection, pedagogy, and practice, in order to broaden personal and social notions of what is choreographically possible, aesthetic, and acceptable embodiment for *all* persons, regardless of biological sex or sexual orientation. These issues are matters of gender equity, which, in regard to embodiment, is the liberty to move freely across a range of gender possibilities, and for an identical embodied performance to not signify differently according to the biological sex of the performer.

OUTCOMES

My autoethnographic investigation revealed the extent to which my habitual ways of viewing and operating in the world around me were compliant with, limited by, and actually reinforcing of gender inequitable heteronormative and gendernormative discourses of embodied performance. Even when a person comes to realize contradictions between ways in which they view and/or do embodiment, and how they may *desire* to embody, past habitus of perceiving and performing in particular ways, embedded-as-nature in the cultures from which one hails, can resurface in current circumstances in the form of 'scar-tissue', which is not easily overcome.

In my ethnographic fieldwork, high school students publicly articulated and rationalized that individuals should be free to embody in masculine and/or feminine ways. However, privately expressed responses, and the ways in which most students engaged in practical embodied workshops, revealed discomfort and anxiety over embodiment that did not align with dominant gendernormative and heteronormative forms of behavior. To a great degree, these anxieties hinged on connections students made between non-normative gender embodiment and homosexuality, both of which were positioned in terms of being 'other', subordinate, undesirable, and unaesthetic. An overwhelming number of student participants anonymously revealed that they did not want to be seen or treated as gay. For me this was confirmation that issues that concerned me retrospectively as a boy are also relevant to contemporary youth.

Educators, performance arts practitioners, and other adult participants shared information and stories that demonstrated concern for the well-being of youth who do not behave in ways that are socially promoted according to biological sex. It surprised me to find that despite these sentiments and perspectives, a number of educators challenged the notion that they could, or should, encourage young people to question norms of gender embodiment. They claimed that to do so would be promoting an agenda, which they contended was not appropriate for schools and educators to take up. This standpoint struck me as being steeped in essentialist assumptions that positioned the education systems in which they operate—and themselves—as politically neutral, *agenda-less,* and beyond interrogation. It also surprised me to find that despite their opposition to notions of gender inequity, a number of participants were oblivious to gendered aspects of their own practices and positioning (such as ways in which they perceived, positioned, and portrayed gendered forms of embodiment that were not normative as being peculiar, amusing, and frequently homosexual). These findings confirmed for me the need to scrutinize and deconstruct that which seems normative and ordinarily escapes notice.

Whereas I acknowledge that my fieldwork findings may have varied had I presented and framed things differently in the sessions I conducted, or had I sought out and selected different fieldwork participant groups (Szarycz 2010), the data gathered from most of the groups, which consisted of individuals from a variety of cultural backgrounds, were relatively consistent.

ARGUMENTS FOR SOCIAL CHANGE

The individual who projects as male and embodies in a feminine manner is likely to be perceived and treated differently from the individual who projects as female and embodies in the same manner. Inversely, the individual who projects as female and embodies in a masculine manner is likely to be perceived and treated differently from the individual who projects as male and embodies in the same manner. It is inequitable that the style of one's embodied expression leads to being perceived or treated differently as a result of one's apparent biological sex. Notions of norms of gender behavior, as they manifest in mainstream Western *viewing* and *doing* of male and female embodiment, reinforce gender positioning and protocol that not only are archaic and divisive but also serve to disempower and marginalize those who do not fit the bill.

Ultimately, it is inequitable to expect individuals' embodiment to be limited to a fixed and restrictive range of possibilities on what is otherwise a continuum of embodied possibilities. My hope is that it becomes broadly acceptable for people to act and deport themselves fluidly in and across any combination or range of gendered manner, without being classified in terms of biology, personality, or sexuality.

ATTENDING TO THE INVISIBLE

Delimitations placed on our bodies in the everyday are very much influenced by the signaling of what has come to be considered normal, and also the aesthetic embodiment for male and female bodies that figure so persistently in mass media, sports, and the arts. Definitive embodied representations of normative heterosexual and homosexual males and females within such mainstream arenas of performance serve to demarcate the discursive space in which individuals in the everyday are able or willing to embody. The machinations of these prevalent representations that have become increasingly and globally common are fundamentally invisible.

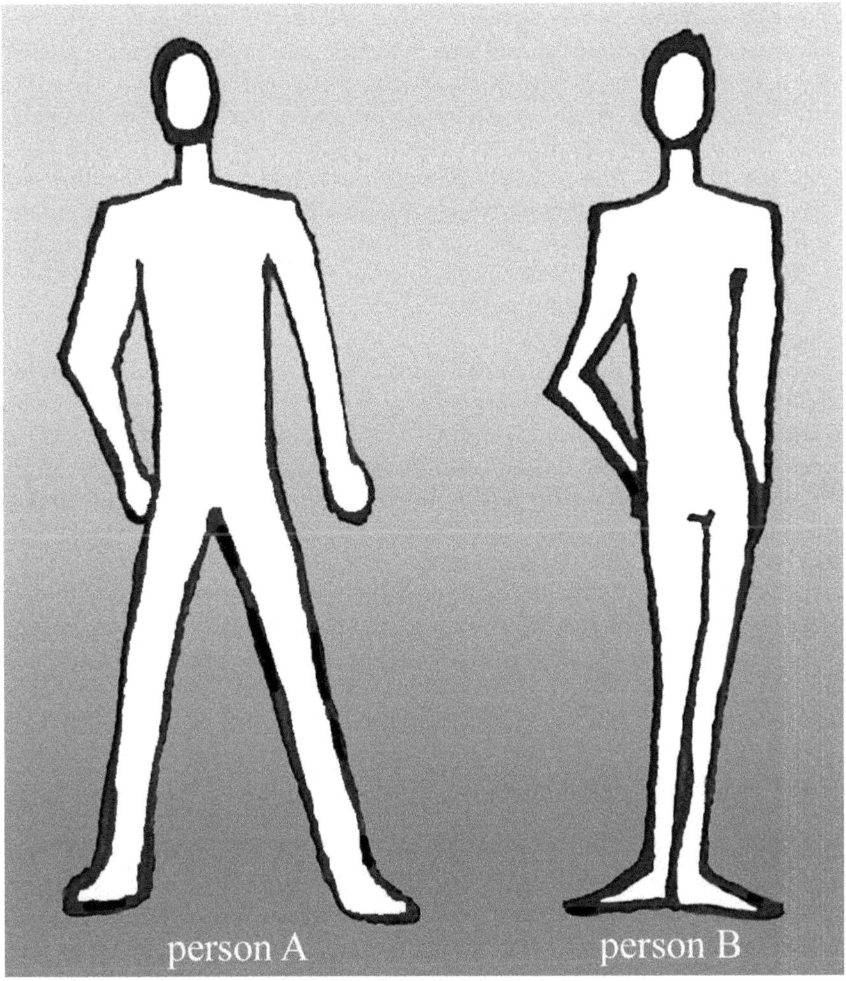

Figure 11.2 Describing person B: not as the 'sissy-boy', 'fag', 'poof', or 'wuss' but as 'the one on the right'. Artwork by Jack Migdalek.

What we regard to be attractive, aesthetic, fitting, and tasteful embodiment for bodies that project as male or female respectively comes to feel as though they are our own rather than externally imposed. Looking back on my work as a director and choreographer, it is not without feelings of guilt that I reflect on the distinctively different ways in which I unwittingly directed and choreographed the bodies of those who presented as males and females respectively. My 'directorial habitus' was reflective of, and dictated by, my already established sense of taste and aesthetic. This was deeply embedded in gendernormative, heteronormative, and patriarchal ideologies, as informed by life inscription and induction to a cultural heritage that prescribes differing norms for male bodies and female bodies. The gendered machinations of my directorial practices were so embedded and invisible that they not only appeared but also *felt* perfectly 'natural'. I was so used to perceiving and operating in particular ways that I was unable to recognize connections between the ways in which I operated and ways in which I had been conditioned. It is precisely because the machinations of habitus and taste (Bourdieu 1990) remain largely invisible to us that essentialist modes of thinking, where a sense of what is 'natural' embodiment for particular bodies is understood to be something fundamental to who we are, have been overlooked and under-problematized in regard to embodied performance of gender.

Unless the machinations of our habitus concerning the viewing and the doing of bodies are made visible, existing gender inequities that marginalize those whose embodiment of gender is not normative will simply continue. Leaving things as they are will sustain discriminatory biases against those whose bodies and deportment do not fit the heteronormative and gender-normative bill. For positive social change to occur in education, popular culture, performance arts, and the everyday, it is vital that all persons, including those who are not oppressed, come to an understanding of how inequitable ideologies and discourses into which we are enculturated influence the way we operate. With education of the young in mind, I present the following recommendations.

PEDAGOGICAL STRATEGIES

Overall, frustrations and discontent at the gendered inflexibility of even very young students, as expressed by educators in this project's fieldwork groups, indicate that changing or challenging rigid behavioral perceptions and practices regarding binary categorizations of male/female, masculine/feminine, and heterosexual/homosexual needs to happen early in a child's enculturation/education. If we are to open people up to the idea that there is a myriad of possibilities for gender embodiment, then there is a need for deconstructive work in the classroom, and indeed within whole school cultures.

The outcomes of my fieldwork indicate that there is a gap between what may be understood through thinking or saying and what is understood through experiencing and embodying. I argue that drawing virtual and actual attention of student bodies and school cultures to embedded and often invisible embodied gender inequities and enculturation processes not ordinarily critiqued in schools is a key toward positive and gender equitable social change. Through educating individuals to deconstruct and question the meaning of fossilized, gendered notions and practices of embodiment, we may be able to expose and overcome existing inequities that continue to dominate. School sites such as drama, dance, or sports classes along with school theatrical productions are sites in which students, and educators, might practically explore, experiment with, disrupt, and transform modes of embodiment that may be restrictive and differential according to biological sex. They are sites in which a more equitable state of embodied gender semiotics may be conceptualized, practiced, and promoted.

I concur with arguments that practical and embodied activities, such as those experienced in the performance arts workshop, may lead not only to an understanding and appreciation of the experiences of others (Sinclair et al. 2009) but also to the disruption of one's own habituated practices (Threadgold 2005). The idea that something staged or explored within a practical workshop, such as the performance arts classroom, is contrived might allow the participant (performer) more license and freedom to transgress norms of behavior, albeit temporarily. However, it needs to be borne in mind that practical exploratory workshops dealing with embodied gender inequity may be more challenging to students than other forms of embodied exploration. In order not to reinscribe inequitable gendered norms, educators need to foster safe environments that are respectful and supportive of embodied expression that is transgressive of embedded patriarchal norms and in which participants feel confident to explore or play, without risk of being ridiculed, being squealed at, or losing face. This work is crucial if we are to promote respect for diversity as prescribed in contemporary staff and student codes of conduct. To this end I advocate the development of teaching strategies, curricula, and resource materials that promote critical inquiry into embodied action. Several of the educational activities and exercises that emerged in my fieldwork with performance arts practitioners/educators lend themselves to such development. For curricula that question entrenched notions and practices of gender embodiment to be effective, they need sensitive guidance, framed by policy and supported by other curricula, as well as a school's public culture.

PROFESSIONAL DEVELOPMENT

Before a change in mindset can occur in and through education of the young, educators themselves need to become mindful of existing and hidden inequities regarding the embodiment of gender within their own habitus, perspectives, taste, and practices. 'Blindspots' such as these were identified in the perspectives and practices of a substantial number of educators and performance arts practitioners/educators in and through my fieldwork and investigation, including myself. As educators, we need to turn a mirror onto ourselves and be open to recognizing, interrogating, and deconstructing aspects of our own positioning toward embodiment that, while being discriminatory and oppressive to some of those under our charge, are so deeply embedded that they are rendered invisible.

To this end, I advocate self-reflexive professional development work with educators (see Ollis 2008) that challenges them to engage with notions of habitus (Bourdieu 1990) and think about the impact that their own routine assumptions, positions, values, and attitudes concerning the embodiment of gender have on their own practices. There is a need for educators to become mindful of and reflexive about ideologies and power relations—many of which stem from arts and other disciplines into which we have been inducted—that impact on the ways in which we educate and influence those under our charge. The prospect that we operate in ignorance of the invisible machinations of ideologies into which we have been enculturated is unsettling, especially to those who hold essentialist personal beliefs that how we educate and how we create art are intrinsic to who we are. If unaddressed, then our own gender inequitable perspectives, blindspots, and practices are likely to be perpetuated and persist in our students' orientations toward gender aesthetics and gender embodiment.

Attention can be directed to these concerns through participation in practical professional development initiatives that apply notions of critical literacy to visual and embodied text, and through focused discussion and analysis of fictocritical works such as *Sugarplum Fairies* (in the Appendix) in which social realities regarding the complicity of adults (carers and educators) in sustaining inequitable norms of gender embodiment can be tackled.

Participant groups with whom I worked included adults and high school students. To inform and enrich the creation and advancement of professional development programs for educators or resource materials for use in schools, it would be beneficial to conduct further fieldwork on the embodiment of gender with participants from a broader range of educational and other sites, including those of earlier childhood education. It would be of interest to undertake comparative studies between participants' attitudes (and also their embodiment of gender) according to age, biological sex, sexuality, race, ethnicity, class, and the composition of participant groups across a broad range of participants and participant groups. Issues of embodiment of gender and the opening and diversifying of possibilities for gender performance are also of relevance to transgender persons, and I advocate further work that spotlights the ways in which issues of embodiment impact on the lives of those who do not identify according to conventional confines of biology and/or gender. In taking up these recommendations I pay heed to postcolonial feminist viewpoints that would caution against the universalizing of groups such as females, males, transsexuals, those who are younger, those who are older, public school students, private school students, and so on.

SOCIAL AND PERSONAL CHANGE

It is not easy to break with corporeal trajectories assigned to us via our social location, habitus, and sense of taste (Shilling 2003). Nor is it easy to combat 'scar-tissue' from the way particular practices resonate in our lives. Delving into and reconstructing the ways in which I operate as a performance arts practitioner and drama/dance educator, and as a person in the everyday, has been both confronting and inspiring. Indeed, as suggested by Ellis (2004), the process of scrutinizing oneself and revealing one's findings can, while insightful, be simultaneously emotionally challenging. In my case, the hope for social change where discrimination pertaining to the embodiment of gender may be exposed inspired me to undertake my auto-ethnographic investigation of Chapters 4 to 8 and gave me the courage to 'put myself out there' and conduct the ethnographic fieldwork described in Chapters 9 and 10. I find it amazing that several participants complimented me on how self-assured they thought I was in this endeavor. Those who commented on my "show of confidence", my "daring", my "not caring about being judged" and "not being scared of how others might regard [me]", were not aware of how uncomfortable and apprehensive I was about 'putting myself out there'. However, looking back on broader and more equitable attitudes toward the embodiment of gender that some of my performances, fieldwork, and discussions have triggered in others has made me see that *doing* this work has had a positive effect on my bearing as well as my resolve to undertake further initiatives in the field. Indeed, the process of having conducted this investigation and fieldwork can be recognized as a means toward fostering, stimulating, and enabling social action (see Lincoln 1995), in that it has been enhancing to me, and also to a number of fieldwork participants who, as a result of their involvement, have come to new understandings surrounding possibilities of gender and embodiment.

This book serves as a provocation to readers via the example of my own reflexivity regarding my own practices and blindspots to gender inequitable machinations of education and performance arts disciplines into which I was inducted, on ways in which educators and arts practitioners train, teach, choreograph, and direct those with whom we work. It is my hope that this book invites further critical interrogation into embodied choreography and performance of gender and inspires further practical exploration and implementation of ways to challenge and deconstruct inherent inequities therein. This should include investigation into the form and composition of performance arts works that both achieve mainstream exposure and are deconstructive of existing gendered notions of embodiment.

The aims of this book were to investigate the situations, well-being, and possibilities of, and for, those whose embodied performance inclinations were not aligned to dominant social norms of gender. In the greater picture, it concerns the well-being of the individual who feels or is treated as *other* in cultures and societies that do not easily accept difference. It is my hope that the sentiments of this book become a historical artifact of social futures in which previously oppressive ideologies are obvious and powerless.

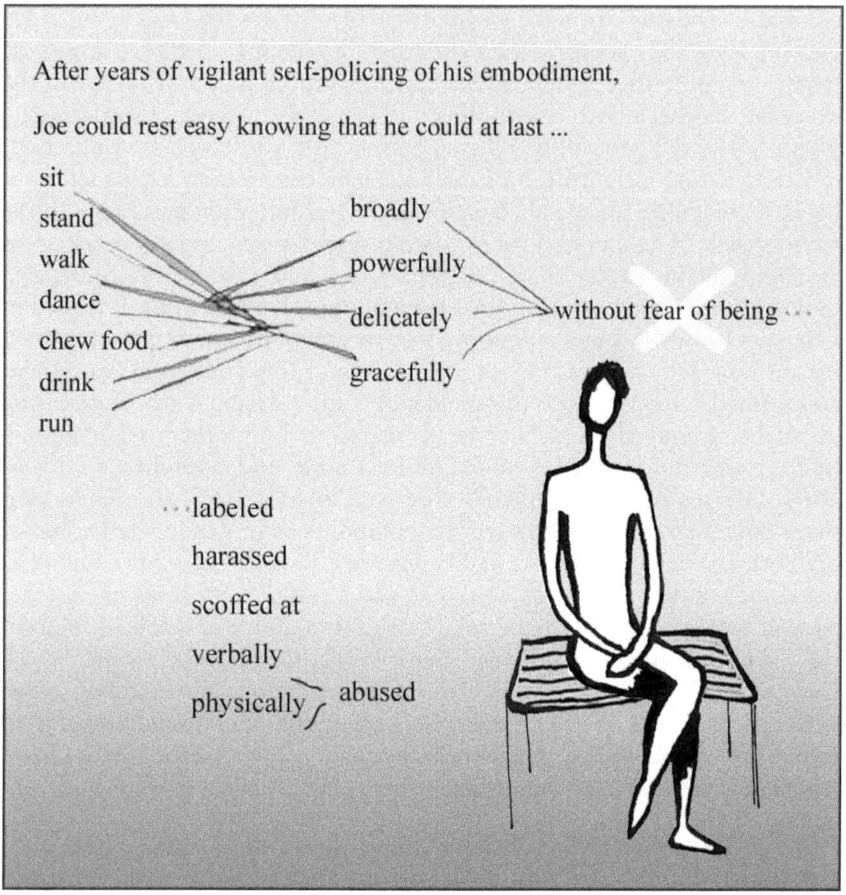

Figure 11.3 Joe. Artwork by Jack Migdalek.

REFERENCES

Bourdieu, P. (1990). *The Logic of Practice*. Oxford: Polity Press.

Ellis, C. (2004). *The Ethnographic I*. Walnut Creek, CA: Altamira Press.

Lincoln, Y.S. (1995). Emerging Criteria for Quality in Qualitative and Interpretive Research. *Qualitative Inquiry*. Vol 1, No 3, pp. 275–289.

Ollis, D. (2008). *Sexualities and Gender in the Classroom: Changing Teacher Practice*. Cologne: Lambert.

Shilling, C. (2003). *The Body and Social Theory*. London: Sage.

Sinclair, C., Jeanneret, N., & O'Toole, J. (2009). *Education in the Arts: Teaching and Learning in the Contemporary Curriculum*. Victoria: Oxford University Press.

Szarycz, G.S. (2010). *Research Realities in the Social Sciences: Negotiating Fieldwork Dilemmas*. New York: Cambria Press.

Threadgold, T. (2005). Performing Theories of Narrative: Theorising Narrative Performance. In Thornborrow, J., & Coates, J. (Eds.). *The Sociolinguistics of Narrative*. Amsterdam: John Benjamins.

Appendix

This book's appendix comprises a fictocritical theater script that can be read for reflection, in addition to discussion topics and practical activity suggestions relating to issues of embodiment and gender. This could be utilized by course facilitators in deconstructive work with educators, youth workers, trainee teachers/youth workers, and/or high school student groups. The theatre script and activity suggestions are relevant for courses that attend to gender, embodiment, sexuality, homophobia, self-image, discrimination, and well-being.

SUGARPLUM FAIRIES

A fictocritical theatre script by Jack Migdalek

SYNOPSIS:

Steven, a boy in Grade 1 of primary school, chooses to be a butterfly in his school's end of year concert. The plot involves the reactions and intervention of Steven's teachers and parents as they grapple with Steven's 'unmanly' choice of role.

Danced interludes are juxtaposed against scenes of the play to highlight and tease out issues of femininity, masculinity, sexuality, and embodiment that arise through the storyline.

CHARACTERS:

ROB:	Grade 1 school teacher, in his twenties
LORRAINE PIERCE:	School librarian, in her forties or fifties
BOBBI:	Mother of Gemma in Grade 1, and newborn Ryan
CLIVE:	Bobbi's husband
ANGIE:	Mother of Steven in Grade 1 (at the same school as Gemma)

LEIGH:	Angie's husband (Steven's father)
TAMARA:	Apparition of aged Russian prima ballerina Tamara Karsavina, reflecting on the events of 1911
MALE DANCER:	Performer for danced interludes

Steven, the protagonist of *SUGARPLUM FAIRIES*, is a role not requiring an actor. His presence is suggested by other cast members.

INTERLUDE 1—'SUGARPLUM FAIRY': MALE DANCER IN BALLET TUTU AND HEAVY MAKE UP PERFORMS A PARODIC REPRESENTATION OF A DAINTY BALLERINA DANCING WITH POUTING LIPS AND FLUTTERING LASHES. THE INTERLUDE LEADS INTO THE OPENING SCENE.

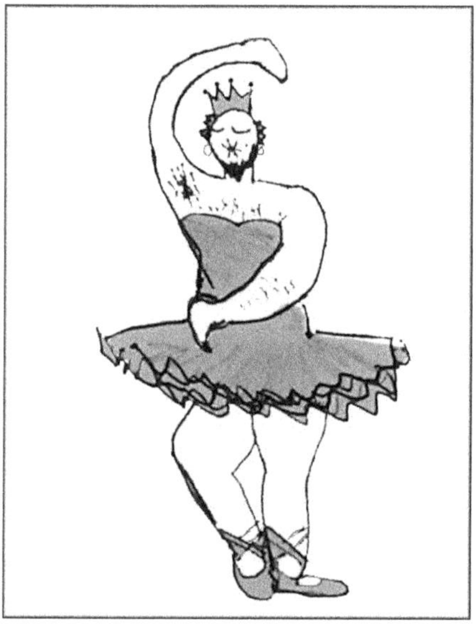

Figure Appendix.1 Burly ballerina. Artwork by Jack Migdalek.

A PRIMARY SCHOOL STAFF ROOM AT RECESS. DURING THE FOLLOWING, THE CHARACTERS OF LORRAINE AND ROB MIME THE PRESENCE OF OTHER STAFF MEMBERS REFERRED TO IN THE SCENE.

LORRAINE: (ADDRESSING FELLOW STAFF MEMBERS) . . . Of course they were anxious, but once the guys donned the costumes, the transformation was incredible. I mean it. Look, I'd been drilling them for what seemed like hours, and to be frank, I was almost ready to pull the plug on the whole divertissement: they weren't concentrating; they were horsing around. Basically they were pissing me off. Then one of them—I think it was Roger—asked what they would be wearing on the night. It wasn't Frank who asked—I know that because he wouldn't have dared: ever since he stage managed for me when I directed and choreographed *Pippin* he knows that is not the way I work. Anyhow, things were going so badly, I relented and explained the costumes that I had in mind. You've got to be flexible when working with amateurs. Well, I sent Frank upstairs to collect valances from the beds and some costume clip-on earrings I had. The transformation was incredible. Once those guys had these makeshift tutus and earrings on, I could hardly hold them back. They were transformed: each trying to outdo and 'out-dainty' one other. That—of course—was just what I needed for this divertissement to succeed. Actually, I had to dissuade them from extra rehearsals, as suggested by Joseph. I didn't let them in on the fact that—in order to work—it had to have a rough edge on the night. I mean, if it were too polished they might look too good doing it. Anyhow, needless to say—and you were there, Andrew—our little divertissement—with the finished fully sequined costumes that I organized for the boys—was the highlight of the night. Did I tell you, Andrew, that Councilor Grafton asked me if I could restage it for the Chamber's Christmas function? I told him: "it's only going to work if you can persuade some of the councilors to volunteer to be in it, including yourself, Councilor". He promised to get me four of the finest . . . including himself. I expect to hear from him end of November. Anyhow—as Andrew can tell you—the performance was a hoot! And when Frank saw the video back, he commented on how amazing he thought his legs looked. I can still see him with Lawrence freeze framing the video and comparing their pegs. Frank does have good calves. Men are so conceited.

ROB HAS ENTERED THE STAFF ROOM.

LORRAINE: Hello, Robert.

ROB ACKNOWLEDGES THE TEACHERS WHO ARE THERE AND HEADS TOWARD THE COFFEE MAKING AREA, WHERE HE CONTEMPLATES THE YEAR PLANNER ON THE WALL. LORRAINE BARELY TAKES HER EYES OFF HIM.

LORRAINE: (TO THE STAFF MEMBERS AROUND HER) Am I right, Ellen? Fiona? Andrew? I can see this is a touchy topic. (ADDRESSING ROB). How are you doing, Rob? You look so intent.

ROB: Oh, I'm just trying to figure out how I'm going to juggle my Grade 1s concert practice with some of the other stuff I've got on. Roland has me rostered on to take Grade 1s and 2s for sports next term.

LORRAINE—REFERRING TO ROB—MIMES 'SO CUTE' TO A FEMALE FELLOW STAFF MEMBER.

LORRAINE: Those lucky things. I'm sure they'll be thrilled to bits about that.

ROB: It's more a case of Roland not wanting the Grade 2 boys to have a female sports teacher two terms in a row: you know, "male teachers as vital role models".

LORRAINE: Actually, I think he's right. I saw those boys running rings around Gabrielle when she took them for sports. And you too, Ellen—no offense. If they don't have a strong male to look up to, they just run amuck.

ROB: I thought Gabrielle was going great guns with them. Oh, and you too, Ellen.

LORRAINE: But those boys idolize you, Robert.

ROB: Thanks, Lorraine. But they play up for me too. Strong female models can be just as significant.

LORRAINE: But not in subjects like sports and P.E. Male models are vital for boys—especially in sports and PE. Anyway, seeing you out there in your sports gear is far preferable to Gabrielle in hers.

ROB: (NOT WANTING TO PURSUE THIS DISCUSSION) The problem is, there's going to be some timetable clashes.

ROB SHIFTS HIS ATTENTION BACK TO THE YEAR PLANNER ON THE WALL. LORRAINE JOINS HIM THERE.

LORRAINE: How do you mean? Let's see if I can help.

ROB: Well, with covering Michael's Grade 5 and Grade 6 PE when he'll be away on the school camp, and with Maria on maternity leave, I can't see how I'm going to put together my kids' end of year concert piece. Maria put it together last year. I thought we were going to get some support staff in to fill in for her.

LORRAINE: Sorry, Robert, are you saying there's no one with arts expertise to replace Maria and direct your kids' concert piece?

ROB: Yeah, that's right.

LORRAINE: Rob, I'd be pleased to help you out with that. Direction and choreography are my specialty. The library audit is already done, so I can easily come across and work with your littlies, and we can use their sessions in the library to work on it too. It is the Grade 1s, isn't it? (HE NODS) Perfect. I love them at that age.

ROB: Are you serious about this? Roland said employing someone else to come in was out of the question, but if the library can spare you . . .?

LORRAINE: Leave it to me. I'll talk to Roland.

ROB: I hate to impose, but it would be a massive help. Putting this kind of thing together is really not my strength.

LORRAINE: And it's my forte. It's going to be a pleasure working together.

ROB: Thank you, Lorraine.

LORRAINE: Do you have anything in mind?

ROB: I was kind of hoping to do something that integrates with what we've been doing in class. Like last year, Maria did this skit about visiting countries of the world.

LORRAINE: Oh, I remember that. (BEGRUDGINGLY) It wasn't bad. Let me talk to Roland, and if he gives us the all clear, we can get moving on this ASAP. In the meantime, you and I can chat about what you've been doing in class this term, and we'll work out some ideas from there. Once we get a theme organized, we can bring June on board to work on props and a set.

ROB: Oh, nothing too fancy. I just want to keep it nice and simple.

LORRAINE: Absolutely. Don't you worry. It's going to be brilliant. I'm really looking forward to this.

ROB: You sure, Lorraine?

LORRAINE: Absolutely. We'll have a great time working on this. And I love the little ones.

ROB: They can sometimes be a handful.

LORRAINE: Relax, Rob. It's going to be a pleasure.

ROB: (WITH SOME DOUBT) Fantastic. Thanks, Lorraine.

BOBBI'S HOUSE. SHE IS HOME FROM THE HOSPITAL AFTER THE BIRTH OF HER SECOND CHILD. A CRIB IS SIDE STAGE WHERE THE NEWBORN BABY SLEEPS SWADDLED IN PINK BLANKETS. A KNOCK AT THE DOOR.

BOBBI: Come in, it's open.

ANGIE: (ENTERS WITH YOUNG GEMMA AND STEVEN—MIMED) Hi, Bobbi. Welcome back. (GIVES HER A CAKE)

BOBBI: Hi, Angie. Oh, thank you. You're so sweet.

ANGIE: No problem.

BOBBI: (TO DAUGHTER GEMMA) Hi, darling (KISSES GEMMA). (TO ANGIE'S SON STEVEN) Hi, Steven (PATS STEVEN). How was school today? (TO ANGIE) And thanks so much for picking Gemma up all week.

ANGIE: That's fine. I had to pick Steven up anyway.

BOBBI: (TO THE CHILDREN, WHO ARE OVER BY THE CRIB) Leave the baby sleep now. You kids want to play in Gemma's room? (USHERS THEM INTO OTHER ROOM) Go on then.

ANGIE: You are looking fantastic.

BOBBI: It's been a lot easier the second time around, . . . so far.

ANGIE: Really? Memories of having Steven are one of the main reasons Leigh and I are hesitant about having a second.

BOBBI: It's been totally different. Just knowing how to physically handle a baby without thinking it's going to break makes all the difference.

ANGIE: And let's see the little one. (GOING TO THE CRIB) Look at you. (NON-PLUSSED) Clive told me you had had a boy.

BOBBI: (AMUSED) That's right. This is Ryan.

ANGIE: Hello, Ryan. Sorry, mate.

BOBBI: (EXPLAINING THE PINK BLANKETS) The blankets and stuff are hand-me-downs from Gemma.

ANGIE: Oh, of course.

BOBBI: You're not the first to have assumed he's a girl.

ANGIE: I can give you some of Steven's old things if you like.

BOBBI: Oh that's OK. It's only a color.

ANGIE: I suppose so.

BOBBI: Anyway, all of Gemma's stuff is still in fine condition. I mean, it's not like I want to treat them any differently from one another, so why not dress them the same?

ANGIE: (PLAYING WITH RYAN, TALKING IN BABY VOICE) That makes perfect sense, doesn't it, Ry'? Whoo! He's got a strong grip there! People are going to know soon enough that you're a boy anyway.

BOBBI: Ha. (OFFERING) Coffee?

ANGIE: Sure.

GRADE 1 CLASSROOM

ROB: Now then people, we are going to prepare a performance for our mums and dads for the end of year concert. And Mrs. Pierce here from the library is going to help us. So, I'd like everyone sitting up really nicely and listening to Mrs. Pierce, okay?

LORRAINE: Thank you, Mr. Johnston.

ROB: No, they call me Rob.

LORRAINE: Oh, okay. Hello, boys and girls. 'Rob' and I have decided it would be a lot of fun to do a performance about some of the things you've been learning about nature, okay? So what we want you to do is to imagine an enormous and amazing garden. Now for the concert, each of you is going to become one of the things that live in that garden. Some of you might be flowers and butterflies. Some of you might be insects and frogs, maybe dragonflies. Alright then. Let's get going! On the count of three, I want to see everyone lying down very quietly on their backs! ONE. TWO. That's it, spread out now.

ROB: Bree and Jacinta, you two can let go of each other's hands, alright.

LORRAINE: THREE. (THEY WATCH THEIR CHARGES SETTLE) I want you all to close your eyes—no talking—for a minute or two. That's right, eyes closed everyone, and let's try to imagine that amazing garden, and what garden creature you might want to be. (ASIDE TO ROB) They are adorable. I think it's going to be great.

ROB: (ASIDE TO LORRAINE) One thing, Lorraine: I don't like to address the kids as 'boys and girls' (LORRAINE ROLLS HER EYES). It's, um, gendered, sexist.

LORRAINE: But they are boys and girls. How do you greet them of a morning?

BOB: Usually 'Good morning, people'. Puts them on a more equal footing.

LORRAINE: Oh.

ROB: 'Boys and girls' is no longer P.C.

LORRAINE: (DISMISSES THIS) Oh. Let's see how they're doing, shall we?

ROB: Alright 'people'. Sitting up now. That's it. Amanda, you want to be a? (LISTENS TO AMANDA'S RESPONSE) Butterfly. And Jarrod? (LISTENS TO RESPONSE) A lizard: Great. And Steven? (LISTENS TO RESPONSE) A butterfly? Wow! Wouldn't you rather be one of the grasshoppers? Or a frog perhaps? No? Okay.

LORRAINE: Steven, do you think your mum would like to make you a butterfly costume for all those people to see you in at the concert? You sure you wouldn't rather be a beetle? No?

ROB: Or a dragonfly perhaps?

INTERLUDE 2—'AMAZING GARDEN': MALE DANCER, HOLDING RODS FROM WHICH GOSSAMER WING-LIKE EXTENTIONS

ARE DRAPED, PERFORMS A GLAMOUROUS AND ELEGANT ZIEGFELD STYLE DEPICTION OF A BUTTERFLY. THE CHOREOGRAPHY IS FEMININE, BUT THE DANCER IS NOT IN DRAG.

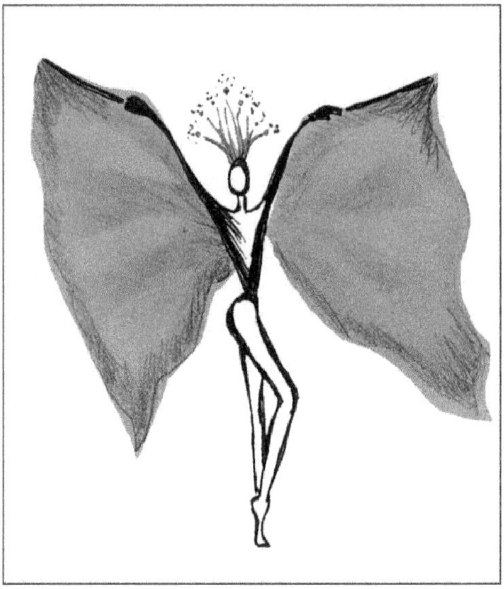

Figure Appendix.2 Gossamer wings. Artwork by Jack Migdalek.

OUTSIDE THE SCHOOL—PICK UP TIME. ANGIE IS SITTING, WAITING FOR HER SON, STEVEN. BOBBI ENTERS WITH NEWBORN RYAN—NOW SWADDLED IN BLUE—IN PRAM OR BASINET. SHE IS WAITING FOR DAUGHTER GEMMA.

ANGIE: Hi, Bobbi.

BOBBI: Hiya. (SETTLES DOWN) Ah, it's good to be back. I see nothing has changed.

ANGIE: (INDICATING BOBBI'S STOMACH) Apart from you.

BOBBI: (LAUGHS) That's right.

ANGIE: How is it all going?

BOBBI: Yeah, good. We actually got a fair bit of sleep last night.

ANGIE: (REFERRING TO RYAN'S BLUE BUNNY RUG) No pink today?

BOBBI: No, I'm afraid not. Clive's parents were over last night and—well, they got very upset that I had him in pink—claimed it was a horrible thing to do to a kid—like I was an abusive parent. They brought this and some blue playsuits over this morning. I didn't have a whole lot of choice.

ANGIE: Wow. Funny, 'cos I couldn't stop thinking about what you said—about pink just being a color. I mean, how stupid is it that we don't put pink on baby boys? Has anyone ever asked, 'Is it a boy or a girl' if a baby is dressed in pink?

BOBBI: The way Clive's parents were going on, dressing a boy in pink made me an unfit mother.

ANGIE: We are so conditioned. And it's not just the colors: we don't dress boys in skirts, or frills, or ribbons . . .

BOBBI: Yeah, true.

ANGIE: And even fibers. I mean, you never see boyswear made in the same materials that stacks of girlswear is made of. You know, those chiffon girlie party dresses.

BOBBI: Yes, Gemma has one of those. She's always laying it out on her bed to wear to school. I've had to limit it to special occasions and fairy parties only . . . along with those frilly edged lacy socks she also loves to wear.

ANGIE: Oh God, I remember wearing those when I was little, and how guilty I'd feel if I ever got them dirty. I remember bursting out in tears once when I got them muddy. I don't know where I got that from. Mum never even bothered putting them in with the whites.

BOBBI: Well, after the fiasco with Clive's folks over the bunny rug, I won't dare handing Gemma's frilly socks down to Ryan.

ANGIE: That would be an interesting experiment. (INDICATING RYAN) I mean, to chart the effects of dressing a little boy in frills and bows. Oh no, I don't mean . . .

BOBBI: (LAUGHING AS SHE CODDLES RYAN) Not on this little guinea pig. Oh here they come.

THEY STAND TO MEET THEIR KIDS.

INTERLUDE 3—MALE DANCER WITH A PINK BOW ON HIS HEAD PERFORMS AN ARTLESS ROUTINE IN CALISTHENICS STYLE. THE BOW IS SEEN TO RESTRICT THE DANCER'S MOVEMENTS IN THAT EVERY TIME HIS BODY PERFORMS A CARTWHEEL OR MOVES FAR OFF CENTER THE BOW FALLS OFF. HE REPLACES THE BOW SEVERAL TIMES, EVENTUALLY LEARNING TO ANTICIPATE WHEN IT MIGHT FALL AND MODIFYING THE DANCE BY EITHER HOLDING ONTO THE RIBBON OR COMPROMISING PHRASES OF THE CHOREOGRAPHY SO AS NOT TO INVERT HIS BODY.

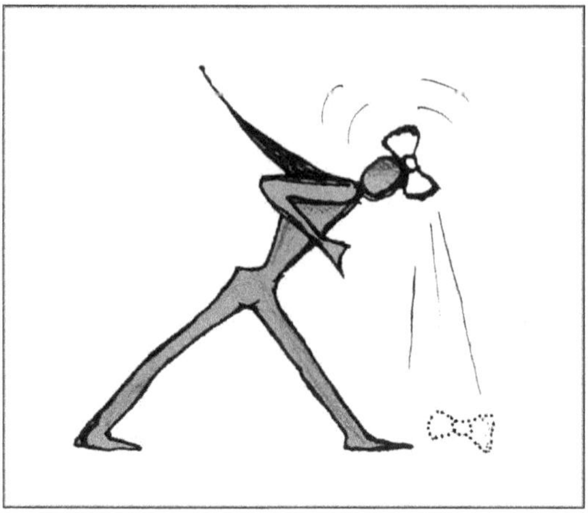

Figure Appendix.3 Off center. Artwork by Jack Migdalek.

ANGIE AND LEIGH'S HOUSE: BOBBI AND CLIVE HAVE BEEN OVER FOR DINNER. ANGIE, BOBBI, AND CLIVE HAVE BEEN WORKING ON COSTUMES FOR THEIR CHILDREN FOR THE END OF YEAR CONCERT. ANGIE IS WORKING WITH NEEDLE AND THREAD AT ATTACHING CHIFFON WINGS TO TWO STICKS (FOR A BUTTERFLY COSTUME). BOBBI IS SEWING SEQUINS ON SOME OTHER FABRIC. CLIVE IS GLUEING PINK AND PURPLE FEATHERS ON A HEAD-DRESS. LEIGH SITS TOYING WITH CRAFT GLUE FROM A TUBE.

ANGIE: Leigh, I wish you'd give me a hand with these wings. I just need you to stand here for me.
LEIGH: (BEGRUDGINGLY OBLIGES) All right then.
ANGIE: Don't make me feel like you're doing me a massive favor, Leigh. Clive's helping with Gemma's costume.
LEIGH: And I'm happy to help with Steven's costume. I just don't know why he has to be a butterfly.
ANGIE: The kids chose for themselves, Leigh. They could choose to be any garden creature they wanted. And Steven chose to be a butterfly.
LEIGH: My son, the butterfly.
ANGIE: Leigh! (TO BOBBI AND CLIVE FOR SUPPORT) Guys?
BOBBI: There are male butterflies.
LEIGH: Great.

CLIVE: You're making too big a deal of it, mate.

LEIGH: You think? What if your pink and purple feather number there was for Ryan and not Gemma?

BOBBI: He'd be fine with it. Not so sure about his parents. (CLIVE GOES TO REACT) No, I'm joking. It'd be fine. You are making too much of this, Leigh. It's a Grade 1 school concert.

LEIGH: Grade 1 or Year 10: I'm not comfortable with my kid prancing around as a butterfly. You think it's not going to have repercussions?

ANGIE: What? That he's going to turn out to be gay?

LEIGH: What? At the age of 6? No! That he's gonna cop a lot of flack. You know how kids get bullied.

ANGIE: They're in Grade 1.

LEIGH: (HOLDING UP THE WINGS) And look what he's going to be wearing . . . in front of the entire school for crying out loud.

CLIVE STIFLES A LAUGH.

LEIGH: (TO CLIVE) What?

CLIVE: Sorry, mate. It's you that I'm laughing at. I have no problem with Steven as a butterfly. You're making this into something much bigger than it really is.

ANGIE: (TO LEIGH) See.

BOBBI: Leigh, I can see where you are coming from, but school culture has changed massively since we were kids. A boy butterfly wouldn't rate in the playground like it would have done in our time.

CLIVE: No one gives a damn.

LEIGH: Are there any other boys being butterflies in this concert?

ANGIE: I've no idea. (A PAUSE) No.

LEIGH: You asked, didn't you? Well? Why ask if it's not a big deal?

ANGIE: Okay, put your arms down now. (TO CLIVE) How is the headdress going?

LEIGH: So, you're telling me you have no concerns about Steven being bullied or teased for being the only boy who's a butterfly in this thing? What about other roles? Did any other boys choose to be flowers . . . or birds?

BOBBI: Yes! Bradley Cooper is a bird.

LEIGH: Sparrow like Gemma? Or something more manly like a crow or a seagull? Well?

BOBBI: Well, he's an eagle. But I think some other boys might be different birds.

LEIGH: Yeah, not flamingos or swans, I bet.

BOBBI: Look, Leigh. When Gemma came home from school and I asked what Steven was going to be in the concert, she just told me "a butterfly". Didn't make a big deal of it . . . like you are, like kids might have done when we were kids.

CLIVE: That's right. Kids don't judge the way they used to, Leigh.

LEIGH: Wearing a girlie butterfly outfit is putting Steven right in the firing line to get labeled the class sissy-boy, and yes, the class poof.

CLIVE: Maybe in our day, mate. But not nowadays. Have a bit more faith in progress, Leigh. Kids are a lot more accepting than they used to be.

ANGIE: Listen, Leigh, at the end of the day, a butterfly is what Steven wants to be. He's obviously comfortable about that. So why aren't you?

LEIGH: Okay. Times have changed; I'm out of touch; Steven will be a lovely butterfly. He is comfortable with that, and so I will be too.

ANGIE: So, there we are.

BOBBI: And on that note, maybe we should pack up our sequins and pipe-cleaners and make a move. Thanks for dinner, guys.

THEY GO TO LEAVE: DURING THE FOLLOWING, THE GIRLS HUG AND KISS ONE ANOTHER, THE GUYS HUG AND KISS THE GIRLS, AND THE GUYS SLAP ONE ANOTHER'S BACKS BY WAY OF BIFFY EMBRACE.

ANGIE: Our pleasure. You sure you don't mind doing Steven's head-dress, Bobbi?

BOBBI: Not at all. Same as Gemma's, but with antennae instead of feathers.

ANGIE: Ta.

BOBBI: No. Thank you.

CLIVE: Yeah, thanks guys. (TO LEIGH) Relax, mate. There's no gulf any-more between boys doing boy things and girls doing girl things. Kids are kids—you treat them the same.

LEIGH: Yeah, I get it, mate. I'm cool.

BOBBI: (COMING TO A REALIZATION) Look at you guys. It's you guys that have the hang ups here. Yes, you too, Clive. "Times have changed"; "boys and girls, it's all the same". You might nod your heads, but you don't really get it. You guys are the root of the problem here. Look at how you just said goodbye. I mean Clive, you and Leigh have known each other for what—fifteen years? You're closer to Leigh than to Angie, yet look at how you say goodbye: You hug and kiss Angie, and then you and Leigh biff one another like this (SHE PARODIES THEIR BIFFY MACHO EMBRACE). Why is that? You nod your heads and pretend there's no 'gulf' between the sexes, but if there is one, it's because you guys keep it that way. Why can't you embrace a friend who happens to be a male in the same way you kiss a friend who happens to be a female? Even your own kids: Clive, when Gemma was newborn, you handled and cuddled her so gently—like you still do. But with Ryan—even at 10 days—you handle him completely differently (SHE PARODIES A GRUFF CUDDLE). "G'day Fella. G'day Mate". Why is that? It's that kind of stuff—treating males and females so differently—that might make little boys like Steven come to think that being a gentle, dainty butterfly is something not on for boys.

ANGIE: Exactly. (TO CLIVE AND LEIGH) Why is it that you don't hug each other goodbye in the same way you hug a female? I mean, what are the biffs and slaps all about? What's an embrace between guys without the biffs or slaps?

BOBBI: Gay.

LEIGH: Yes, it would be.

CLIVE: What are you on about? If we 'biff' and 'slap' it's just a reinforcement of a hug, . . . as a show of affection.

ANGIE: Yet you never embrace a woman with that kind of affection.

BOBBI: If you see a non-biffy, sustained embrace between guys as gay, then isn't it also gay when Angie and I do it? (HUGS ANGIE—SUSTAINED)

LEIGH: No it's not. But you tell me: you don't see it as queer if you see that hug on two guys?

BOBBI: Do you? (DIRECTED AT CLIVE) If what you are saying about there no longer being a difference between boy things and girl things is true, then a soft, non-biffy embrace between two guys shouldn't be a problem.

CLIVE: No, it shouldn't. (TO LEIGH) Come on, mate. Let's put this to rest.

LEIGH: This is ridiculous. You think we can't do it? You think we won't do it? Okay, you are on. No biffs then. (TO CLIVE) G'night mate.

CLIVE: 'Night. (LEIGH AND CLIVE EMBRACE—NO BIFFS OR SLAPS)

THE POSE IS SUSTAINED. DISCONCERTED, ANGIE GOES TO OPEN THE DOOR FOR BOBBI AND LEIGH TO LEAVE.

ANGIE: Okay, good night.

CLASSROOM. ROB IS TURING OFF A VIDEO RECORDER AND TURNING UP THE LIGHTS. LORRAINE AND ROB ARE TALKING TO THE CHILDREN IN REGARD TO A NATURE-VIDEO RECORDING THEY HAVE JUST VIEWED.

ROB: Let's thank Mrs. Pierce for organizing that great video for us. (LEADS APPLAUSE) It was interesting, wasn't it? Now we can really see how some of our garden creatures move, can't we? And we might be able to use some of that new knowledge in how we find ways to move as the creatures we've each chosen to be for the end of year concert.

LORRAINE: Alright then. Let's get on with things, shall we? Do you remember what we did in our last rehearsal? When I count THREE, I want you all to go and sit in your groups: (DIRECTING EACH OF THE FOLLOWING GROUPS TO DIFFERENT AREAS OF THE CLASSROOM, LEAVING A CENTRAL AREA CLEAR) my beautiful flowers over here; jumping frogs and grasshoppers here, my slow and incredible caterpillars here, my butterflies here, my flocks of birds here, beetles here, my monster dragonflies here, and my creepy crawly lizards over here. Ready? ONE, TWO, THREE. (TO ROB, AS THE CHILDREN ARE MOVING) I'm still uncomfortable about that boy being in the butterfly group. It really messes up my ideas for the choreography.

ROB: I want for the kids to do whatever parts they want.

LORRAINE: Actually, I was hoping we might have a little chat with him. See if we can coax him into joining one of the other groups.

ROB: No, Lorraine, I'm uncomfortable about that. He chose to be a butterfly, and unless he's unhappy about that, that's what he should be.

LORRAINE: (TO THE CHILDREN) Very good boys an' . . . 'people'. In a moment I'm going to play some music, and when I call your group of garden creatures, I want you to come into the center here and move with me. Okay?

ROB: (TO THE CHILDREN) And while you're moving, remember the way you just saw some of those creatures moving in the video.

LORRAINE: And by the way, if anyone wants to change from being the creatures that they've chosen, that's still alright. You just come and see me, or Rob, afterwards, and we will let you change. Alright then?

LORRAINE TURNS ON A CD PLAYER. THE FOLLOWING IS SPOKEN OVER THE MUSIC, WHICH IS A COMPILATION OF MUSICS THAT ARE TYPICAL OF THE CREATURES BEING SUGGESTED, E.G. DAINTY AND CLASSICAL FOR FLOWERS AND BUTTERFLIES; STRONG AND PERCUSSIVE FOR BEETLES; CREEPY FOR LIZARDS, ETC. LORRAINE DANCES IN THE CENTER OF THE CLASSROOM SPACE, REPRESENTING EACH CREATURE AND ENCOURAGING STUDENT GROUPS TO COPY HER MOVEMENT STYLE.

LORRAINE: Let's begin with my beautiful flowers (MOVES DELICATELY, DAINTILY, AND GRACEFULLY). That's right. Come on, moving your petals in the breeze, and twirling around to show the gorgeous colors of the costumes that your mums are going to make for you. Lovely. What's your name again, my lovely? Fiona. Let's move like Fiona here. Do you learn ballet, dear? That's wonderful. And let's have all my beautiful daffodils and roses and tulips and pansies smiling up toward the afternoon sunshine as we do these entrechats. (DANCES) And let's have all the flowers do a little curtsy, like this, that's it. And now, when the music changes, up on your tip-toes, and all the flowers go back to your places. And let's have the monster lizards crawl out onto the stage. Let's hear a big roar. (MOVES AND ROARS LIKE A MONSTER WITH CLAWS) Come on, let me see my terrible lizards. Oh boys, that's fantastic. Let's all chomp at the grass, snap snap snap to the right, and snap snap snap to the left.

ROB: (ADDRESSING THE STUDENTS BUT TRYING TO GET HIS MESSAGE TO LORRAINE) Some of those lizards in the video moved very slowly and gracefully too, do you remember?

LORRAINE: Okay, let's try that too. (DOES EXACTLY THE SAME AGGRESSIVE ACTION SHE HAS BEEN DOING BUT SLOWER) And lizards go back. Now, who comes next? Ah, the frogs. Come on frogs, and grasshoppers too, jumping into the center. Come on you grasshoppers, jumping as high as you can.

ROB: And remember how in the video the frogs legs bent right into their bodies when they jumped up?

LORRAINE: (ASIDE TO ROB) They won't be able to do that in the costumes I've asked the mums to make. (TO THE CHILDREN) And sitting still. And jumps. And sitting still. And jumps. Let's see if we can sit very still until I say, and then we'll do four big jumps all together. Sitting still. And jump: to the right, to the left, to the right, and to the left. Very good. And let's have our frogs and grasshoppers go back to their places. And listen to this music now. Who's that? Look up. It's the butterflies. Come on my butterflies, let's float down from the sky, landing beautifully on a blade of grass. Let's enjoy opening and closing our wings. (MOVING ELEGANTLY, STRIKING CLASSIC POSES IN A BALLETIC STYLE, LORRAINE IS DISCONCERTED AT STEVEN BEING PART OF THIS GROUP BUT CONTINUES ON) And let's see you all balance along the blade of grass on your tippy toes. Open your arms, and show everyone your stunning wings.

ROB: (ANGRY AT TWO CHILDREN WHO ARE SNIGGERING AT STEVEN PERFORMING THESE ACTIONS) Ashley! Craig! Something bothering you?

LORRAINE: And as we balance, we raise and lower our wings, smoothly and beautifully like a ballerina . . . like a ballet dancer.

ROB: Those butterflies need to be amazingly strong to move their wings. And didn't some of the butterflies we just watched on the video sometimes move their wings in a jerky way too?

LORRAINE: (GOES TO ROB AND SAYS THROUGH HER TEETH WHILE STILL OPENING AND CLOSING HER WINGS) If you insist on letting that boy go ahead and dance this part I think you'd best join in, or those other boys are going to eat him for lunch. (FOR THE WHOLE CLASS TO HEAR) Come on Rob, can you join us too please? Show us how you mean.

ROB: (UNCOMFORTABLE) Oh, sure. Um . . .

ROB JOINS THE GROUP IN THE CENTER AND DANCES AWKWARDLY WITH THEM.

LORRAINE: (ENJOYING HIS DISCOMFORT) And now let's bend our knees and turn to the right, spreading our beautiful wings in the sunshine. And now to the left. That's just lovely. Very good. Alright butterflies, take off, and fly gracefully up, up, up into the sky . . .

ROB: And butterflies can go back now.

LORRAINE: . . . as we have our beetles marching in now, marching like little soldiers with big heavy boots. (ASIDE TO ROB AS SHE CONDUCTS THE BEETLES) We have to do something about this. (TO THE BEETLES) Marching, marching, marching, making lots of noise with those arms and legs. (TO ROB) Robert, do beetles have arms?

OUTSIDE SCHOOL AT THE END OF THE DAY. BOBBI IS STANDING, THE BABY PRAM NEARBY. SHE IS LEANING AGAINST A WALL IN A FEMININE MANNER: HIP COCKED AND KNEE BENT, ONE ARM DOWN, THE OTHER HAND HOLDING THE OUTSIDE OF HER ELBOW. LEIGH ENTERS, UNSEEN BY BOBBI, AND TAKES IN HER FEMININE POSE.

LEIGH: Hi there (EMBRACES HER, MAKING A SHOW OF SLAPPING HER SHOULDER AS HE DOES) Just so you know I embrace everyone the same.

BOBBI: (LAUGHS) I'm impressed. How are things going?

LEIGH: Good. (HE ADOPTS THE SAME FEMININE POSE THAT BOBBI WAS IN)

BOBBI: What are you doing?

LEIGH: Waiting for the kids.

BOBBI: (AMUSED) Come on. Stand up properly.

LEIGH: What do you mean?

BOBBI: You look ridiculous. People are staring.

LEIGH: This is exactly how you were standing—just a moment ago. Okay for you but too feminine on a guy? Do you think it makes me look gay? (BOBBI IS FLABBERGASTED) So just like Clive, and just like me, you too haven't really changed with the times. Why aren't you okay with me standing like this then? You and Angie went on and on the other night about how I wasn't able to see my boy in a butterfly outfit as being okay. But what's going on when it comes to how a man in this pose—in a public place—might come across to others? What's the problem?

BOBBI: Okay Leigh. I get your point. You can drop the pose now.

LEIGH: Actually, I think I'm on a roll here. What do you think all these mums are going to make of me in this pose—as I wait for my kid—that's different from what they might have made of you in the same pose yourself? They wouldn't have noticed it on you, not at all. But the same pose on a male? How odd is that? But why, Bobbi, if times and attitudes have changed? Or is it just me who's not changed? (ACKNOWLEDGING A PARENT WHO IS LOOKING AT HIM) Hi. How's the kids? (TO BOBBI) Why do you suppose they are staring at me?

BOBBI: 'Cos you're making an ass of yourself, Leigh.

LEIGH: In what way, Bobbi? Too feminine for a man?

BOBBI: It's not that it's feminine, it just looks ridiculous.

LEIGH: And on you? Double standards, Bobbi. (DURING THE FOLLOWING, LEIGH ASSUMES OTHER FEMININE POSES) You said yourself how it disheartened you that Clive would cuddle Gemma in one way and Ryan in a completely different way. But here, all these people are staring at me—a male—in a completely different way from how they *weren't* staring at you—a female—just moments ago. Even you find it uncomfortable. What's that all about?

BOBBI: I'm uncomfortable for you. Come on, Leigh, the kids will be out any time now.

LEIGH: And when the kids come out of school today, do you think they'll also notice this 'strange' man over here? Why is that? "Oh, that's okay, it's Steven's dad. He must be the reason that Steven wants to be a butterfly in the concert". I've changed my tune on this, Bobbi. Perhaps I'm on the same wave length as you were the other night now. Perhaps I agree with you: that Steven should be able to be a butterfly. But perhaps I also think that I should be able to stand here like this . . . But you don't.

BOBBI: The problem is how other people see things.

LEIGH: . . . which is exactly why I feel how I feel about Steven being a butterfly in that performance. Not just old adults but also the kids of those adults are going to point him out as different, and label him—possibly as weird, probably as a poof—neither of which—at 7 years old—is in his best interests. Why wouldn't I want to protect him from that?

BOBBI: Here they come now, Leigh. Just let it go.

LEIGH: Sure.

BOBBI: (TO GEMMA AS SHE TAKES HER HAND AND TURNS THE PRAM TO GO) Hey, Gemma. How was today?

LEIGH: See you later. (TO STEVEN) Hey, mate, how's the butterfly going? (THEY EXIT. BOBBI LOOKS ON AS THEY DO SO)

BOBBI: See you, Leigh, Steven.

INTERLUDE 4—'JAZZ ROUTINE': MALE DANCER PERFORMS A JAZZ ROUTINE, ALTERNATING STRONG EXPANSIVE MASCULINE ACTION AND RUGGED FACIAL EXPRESION WITH SLINKY FEMININE ACTION AND SULTRY, VAMPY FACIAL EXPRESSION.

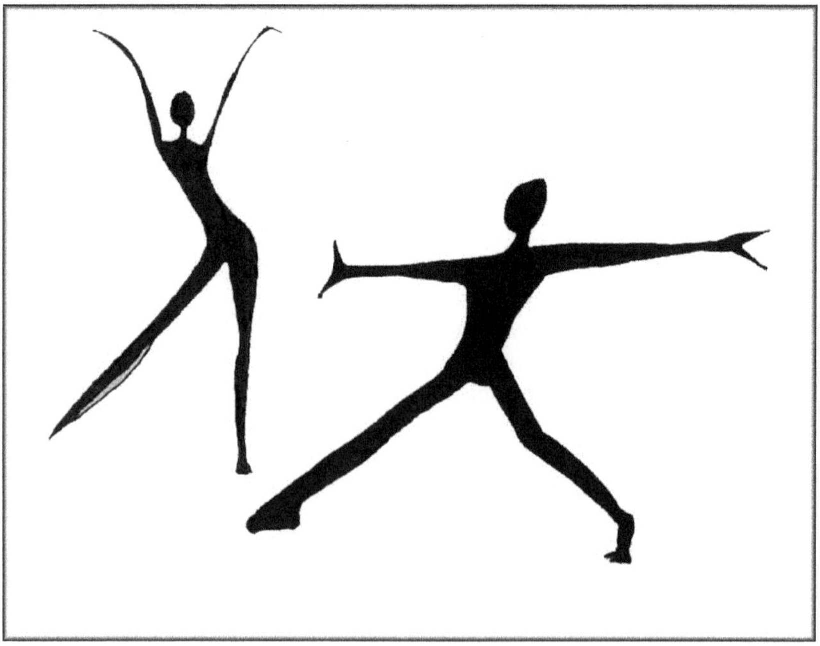

Figure Appendix.4 Jazz. Artwork by Jack Migdalek.

ROB'S HOUSE. ROB IS LABELING A STACK OF CDs (FOR HIS STUDENTS). HIS PARTNER KEVIN (MIMED) ENTERS.

ROB: Hi, babe (KISSES/HUGS KEVIN). I'm just burning copies of the music for the concert. You should have seen Lorraine at today's session. She wore these gold jazz shoes and a turban, you know, like what's her name wore in those backstage musical movies. You would have loved it. I swear if she were a guy, she'd have been a drag queen. (IN ANSWER TO A QUESTION FROM KEVIN) Yeah, it's going to be alright—I think. Lots of color and movement, as Lorraine keeps emphasizing. She's got these big ideas for costumes, and has somehow heavied the parents into making them, which was a total impossibility last year. (ANSWERING KEVIN) Yes, Steven the boy butterfly is still amazing. Lorraine keeps on doing these guided improvisation things with the kids, and I tell you, he's so responsive, it's actually really touching to see him move. He gets up there, and, like he's basking in the sun, opens up his wings, and you should see: his arms—all the way to his little fingers—just flitter, as he crooks his neck toward the sun. It's very cute. (RESPONDS TO KEVIN) Oh, come on. That doesn't mean he's gay at all. He's a kid! It's not fair to label people for something like that. I hate that. Mind you, I'm sure they've all labeled me as a poof. No, not the kids. The staff. Ironic, seeing as I'm the only male staff member who gets out there and kicks a footy. Maybe I'm wrong. Although I think Lorraine may think I'm straight. Anyhow, I just hope little Steven doesn't get any flack when it comes to dressing up as a butterfly. (ANSWERS KEVIN) Tights, sequins, wings: Lorraine's directive. (RESPONDS TO KEVIN) Really? Well, if you want to . . . though I think it'll bore the socks off you. I think you'll hate being there otherwise. I mean, I'll be backstage, and then afterwards I'll have to mingle with the parents. Why don't I get two tickets, and we can ask Dena to come with you? I'd prefer it if you weren't there alone.

THE FOLLOWING ARE SPLIT SCENES THAT TAKE PLACE BETWEEN ANGIE DRIVING WITH STEVEN IN THE CAR, AND LEIGH WITH STEVEN AT THE DOOR TO STEVEN'S ROOM. (IN EACH CASE STEVEN'S PRESENCE IS MIMED.)

ANGIE: You're very quiet today. (PAUSE AS SHE WAITS FOR STEVEN TO RESPOND)

LEIGH: Hey. How's things, mate? (PAUSE AS HE WAITS FOR STEVEN TO RESPOND)

ANGIE: Steven? How did school go today? (PAUSE AS SHE WAITS FOR STEVEN TO RESPOND)

LEIGH: You feeling alright, Steve? (PAUSE AS HE WAITS FOR STEVEN TO RESPOND)

ANGIE: What's up, hey? (PAUSE AS SHE WAITS FOR STEVEN TO RESPOND)

LEIGH: Everything okay? (PAUSE AS HE WAITS FOR STEVEN TO RESPOND)

ANGIE: Bub? (PAUSE AS SHE WAITS FOR STEVEN TO RESPOND)

BOTH ANGIE AND LEIGH SNAP OUT OF SPLIT SCENE LOCATIONS AND ADDRESS ONE ANOTHER:

ANGIE: He hasn't been himself lately.

LEIGH: I know.

THE FOLLOWING ARE SPLIT SCENES THAT TAKE PLACE BETWEEN LORRAINE AND ROB IN THE STAFF ROOM, AND BOBBI AND ANGIE AT ANGIE'S HOUSE.

LORRAINE AND ROB ENTER STAFF AREA IN MID-CONVERSATION.

LORRAINE: I couldn't be happier Robert, and I think it's the best thing for everyone.

ROB: I don't like that he's changed his mind at this late stage.

LORRAINE: It's for the best, Robert. The boy came up to me at the end of yesterday's rehearsal and asked if he could change roles. He asked if he could be one of the beetles instead. So I told him 'yes'.

ROB: Well, why do you suppose he changed his mind, Lorraine?

SPLIT SCENE TO ANGIE'S HOME. ANGIE IS FOLDING UP THE BUTTERFLY WINGS' FABRIC. BOTH ANGIE AND BOBBI SPEAK IN LOW TONES, INDICATING THAT STEVEN IS WITHIN EARSHOT.

ANGIE: Steven told me he decided to be a beetle instead, and that Mrs. Pierce said okay.

BOBBI: No other reason? You don't you think the kids were giving him a rough time over being a butterfly?

ANGIE: I honestly don't know. If they did, he didn't let on to me. Did Gemma say anything?

BOBBI: No, nothing. This is the first I've heard of it.

ANGIE: I don't want to grill him over what made him change his mind, though I wish I knew.

BOBBI: You don't think his dad has been wording him up on how he feels about a boy being a butterfly? Just I know how tetchy Leigh was about all this.

ANGIE: No, I'm pretty sure he wouldn't have said anything, even if he did think that . . .

SPLIT SCENE TO STAFF ROOM

LORRAINE: . . . being a butterfly is not an appropriate role for a boy. In some ways I blame you, Robert. I would have spelled out the students' options much more clearly from the start. Who knows what teasing he got from the other kids. You heard the boys giggling at him at rehearsals.

ROB: And you don't think you made it rough on him? Don't get me wrong, I'm really grateful that you came on board and are directing this project, but you're the one who choreographed the butterflies to be so dainty and graceful. You could have catered more sensitively to the fact that we had a boy as one of the butterflies.

LORRAINE: And what does that mean? Exactly how would you have had me choreograph them?

ROB: Well, I've certainly never seen a butterfly twirl in circles or dance on its tippy toes.

LORRAINE: Oh don't be ridiculous, Robert. Ask anyone. Go back into ballet history. That's how butterflies—and flowers and fairies—are represented. It's universal.

ROB: Well, maybe that needs some radical revision.

LORRAINE: I have choreographed and directed for years now Robert, and I know my craft. You think you're so modern, making out that I'm 'Ms. Out of Date' on this. I've seen some of the 'wanky' experimental performances that pop up from time to time, . . . you know, where men wear skirts, or roles are reversed, or where everyone moves around like cyborgs with no gender. But take my word for it, in the scheme of things, that kind of stuff is a fleeting oddity and nothing more. Theatre has universal precedents that are not to be tampered with. Unless you're going for a comic element, males do the masculine parts and females do the feminine ones. That's nature, and you would do well to stop encouraging your students—especially boys like Steven—to overstep the mark of what is natural and expected of them—and for them. Boys need to aspire to masculine models. Encouraging them to do girlie things is hardly what the Department of Education had in mind when they were trying to encourage male teachers back into primary schools.

ROB: (CHANGING TACTIC) All the parents were asked to start on costumes weeks ago. How do you suppose Steven's folks are going to react to us telling them to dump the butterfly costume they've been working on and turn it into a beetle outfit?

LORRAINE: I've already sent a note home to them. I'm sure they'll be fine.

SPLIT SCENE TO ANGIE'S HOME

ANGIE: (DISPOSING OF BUTTERFLY WING FABRIC) At least Leigh will be thrilled about the change over.

INTERLUDE 5—'CYBORG GENDERLESS DANCE': MALE DANCER PERFORMING IN AN EXPRESSIONLESS, ALMOST MECHANICAL STYLE THAT IS NEITHER FEMININE NOR MASCULINE.

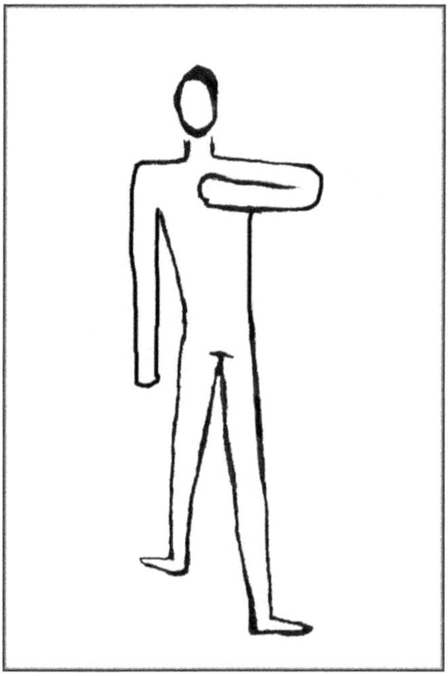

Figure Appendix.5 Automaton. Artwork by Jack Migdalek.

SCHOOL. LEIGH HAS MADE AN APPOINTMENT TO SEE ROB. HE IS HOLDING A LARGE BOX. ROB ENTERS IN SPORTS GEAR.

ROB: Mr. Anders, sorry to keep you waiting: sports club.

LEIGH: No problem. Call me Leigh.

ROB: (SHAKING HANDS) Cheers. What can I do for you?

LEIGH: I wanted to talk to you about the concert, and Steven changing roles.

ROB: Mmm. It was Mrs. Pierce—the director—who Steven approached last week to see if he could change his role.

LEIGH: I've got to tell you, I wasn't thrilled about him choosing to be a butterfly in the first place.

ROB: I see.

LEIGH: But, when it comes down to it, I hate the idea of letting a kid change their mind once they've made a decision on something. It's like, when a kid decides on a sport they want to do, and you go ahead and enroll them and buy all the stuff, and then the kid suddenly decides that they want to do something else. If you let them back out of something, it doesn't teach them anything . . . just that they can change their mind at the drop of a hat.

ROB: So, you're wanting him to stick with his initial choice. You want him to continue to be a butterfly?

LEIGH: What do you think? Unless some of the kids've been giving him a rough time . . .?

ROB: No. Not really. Not as far as I know.

LEIGH: If that's the case, I think he needs to know that people should stick to decisions they make.

ROB: Mmmm. I'll talk to him, see if I can convince him to change back again.

LEIGH: I'm still not thrilled about him being a butterfly, but I've been thinking: If it's okay with you, I've got some ideas about the costume. Angie had already made the wings and antennae, and what I was hoping we could do is to take some of the girliness out of the whole look of the thing. (DURING THE FOLLOWING HE TAKES MATERIALS OUT OF THE BOX HE HAS WITH HIM AND DEMONSTRATES IDEAS AS HE OUTLINES THEM) I've spoken with a mate of mine, who's an electronics genius, and we think—with some adjustments—we could rig the antennae with some of these chaser lights and even a couple of these red laser pen things you can get nowadays. So wherever he faces, these laser lights would hit. Imagine how it would be when they scan across the faces in the audience. Not just for Steven: We could do this for all the butterflies. How many are there?

ROB: Um, 6, I think.

LEIGH: No problem.

ROB: It wouldn't be too heavy?

LEIGH: No, I don't think so . . . not for a short performance. I'll try the weight out at home with Steven and get back to you on that. If it does turn out to be too heavy we could always cut the chaser lights and just go with the laser pens. Now, my other idea is with the wings: The design Angie received in the school notice just had the wings tied to the kids' wrists . . .

LORRAINE ENTERS UNNOTICED

LEIGH: . . . but I thought, if we took this further and extended the arm-span like this (DOES SO WITH FABRIC ON STICKS) these things could look awesome (SWOOPING HIS ARMS).

ROB: Oh Lorraine, this is Mr. Anders, Steven's father. Lorraine is directing the performance.

LORRAINE: Oh, Mrs. Pierce. Nice to meet you.

LEIGH: Leigh. Nice to meet you. (EXTENDS A WINGED ARM TO SHAKE HANDS)

ROB: Lorraine, Leigh doesn't want Steven to change his role in the concert. Leigh has been telling me about some ideas he has . . . which I think could be fantastic actually. (TO LEIGH) Perhaps I can get you to run us both through what you were explaining to me.

LEIGH: Pleasure. I think you'll find this will make the role a lot more satisfying for a boy to perform, and as I said to Rob, I'm more than pleased to help out with adjusting the costumes for all the butterflies, which to tell the truth, were just way too typical.

LORRAINE PREPARES TO LISTEN THROUGH CLENCHED TEETH, UNIMPRESSED.

LEIGH: Now, cut me off if you think this is too much, but I've also had this pretty daring idea of how—if we could rig up a simple pulley system—we could fly Steven onto the stage. You'd just need a couple of dads backstage, and I reckon the effect would be dynamite . . . (LAUNCHES INTO HIS EXPLANATION)

INTERLUDE 6—MALE CLASSICAL BALLET DANCER PROMENADES EXPANSIVELY AROUND THE STAGE IN A GRAND, STATELY, AND NOBLE STYLE, AS THOUGH DISPLAYING, PRESENTING, POSITIONING, GUIDING, TURNING, AND LIFTING A BALLERINA (MIMED).

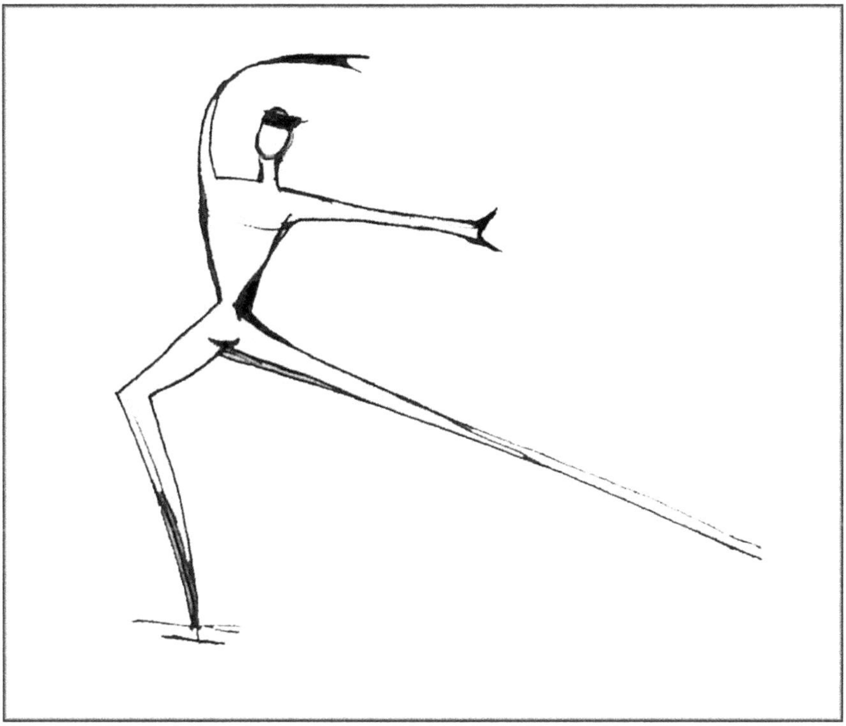

Figure Appendix.6 Majestic. Artwork by Jack Migdalek.

A BARE DANCE STUDIO, AS TAMARA KARSAVINA, A RUSSIAN PREMIER BALLERINA OF THE EARLY 1900s, REMINISCES ON HER CAREER AND THE EVENTS OF 1911. DURING THE FOLLOWING TAMARA IMPERSONATES THE DANCERS AND DANCES SHE REFERS TO.

TAMARA: Tamara Karsavina, Russian born, premier ballerina. I have been dancer with many of greatest artists Europe did produce. I have made long association with Marlinsky theatre and also Ballets Russes. Of course you know Ballets Russes' impresario Sergei Diaghilev. He bring together all kind of artist to collaborate of many wonderful and also avant garde new works. I was in demand as dancer, not only for choreographers who has been doing established repertoire—*Swan Lake, Sleeping Beauty, Giselle*—but also for choreographers when they has been making new works. I has been in some pioneer dance works what was so radical at this time, they was considered extreme and outrageous. *Spectre de la Rose* was original new work: choreography by Michel Fokine for Diaghilev's Ballets Russes. *Spectre de la Rose* story was like this: (EMBODIES AS SHE EXPLAINS) Beautiful girl comes home from party. She has rose in her hand, probably given to her from eligible gentleman at party. She is excited from party, and fatigued. She sits, and falls to sleep, and is dreaming of wonderful evening, at party. Choreographer Fokine, and Diaghilev too, has wanted me for original cast of *Spectre de la Rose* to dance role of young beautiful girl. Michel Fokine was becoming famous choreographer, and dancing duet in original Fokine ballet is very good thing for dancer's career. Anyway, choreographer Fokine's idea is that comes to young girl a specter, spirit of the rose—like symbolic representation of gentleman from party—and Fokine plans this rose character will be played by male dancer. We was all thinking, oh is lovely idea, and man would be look like man from party. But then Fokine tells us his idea, and we see designs what he has chosen. These are by famous artist Leon Bakst. Designs Bakst made is man dancer not just represent rose, but, IS rose. Design is pink headdress and petals around head—like rose bud—with lower body like stem of rose. How can this be costume for role for man we was all thinking. Original idea was for young dancer Nikolai (SEARCHING FOR HIS SECOND NAME) Sze . . ., Szye . . . Never mind second name; he did not become famous. Anyway, Nikolai is chosen to dance rose character in ballet. Beautiful dancer. Body is svelte, and movement very graceful, very good for Suitor in *Sleeping Beauty*. But I am thinking, in this ballet, impression will be very bizarre. I have been thinking how audience will react to this man in rose outfit. Of course, I am dancer, not choreographer, so must only dance steps what choreographer makes for me. But already, in rehearsal, I am feeling like this man Nikolai, dancing rose in such costume, and with such soft style, will not be working. Nikolai's dancing style—and slim body too—looks like body of woman. Not just me, but everyone is thinking like this. Impression will be very strange, maybe comedy for audience. Even repetiteur Boris—who hardly never make comment for no-one, also I hear comment that man dancing rose is not working. Boris is suggesting music be played more fast, more heavy to make rose more stronger, more manly. We all thinking that costume looks . . . ridiculous, and that—

really—svelte Nikolai will look like female. But of course, Fokine is modern choreographer. He is not interested in what we are thinking. But I am not happy because this ballet—big opportunity for me—will maybe become like comedy. We dance once rehearsal for company members, and Diaghilev is here, with young boyfriend Nijinksy. Well, we are hearing titter laughing from some members when we are dancing. Is really bad feeling for us. My friends from corps de ballet says Nikolai in this costume is not manly for beautiful girl who is dreaming of man from party. I am hating this ballet. Actually I am hoping that it is going to be cut from coming program. But then something wonderful happen: Impresario, Diaghilev announce cast change. Nijinsky will dance character of rose, not Nikolai. Well, Nijinsky dancing rose is something completely different. Nijinsky's body, and dancing, is sublime, not like Nikolai. Nijinsky shows how real man does dance. As you know, Nijinsky's body is very strong—legs and thighs and chest is very solid. Even in rose costume he looks manly. And more. When Nijinsky jumps—as you know—is amazing. His elevation . . . is something unbelievable. I have not seen nothing like that: so majestic. So now, impression of this ballet is totally something different. Of course Nijinsky can dance very soft and delicate for rose, but also something what is strong and masculine as manifestation of romance from party in imagination of beautiful girl. Choreographer Fokine now makes new ideas in choreography: Nijinsky as rose enters stage with huge leap through window near sleeping girl. This is leap what is something so incredible it did make audiences gasp (GASPS). Of course, when this happens, beautiful girl is asleep with eyes closed, but I can hear this reaction from audience in every performance. His leap is so athletic, so masculine. This is way for male to dance. Men must dance only in this way: Spectacular, athletic, proud, strong, powerful. As real man. Of course Nijinsky was homo. We all know he is Diaghilev's lover, and yes, did sometimes move very graceful and soft. But even so, his leaps and jumps and power is what makes him such perfect male dancer. This makes possible to raise status and impression for male dancer as something absolute wonderful. Dancing with Nijinsky was highlight from my career.

INTERLUDE 7—'SUPER-HERO BUTTERFLY DANCE': MALE DANCER PERFORMS A DANCE AS A POWERFUL, HYPERATHLETIC, HYPERMASCULINE BUTTERFLY.

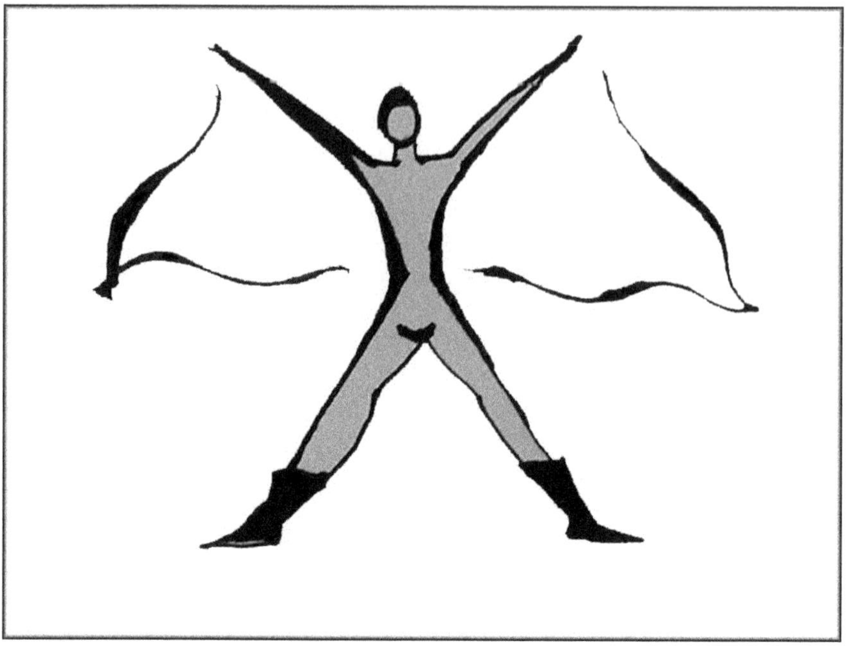

Figure Appendix.7 Superhero butterfly. Artwork by Jack Migdalek.

THE FOYER OF THE SCHOOL, FOLLOWING THE SCHOOL CONCERT.

ANGIE, BOBBI, LEIGH, AND CLIVE ENTER FROM THE AUDITIORIUM, TOTING CAMERAS. THERE ARE OTHER PARENTS AND FAMILIES MILLING AROUND, WHOM THEY NOD TO AND EXCHANGE PLEASANTRIES WITH DURING THE SCENE (MIMED).

CLIVE: (TO LEIGH) That was pretty fantastic, man!
LEIGH: Yeah, it was, wasn't it?
ANGIE: What a relief.
CLIVE: Best end of year concert I've ever seen.
BOBBI: Brace yourself my darling, 'cos we've got years and years more of the same.
ANGIE: We should all be very proud of our little troupers.
CLIVE: Did you see that little one who wet her pants?
BOBBI: What? Who?
LEIGH: One of the little girls in the first group.
ANGIE: The girl who was the lollypop. Probably just overwhelmed by the whole evening.
BOBBI: Oh, I wondered why everyone was laughing during that section.
ANGIE: She didn't seem to notice it herself, so that was good.
CLIVE: I'd say that on that girl's 21st, there's going to be some photographs circulating that she's not going to be too happy about.

BOBBI: I'm sure she'll get over it.
ANGIE: Gemma was adorable.
BOBBI: And so was Steven. Everything worked out pretty well in the end.
CLIVE: Looks like all that fuss was a storm in a tea-cup, hey.
LEIGH: I wonder how Steven will feel about tonight's photographs of him on his 21st.
BOBBI: I should think he'll feel pretty terrific. He looked spectacular.
CLIVE: (TO LEIGH) Great job, man.

ROB ENTERS AND SEEKS LEIGH OUT, ACKNOWLEDGING OTHER PARENTS ON HIS WAY OVER (MIMED).

ROB: Congratulations Leigh. Thought that went brilliantly.
LEIGH: Yeah, it did go well, didn't it? Thanks for your support.
ROB: No worries. I've got to tell you, the way that costume looked with the mechanical arms and spinning antennae, I think half the other boys in the school wish they could have been butterflies too.
ANGIE: Yes, I'm so glad we managed to talk Steven out of changing roles.
ROB: Yeah, I'm glad he saw it through, (TO LEIGH) which I don't think would have been all that easy looking back at how things were progressing three weeks back.
ANGIE: (TO ROB) Congratulations, Rob. (INTRODUCES SELF) Steven's mum. That was great.
ROB: Thank you very much. Always nice to end the year on a high.
ANGIE: And these are Gemma's parents.
BOBBI: (TO ROB) Bobbi. Gemma had a ball.
ROB: I'm glad. She's not without confidence, is she?

AN EFFUSIVE LORRAINE HAS ENTERED, THANKING AND ACKNOWLEDGING PARENTS AND AUDIENCE MEMBERS (MIMED).

CLIVE: (TO THE OTHERS) Is that the bird who directed?
LEIGH: Yeah. Lorraine. I think she looks pretty satisfied.
ANGIE: So she should be.
LEIGH: She hated the ideas we pitched to her.
ROB: Let's just say she preferred her own.
ANGIE: (CATCHES LORRAINE'S EYE AND ENGAGES HER IN CONVERSATION) Congratulations. That was wonderful.
LORRAINE: Oh, thank you. We are proud of our wonderful little ones.
ANGIE: I'm Steven's mum, and these are Gemma's parents.
BOBBI: Hi. Congratulations (IT SEEMS LORRAINE DOES NOT RECOGNIZE THE CHILDREN'S NAMES) . . . Gemma was one of the sparrows.

ANGIE: And Steven was one of the butterflies . . . the boy butterfly.

LORRAINE: Oh. (SEEING LEIGH NEARBY) Oh, yes. I met your husband . . . who was a great help. (CALLING LEIGH OVER) Leigh, thank you. It went terrifically.

LEIGH: Yeah, sure did. Though, if I would've gotten clearance to fly Steve in on a pulley system, we could have really brought the house down. Anyhow, thanks for going with the changes.

LORRAINE: Oh, one needs to be flexible in the theatre . . . and accommodate according to the needs of one's performers—and their parents. Excuse me. (SHE SWANS OFF TO BE CONGRATULATED BY OTHER PARENTS IN THE FOYER)

BOBBI: What was that all about?

ROB: (SHRUGS) I'll move off now too. We've got to be out of here by 9:30. Good night.

THE OTHERS WISH ROB A GOOD NIGHT.

ANGIE: (TO LEIGH) Thanks, Leigh.

LEIGH: What?

ANGIE: For protecting our boy. I realize that—had it not been for sensationalizing his costume—Steven might have stood out in ways far more demeaning than the little girl who had wet herself.

LEIGH: Yeah. So far as boy butterflies go, ours stood out for all the right reasons.

SLIDE SHOW OF STEVEN AS BUTTERFLY IN THE SCHOOL CONCERT. HIS COSTUME IS DARK AND FIERCE LOOKING, COMPLETE WITH LASER LIGHT ANTENNAE.

STAFF AREA. LORRAINE IS PACKING UP ELEGANT LOOKING MASKS. ROB IS BOXING SOME OTHER GEAR FROM THE CONCERT.

LORRAINE: (REGARDING PACKING UP) How unglamorous: the reward for all our efforts.

ROB: Do you want me to finish up for you?

LORRAINE: No, no. I'm almost done. (REFERRING TO THE MASKS SHE IS PACKING) We bought these when we were in Venice. Frank thought I was crazy, but I knew they would come in handy. This must be the fourth time I've used them at least. And now it's back to the walls above our piano.

ROB: I hope none of them were damaged. The kids weren't exactly gentle with them.

LORRAINE: No, all fine.

ROB: Good. (AFTER A PAUSE) Steven's parents seemed very pleased with how things went.

LORRAINE: (NOT HAPPY HEARING ROB SPEAK OF STEVEN) Yes.

ROB: It did work out well for him after all.

LORRAINE: Yes. (AFTER A PAUSE) You're gay, aren't you? (ROB IS TAKEN ABACK—AND REMAINS GOBSMACKED THROUGH THE REMAINDER OF THE SCENE) Not that it would worry me . . . ordinarily. I do need to tell you, Robert, that I think you giving that boy the option—and then actually encouraging him—to be a butterfly was highly inappropriate, even if the boy does have a gentle and effeminate inclination. (ACCUSING) A male teacher in a primary school should be a male role model, not someone who promotes alternative . . . contrary behavior. It was not your place, Robert, to encourage that boy to be a butterfly, especially if you are a homosexual—or pedophile—yourself. (SHE STOPS ROB FROM REPLYING) I don't want to get into a discussion over this, Rob, but I do want you to be aware that I've spoken about my concerns to the principal, so just know that you should be watching yourself in future. If you are gay, I seriously advise you—for your own protection—not to interfere with these children. They are children, so—leave—them—be. (EXITING WITH HER MASKS) I'll see you next week. Good night.

ROB IS GOBSMACKED. ANGIE APPEARS HAND IN HAND WITH STEVEN (MIMED). SHE IS HOLDING A GIFT.

ANGIE: Can we come in?

ROB: Yes, . . . sure.

ANGIE: Sorry to disturb you. Steven wanted to give this to you. Steven?

SHE PROMPTS STEVEN TO PASS THE GIFT TO ROB AND TO THANK ROB (MIMED).

ROB: (KNEELING DOWN TO STEVEN'S LEVEL TO ACCEPT THE GIFT) Thanks, Steven. And you made it yourself? That's great. Thank you.

STEVEN HUGS ROB, WHO RECIPROCATES.

ROB: (DISENGAGING) Thanks, Steven. Good night.

ANGIE: Good night, . . . and thanks.

ANGIE AND STEVEN EXIT.

ROB SITS ON THE FLOOR AND OPENS THE GIFT. IT IS AN OVERSIZE EXQUISITE, DELICATE, AND COLORFUL BUTTERFLY WITH MOVEABLE WINGS. HE EXAMINES THE GIFT DURING THE FOLLOWING.

INTERLUDE 8—'BUTTERFLY': MALE DANCER IN UNITARD PERFORMS A SERIOUS AND SENSITIVE DANCE AS A DELICATE, EXQUISITE, GRACEFUL CREATURE THAT CHOOSES A SPOT IN WHICH TO BASK MOMENTARILY IN THE COMFORT OF THE SUN—AND THEN FLITTER OFF TO WHERE LIFE LEADS HIM.

AS THE DANCE ENDS ROB MANIPULATES THE BUTTERFLY TO PERCH ON HIS OUTSTRETCHED ARM AND EXITS.

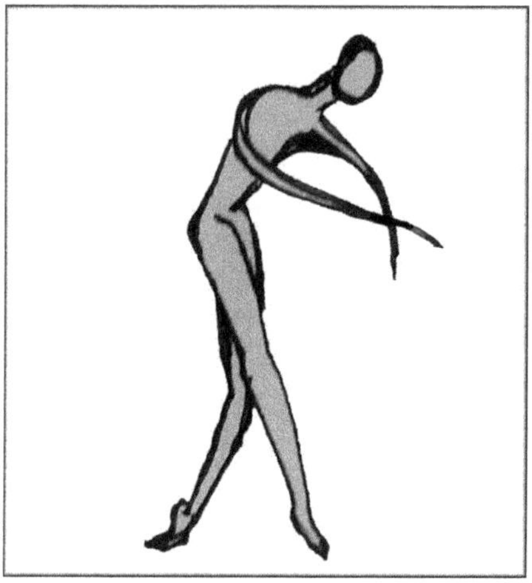

Figure Appendix.8 Solo. Artwork by Jack Migdalek.

DISCUSSION TOPICS

In the first scene of the play, Lorraine raves about a drag routine that she choreographed on her husband and his buddies. Why do people tend to regard men in drag as humorous? Why are males in drag regarded differently from females in drag?

Lorraine refers to male teachers as being vital role models for boys. Debate whether and why role models for boys should necessarily be masculine or male.

Angie assumes that a baby swaddled in pink is a girl. Why? What is at stake for the boy or girl not clothed according to socially promoted norms of sex appropriate children's clothing? Debate the extent to which individuals are free to style themselves in a masculine/feminine manner.

Steven was encouraged to perform the role of a grasshopper or a beetle instead of a butterfly. Why are boys generally not encouraged to follow 'feminine' pursuits?

Rob states that it is gendered and sexist to address children as 'boys and girls'. Loraine reasons that they *are* boys and girls. Debate the importance or irrelevance of differentiating between boys and girls in education and other settings.

Angie observes that males are unable to embrace one another in the same way as they are able to embrace females or that females are able to embrace one another. Discuss whether, to what extent, and why this is so.

Rob chooses not to disclose to his fellow staff members that he is gay. Under what circumstances might individuals withhold such aspects of who they are? In what ways might school contexts differ from other contexts?

The majority of characters in the play would probably claim not to be gendered. Consider if and why gendered positions that we occupy are often beyond our consciousness.

Lorraine refers to universal precedents in the theatre in defense of her gendered choreography for specific roles in the school concert. Discuss connections between mainstream choreography of male and female bodies in public performance arenas and the kinds of embodiment deemed appropriate and aesthetic for male and female bodies in the everyday.

Vaslav Nijinsky's portrayal of a rose was lauded due to his palpable strength and muscularity. Consider why males/females involved in 'feminine/masculine' pursuits (such as rhythmic gymnastics or boxing) may be lauded/denigrated.

In the final scene Lorraine implies that encouraging young Steven to play a feminine role in the school concert can be seen to be recruiting the child to alternative behaviors such as homosexuality. Discuss connections that Lorraine makes between feminine behavior in males and homosexuality. How widespread are these perceptions, and in what ways are they true/untrue/harmful?

PRACTICAL ACTIVITY SUGGESTIONS

Monologues

Conceive and stage monologues of Steven's thoughts at various points in the *Sugarplum Fairies* plot: on choosing to be a butterfly; on Lorraine's direction; on interactions with his teachers/parents/classmates; on his costume. Conceive a monologue as spoken by an adult Steven reflecting back on the events of the play.

Dramatized Scenes

Conceive and stage scenes that feature situations and outlooks of peripheral characters of *Sugarplum Fairies:* the males who appeared in Lorraine's drag routine; Bobbi's parents-in-law on their grandson being swaddled in pink hand-me-downs; Steven's classmates on Steven's role in the school concert; audience members on seeing Steven's performance.

Action Types

Physically explore, compare, and contrast what it is to glide, stride, float, stomp, and dart across an empty space. Consider when and why the impressions of various action types mean differently according to the perceived biological sex of the person performing them.

Dance Sequences

Choreograph non-parodic dance sequences that are intrinsically masculine or feminine in movement quality and designed to be aesthetically pleasing when performed by male or female bodies. Consider whether and why there may be variations in audiences' aesthetic appreciation of the same dance sequence according to whether it is performed by male or female bodies.

Costume Design

Design 'Garden Creature' costumes, such as butterflies, grasshoppers, flowers, beetles, and slugs, that are intrinsically masculine or feminine and designed to be aesthetically pleasing when worn by male or female bodies. Consider whether and why there may be variations in audiences' aesthetic appreciation of the same costumes according to whether they are worn by male or female bodies.

Scenario Improvisation

Divide participants into three groups, and allocate each group one of the following scenarios (unseen by other groups):

- Group 1: A *Fairy Princess* is flitting through an enchanted forest. She comes across three dormant flowers and casts a spell to make each bloom.

- Group 2: A *Champion Gladiator* resolves to defeat an arrogant opponent. Determined to be victorious, he puts on his helmet, chooses weapons, and enters the arena, prepared to kill.
- Group 3: A *butterfly* metamorphoses into a *bulldog*.

Each group is to work as composers and create a short soundscape to represent its given scenario. Soundscapes may include voice and sound making implements (but no lyrics).

As each group of composers performs their soundscape, have another group, working as actors, physically improvise to it. The third group can observe as audience. Rotate so that each group has a turn at each task.

Following each performance, invite audiences to speak about how they interpreted both the soundscape they heard (as performed by composers) and the physical action that they viewed (as performed by actors). Did soundscapes and/or performed movement qualities evoke images or feelings that were particularly masculine or feminine, or pertinent to males or females? If so, is it possible to pinpoint what evoked these responses?

Next, invite actors to speak about how they interpreted the soundscape to which they improvised. After having composers reveal what their scenario briefs had been, invite groups to discuss common readings, especially in regard to images or feelings that were understood to be particularly masculine or feminine and/or pertinent to male or female character and/or embodiment. Consider whether and why individuals may be more comfortable or uncomfortable moving in some ways as opposed to others.

Have participants comment on the semiotics of certain sounds and certain styles of embodiment from their own personal, cultural, and professional perspectives, and pose the question of whether common readings of embodied gender are natural or learned (Migdalek 2014).

Embodied Characterization

Teach all participants the following simple sequence to be performed as a mimed solo set in a café:

- A figure is facing the café counter as they wait for an order of coffee and a pastry
- The figure receives their coffee and pastry, walks to a table, puts the coffee and pastry on the table, and sits down
- The character eats and drinks

Working in groups that include male and female participants in each, allocate each group one of the following briefs by which to cast and block the learned sequence as a solo mimed scene for a male or female character (as prescribed). Encourage groups to be detailed in their blocking so that their actor's performance of the blocking will project their character's disposition and state of mind as outlined in the briefs.

Character Brief for Character X (Male)

X is a successful, aggressive manager of a major corporation. X commands space, respect, and admiration.

Scenario: X is in a café between appointments. X is civil yet disinterested in fellow patrons and staff in the café. X finds the pastry is delicious, but the coffee is bland.

Character Brief for Character Z (Female)

Z is a successful television journalist. Z is well heeled and likes to be regarded positively by others.

Scenario: Z is in a café prior to a scheduled interview with a high-profile public figure. Z finds the pastry is delicious, but the coffee is bland.

Have groups spend time preparing and rehearsing these short mimed scenes. However, prior to performing the scenes, ask for each group to enlist an actor of the opposite biological sex from their group who is to also learn the blocking as directed on the body of the original actor. After some rehearsal time, have each group's two actors perform their *identically* blocked mimed scenes for the entire group (Migdalek 2014).

After watching both groups, initiate discussion on the following:

- Did the same blocking read differently on the bodies of a male actor and a female actor? If so, explain any variation in how the characters of both figures projected.
- When and why might characters with identical character descriptions (e.g. gay, evil, psychotic) be cast/directed/depicted differently according to whether they are male or female?
- For those who teach or direct drama: Do you think you direct the bodies of males differently from the bodies of females? If so, when and why? In what ways might this impact on actors'/audiences' perspectives toward gender embodiment?
- Consider and comment on how much information on the sexuality of characters in movies or television programs is gleaned via characters' embodiment prior to the unfolding of storyline or the speaking of dialogue.
- Consider and comment on the impact that recurring valorized images of masculine-embodying males and feminine-embodying females may have on the social and emotional well-being of those inclined to

perform gender differently from what is deemed socially appropriate to their biological sex.

- To what extent are performance arts practitioners complicit in the repetition of oppressive and restrictive gender representations? Consider and comment on whether and how gendered standards of embodiment may be directed/choreographed without reinscribing dominant patriarchal, masculinist, heterosexist, and gender oppressive norms. How can performance arts practitioners/educators work to disrupt the ways we view and perform dominant ideologies of gender?

REFERENCE

Migdalek, J. (2014). Challenging Gendered Practices through Drama. In Meyer, E.J., and Carlson, C. (Eds.). *Gender and Sexualities in Education.* New York: Peter Lang.

Index

For Product Safety Concerns and Information please contact our EU representative GPSR@taylorandfrancis.com
Taylor & Francis Verlag GmbH, Kaufingerstraße 24, 80331 München, Germany

www.ingramcontent.com/pod-product-compliance
Ingram Content Group UK Ltd.
Pitfield, Milton Keynes, MK11 3LW, UK
UKHW022116190926
475702UK00013B/1483
* 9 7 8 1 1 3 8 3 7 9 4 7 3 *